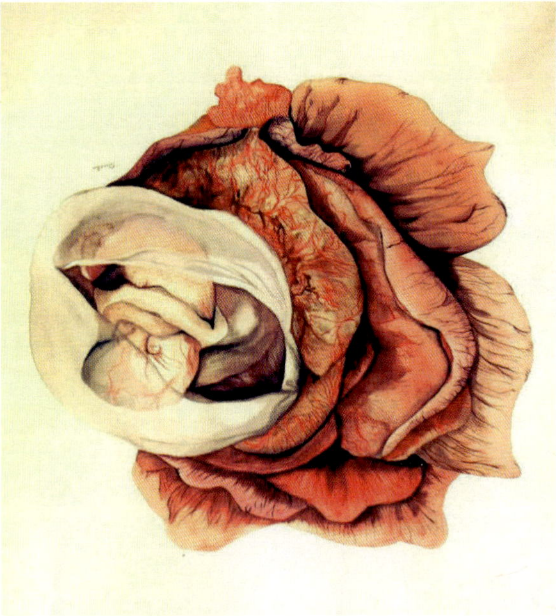

In Utero 2013

Watercolour and pencil on paper

Description: This painting depicts the birth of new life in the form of a blooming flower.

Practical Obstetrics and Gynaecology Handbook

For O&G Clinicians and General Practitioners

2nd Edition

PRACTICAL OBSTETRICS AND GYNAECOLOGY HANDBOOK

For O&G Clinicians and General Practitioners

2nd Edition

A/Prof. Tan Thiam Chye
KK Women's and Children's Hospital, Singapore

Dr. Tan Kim Teng
KK Women's and Children's Hospital, Singapore

Dr. Tay Eng Hseon
Thomson Women Cancer Centre, Singapore

Chief Editor
Dr. S. P. Chonkar
KK Women's and Children's Hospital, Singapore

KK Women's and Children's Hospital
SingHealth

World Scientific

NEW JERSEY • LONDON • SINGAPORE • BEIJING • SHANGHAI • HONG KONG • TAIPEI • CHENNAI

Published by

World Scientific Publishing Co. Pte. Ltd.

5 Toh Tuck Link, Singapore 596224

USA office: 27 Warren Street, Suite 401-402, Hackensack, NJ 07601

UK office: 57 Shelton Street, Covent Garden, London WC2H 9HE

and

KK Women's and Children's Hospital Pte. Ltd.
100 Bukit Timah Road
Singapore 229899

Library of Congress Cataloging-in-Publication Data
Tan, Thiam Chye, author.
[Practical obstetrics and gynaecology handbook for the general practitioner]
Practical obstetrics and gynaecology handbook for O&G clinicians and general practitioners / Tan Thiam Chye, Tan Kim Teng, Tay Eng Hseon ; chief editor, S. P. Chonkar -- 2nd edition.
p. ; cm.
Preceded by Practical obstetrics and gynaecology handbook for the general practitioner / Tan Thiam Chye, Tan Kim Teng, Tay Eng Hseon. c2006.
Includes bibliographical references and index.
ISBN 978-9814522939 (hardcover : alk. paper) -- ISBN 978-9814579308 (pbk. : alk. paper)
I. Tan, Kim Teng, author. II. Tay, Eng Hseon, author. III. Chonkar, S. P. (Sonali Prashant), editor. IV. Title.
[DNLM: 1. Obstetrics--methods--Handbooks. 2. Genital Diseases, Female--Handbooks. 3. Gynecology--methods--Handbooks. 4. Pregnancy--physiology--Handbooks. 5. Pregnancy Complications--Handbooks. WQ 39]
RG531
618.2'07543--dc23

2013039769

British Library Cataloguing-in-Publication Data
A catalogue record for this book is available from the British Library.

Typeset by Stallion Press
Email: enquiries@stallionpress.com

Printed by FuIsland Offset Printing (S) Pte Ltd Singapore

FOREWORD TO THE 2ND EDITION

Let the young know they will never find a more interesting, more instructive book than the patient himself.

Giorgio Baglivi (1668–1707)

Who dares to teach must never cease to learn.

John Cotton Dana (1856–1929)

The best-selling 1st edition of the *Practical Obstetrics and Gynaecology (O&G) Handbook for the General Practitioner* was successful in many ways. I quote Adjunct A/Prof Lim Lean Huat, Past President of the College of Family Physicians: "[It] is an essential textbook for primary-care doctors as well as graduate doctors preparing for their postgraduate degrees or diplomas in Family Medicine. The practising general practitioner or family physician will be able to find ready answers to the problems they face during difficult consultations in O&G."

Seven years on, much in obstetrics & gynaecology has changed. Keeping in line with the latest trends in patient management and the development of new drugs, the authors have come together again to bring you the 2nd edition of this handbook.

Many GPs have told us that they wanted an insider's perspective of how O&G specialists manage their patients. They wanted to be able to provide advice to their patients on what to expect when they are referred to us for further management.

Therefore, the authors have reworked this book from the ground up. Many new chapters have been added while existing chapters have been expanded and revised for clarity and brevity. For easy comprehension many clear and easy-to-read charts and tables have been included. Indeed, the new edition surpasses the last in many ways, and I would strongly recommend it to all practising O&G specialists as well.

In writing this book, the authors have sought the opinions of many expert members of the medical community and allied health specialties, from both KK Women's and Children's Hospital and the wider healthcare community. Drawing on their wide experience as well as the fresh insights, the authors now put forth an updated, comprehensive and clear book. On the authors' behalf, I would like to say: thank you.

We hope that this book will continue to be a mainstay on the shelves of many clinics and that you will find it a most useful guide.

A/Prof John Tee Chee Seng
Director of Education (Undergraduate)
Senior Consultant
KK Women's and Children's Hospital

Past Division Chairman
Division of Obstetrics and Gynaecology

HISTORY OF KK WOMEN'S AND CHILDREN'S HOSPITAL

Since its founding in 1858, KK Women's and Children's Hospital has evolved over the decades, having become a regional leader in Obstetrics & Gynaecology (O&G), Paediatrics and Neonatology.

The story of KK Women's and Children's Hospital is the story of maternal and foetal care in Singapore. It is also a story of significant medical highlights.

Before KK Hospital became a maternity hospital, it was a general hospital in the Kandang Kerbau District.

On 1 October 1924, Kandang Kerbau Hospital (KKH) was opened with 30 beds and 12 children's cots. The hospital was led by Professor J S English, Singapore's first Professor of O&G. The hospital's mission then was to provide good maternity care and midwifery training for medical students and pupil midwives to bring maternal and infant mortality rates down.

In 1952, the School of Midwifery was set up.

The annual "birthquake" of over 26,000 babies referred to in the 1960 edition of the Guinness Book of Records appeared to be based on KKH's 1956 birth statistics. KKH was the busiest maternity hospital in the world. Then, KKH broke this record year after year until 1966 when it achieved a peak delivery number of 39,856.

Over the years, the medical undergraduate curriculum has seen radical changes. Partial accreditation of KKH's postings for membership examinations for The Royal College of Obstetricians and Gynaecologists (RCOG) was given in 1963 and full accreditation was awarded in 1967.

Until 1978, KKH was the only training hospital in obstetrics & gynaecology. It has a unique concentration of clinical material. As an academic healthcare institution, KKH believes that world-class training and research are imperative in raising the standard of patient care.

On 1 April 1990, KKH ended its 132-year history as a government hospital and became a Restructured Hospital.

In 1997, KKH shifted its premises to 100 Bukit Timah Road, where it currently stands, with state-of-the-art facilities.

In 1999, the Department of General Obstetrics & Gynaecology (GOG) in KKH was created under Dr John Tee Chee Seng to focus on enhancing service commitments to patients. Since then, KKH has built on its leading role in teaching, training and research, and continues to produce most of the O&G specialists in Singapore.

In 2001, the first RCOG part 2 examination course was held at KKH. This was the first time the RCOG co-hosted an examination course in Asia to develop and accredit aspiring O&G trainees from the region.

Today, the institution continues to raise the bar on clinical excellence while providing quality care for patients. More than 400 specialists adopt a multi-disciplinary and holistic approach to treatment and harness the latest innovations and technology for the best medical care possible for our patients.

PREFACE

In obstetrics & gynaecology, it has always been our practice to place the interests of our patients as first. With the advent of evidence-based medicine, we face the greater challenge of providing the most cost-effective services in meeting the healthcare needs of our patients based on current evidence in management.

*Incorporating the latest research in various topics, **Practical Obstetrics and Gynaecology Handbook for O&G Clinicians and General Practitioners, 2nd Edition*** aims to provide simple, practical and yet cost-effective guidelines in the management of common O&G problems.

We hope that the information in this book will help our colleagues in the primary healthcare setting make the right and cost-effective decisions for the patients. Guidelines for referral to a tertiary centre have also been included. The first edition has been well received and many medical students, trainees and general practitioners have found our book useful as a quick reference text in the clinics.

In this second edition, we have included many new updates in recent years such as Human Papilloma Virus Vaccine, new contraceptive pills as well as the recent FIGO recommendations for abnormal uterine bleeding.

Thank you for your encouragements and comments in this edition!

TAN Thiam Chye
MBBS (Singapore), MMed (O&G) (Singapore)

TAN Kim Teng
MBBS (Singapore), MMed (O&G) (Singapore), MRACOG (RANZCOG), FAMS (Singapore)

TAY Eng Hseon
MBBS (Singapore), FRCOG (United Kingdom), MMed (O&G) (Singapore), DGO (RANZCOG), FAMS (Singapore)

Chonkar Sonali Prashant
MBBS (Mumbai), MD (O&G) (Mumbai), MRCOG (London)

ABOUT THE AUTHORS AND CHIEF EDITOR

AUTHORS

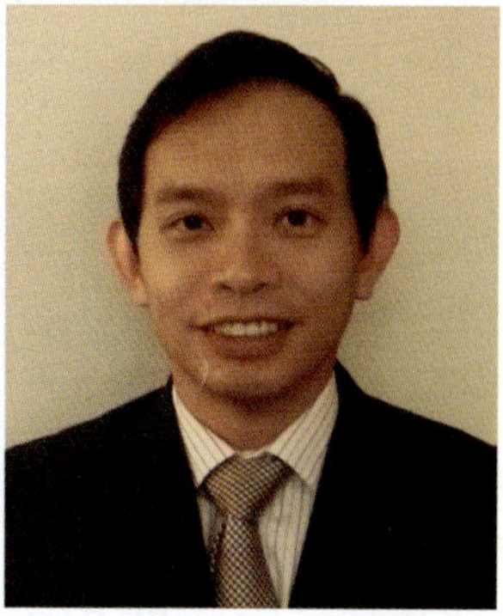

MBBS (S'pore), MMED (O&G)(S'pore)

Associate Professor TAN Thiam Chye is Deputy Director for Education and Senior Consultant Obstetrician and Gynaecologist in KK Women's Hospital. He co-authored "The New Art and Science of Pregnancy and Childbirth" in 2008. He is also the founding Clerkship co-ordinator for Obstetrics and Gynaecology Clerkship in the Duke-NUS Graduate Medical School and developed the entire curriculum from scratch with his faculty. He was awarded the inaugural SingHealth Golden

Apple Award for Outstanding Educator in 2011. He publishes extensively and is a reviewer in medical journals such as Singapore Medical Journal and Saudi Medical Journal. He is also the co-editor for Singapore Journal of Obstetrics and Gynaecology, KK Review and Proceedings of Singapore Healthcare. He is currently serving as a Board Member in both KKH Executive Committee and Medical Board (2013–2014).

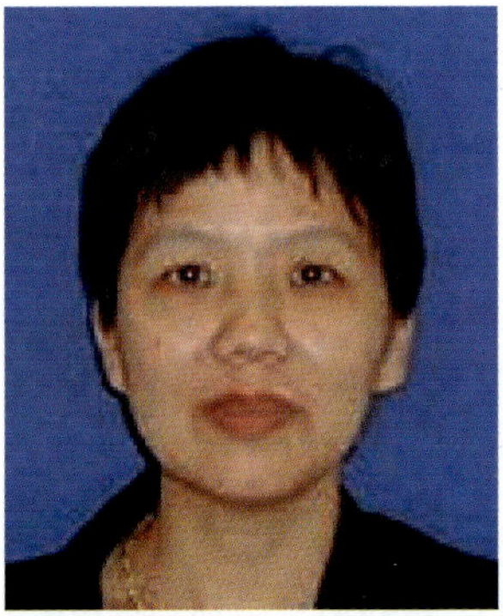

MBBS (S'pore), MMED (O&G) (S'pore), MRACOG, FAMS (S'pore)

Dr TAN Kim Teng (Dr KT Tan) is a Senior Consultant in the Division of O&G in KKH. She was the Head of the Department of General O&G in KKH from 2005 to 2007. A medical practitioner since 1987, she runs a busy clinical practice seeing both obstetrics and gynaecological patients. In addition, she co-authored the "The New Art and Science of Pregnancy and Childbirth" in 2008. She is also an Adjunct Assistant Professor in the Duke-NUS Graduate Medical School and is constantly involved in imparting her valuable knowledge and experience to the next generation of doctors.

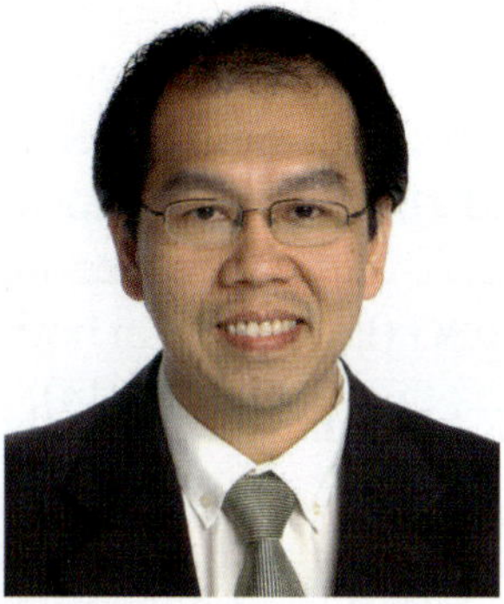

MBBS (S'pore), FRCOG (UK), MMED (O&G)(S'pore), DGO (RANZCOG), FAMS (S'pore)

Dr TAY Eng-Hseon is a gynaecologist who sub-specialises in gynaecological oncology. After spending 22 years in government institutions, he started private practice in 2009 as the Medical Director of Thomson Women Cancer Centre and an associate with WC Cheng & Associates. Dr Tay served as the Chairman, Medical Board, KK Women's & Children's Hospital (2004–2009), President, O&G Society of Singapore (2006–2008), Chairman, Gynaecological Oncology Committee, Asia-Oceania Federation of O&G (2007–2011) and Chairman, Gynaecological Oncology Section, College of O&G of Singapore (2007–2009). Presently, Dr Tay is the Chairman, Medical Advisory Board, Hanh-Phuc International Hospital (Vietnam), Executive Medical Director, Delphi Bioscience Asia Ltd (Asia-Pacific), and the Founding Member & Honorary Treasurer of Asia-Oceana Organization for (Research), Genital Infection, and Neoplasia.

CHIEF EDITOR

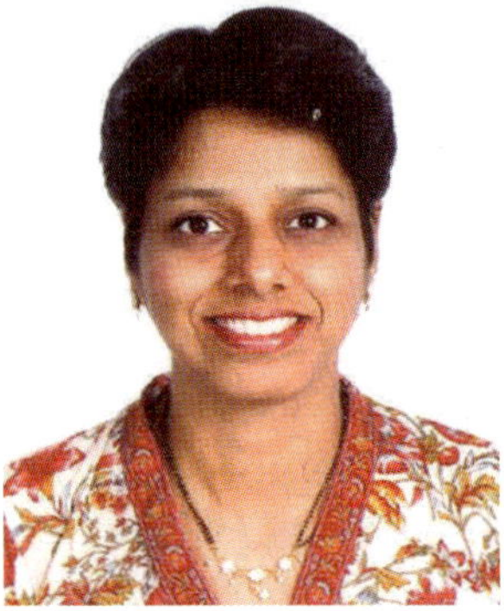

MBBS (Mumbai, India), MD (O&G) (Mumbai, India), Diplomate National Board (India), DGO (Mumbai, India), MRCOG (London)

Dr CHONKAR Sonali is currently working as a Senior Staff Registrar in KK Women's and Children's Hospital. She graduated from Seth G S Medical College in India and did her postgraduate studies with the KEM Hospital in Mumbai. Later, she joined the St Johns Medical College in Bangalore as a faculty member and worked as an Associate Professor at the Padmashree DY Patil Medical College in Mumbai. After she came to Singapore, she became an Associate in Education at the Duke-NUS Graduate Medical School and Clinical Lecturer with the Yong Loo Lin School of Medicine in NUS. She is actively involved in teaching at KKH. She is recipient of the Duke-NUS Graduate Medical School Faculty Appreciation Award 2012 for being an outstanding faculty member for development (O&G) and was also awarded The Best Registrar Educator Award at the ACP Education Day, 2013. She is currently the Deputy for OBGYN clerkship at Duke-NUS Graduate Medical School.

ACKNOWLEDGEMENTS

Contributors from the Division of Obstetrics and Gynaecology KK Women's & Children's Hospital.

Faculty

1. Dr Chin Pui See, Janice	—	Consultant
2. Dr Chonkar Sonali Prashant	—	Senior Staff Registrar
3. Dr Hong Sze Ching	—	Associate Consultant
4. Dr Lau Sie Kuei, Matthew	—	Consultant
5. Dr Mulik Varsha	—	Senior Consultant
6. Dr Phoon Wai Leng, Jessie	—	Associate Consultant
7. Dr Rama Padmavathi Namuduri	—	Senior Staff Registrar
8. Dr Suzanna Sulaiman	—	Consultant
9. A/Prof Tan Thiam Chye	—	Senior Consultant
10. Dr Tan Kim Teng	—	Senior Consultant
11. A/Prof Tee Chee Seng, John	—	Senior Consultant
12. Dr Wee Wei-Wei	—	Associate Consultant

ASTs/Residents

1. Dr Chua Ka-Hee	—	Resident
2. Dr Ho Weng Yan	—	Resident
3. Dr Hui Yan Yan, Celene	—	Resident
4. Dr Lee Cheng Sim, Jill	—	Resident
5. Dr Lim Hui Ping, Michelle	—	Resident
6. Dr Liu Shuling	—	AST
7. Dr Tan Yu Fen, Pamela	—	AST
8. Dr Tan Shu Qi	—	Resident
9. Dr Wang Peiying, Candice	—	AST

Ms Ong Phei Hong — Executive, Division of Obstetrics & Gynaecology

Invited Guest Contributors

1. *Associate Professor Chan, Roy*
   Director, National Skin Centre

2. *Dr Chen, Helen*
   Head & Senior Consultant, Department of Psychological Medicine, KK Women's & Children's Hospital

3. *Dr Chia Yin Nin*
   Senior Consultant Gynaecologist and Certified Gynaecological Oncologist, Gleneagles Hospital
   Visiting Consultant, KK Women's & Children's Hospital

4. *Clinical Associate Professor Giam Yoke Chin*
   Senior Consultant, National Skin Centre

5. *Dr Law Hai Yang*
Chief Scientific Officer, DNA Diagnostic and Research Lab, Genetics Service, Dept of Paediatric Medicine, KK Women's & Children's Hospital

6. *Mr Lee Kwok Hao*
Undergraduate, Washington University, St Louis, USA

7. *Ms Lim Kae Shin*
Pharmacist (Drug Information), Pharmacy, KK Women's & Children's Hospital

8. *Ms Pang, Cynthia*
Lactation Consultant, KK Women's & Children's Hospital

9. *Ms Stephaine Jamie*
Pharmacist (Drug Information), Pharmacy, KK Women's & Children's Hospital

10. *Dr Tan Yah Yuen*
Consultant, Breast Surgeon, PanAsia Surgery, Mount Elizabeth Medical Centre

11. *Dr Tay Eng Hseon*
Senior Consultant, Thomson Women Cancer Centre

12. *Dr Teh, Marina*
Consultant Orthodontist, Pacific Healthcare

13. *Dr Toh HanWei, Luke*
Consultant, Dept of Diagnostic Interventional Imaging KK Women's & Children's Hospital

14. *Dr Tseng Leng Aun, Arthur*
    Consultant, Obstetrician & Gynaecologist, Gleneagles Medical Centre

15. *Dr Vytialingam Atputharajah*
    Visiting Consultant, KK Women's & Children's Hospital

Sponsors

Bayer Healthcare
Hyphens Pharma
Glaxo Smith Kline (GSK)

CONTENTS

Part 1

OBSTETRICS

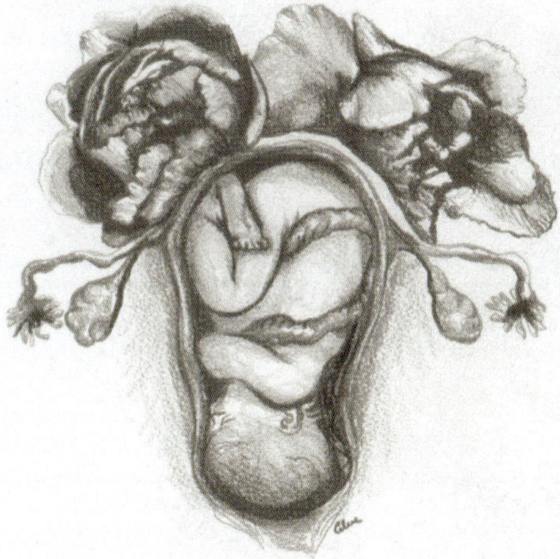

"The Dream" 2013

Description: "For the womb has dreams" — Anais Nin.

Chapter 1

PRE-CONCEPTION PREPARATION

OBJECTIVES:
TO IMPROVE PREGNANCY OUTCOME

1) Optimising medical conditions prior to pregnancy
2) Avoid teratogenic drugs
3) Screen for infections and genetic blood disorders
4) Encourage appropriate counselling sessions

1. Optimising Medical Conditions Prior to Pregnancy — to Improve the Prognosis for both Mother and Baby

a. Diabetes mellitus

- Use contraception until glucose control is achieved.
- Self-monitor glucose level
- Refer to dietician for diabetic diet control
- Check for retinopathy, nephropathy and coronary heart disease.

- HbA_1c — aim for <6%
- Achieve good glycaemic control before conception to reduce the risk of miscarriage, congenital malformation and stillbirth
- Attend counselling on risks of pregnancy, frequency of follow up and need for close monitoring
- Take the required amount of folic acid — 5 mg per day

b. Hypertension

- Ensure optimal blood pressure control (maintain below 140/90 mmHg).
- Take antihypertensives as required
- Stop ACE inhibitors, angiotensin II receptor antagonists, Thiazide diuretics. Change medication to safe antihypertensives once the patient becomes pregnant (e.g. Methyldopa, Labetalol, Nifedipine)

c. Cardiac Disease in pregnancy

- Optimise maternal status
- Co-manage with cardiologist. Include a complete evaluation including an echocardiogram.
- Patients need to understand maternal and foetal risks
- Maternal risks include pulmonary oedema, arrhythmias, stroke, cardiac arrest, aortic aneurysm/dissection, venous thromboembolism and death

- Discussion of foetal risks – increased perinatal morbidity and mortality (intrauterine growth restriction, preterm labour, foetal acidosis and foetal death)
- Awareness of risk of transmission of cardiac defect to off-spring — risk of recurrence varies with specific parental defect. The frequent recurrent lesions include: Ventricular septal defect, coarctation of aorta, hypoplastic left heart syndrome.
- Cardiac surgery improves fertility. Repair defects prior to pregnancy if indicated, do necessary medication adjustments. If condition can be cured, do so before pregnancy (ASD, PDA, some forms of coarctation). If condition can be ameliorated, do so before pregnancy (MS, MR, AS, Tetralogy, VSD with mild pulmonary hypertension, PS)
- Pregnancy before valve replacement (prosthetic) should be advised
- Patients with valve replacements should be aware of the need for continuous monitoring and therapeutic anticoagulation. In women on long-term Warfarin who are planning to conceive, pregnancy tests should be done if patients miss their menses, to ensure prompt adjustment of anticoagulation therapy if needed.
- Predictors for adverse cardiac events include:
  - Pulmonary hypertension
  - Maternal cyanosis
  - Poor maternal functional class (NYHA 3/4)
  - History of arrhythmias
  - Maternal anticoagulants

- High risk lesions include:
  - Severe aortic stenosis
  - Symptomatic mitral stenosis (NYHA class II-IV)
  - Aortic or mitral regurgitation (NYHA class III-IV)
  - Aortic or mitral valve disease with left ventricular dysfunction (left ventricular ejection fraction <40%)
  - Severe pulmonary hypertension (Pulmonary artery pressure >75% of systemic pressure)

(Key: MS- mitral stenosis, MR- mitral regurgitation, AS- aortic stenosis, VSD-ventricular septal defect, PS-pulmonary stenosis)

d. Thyroid disorders

- Optimise control
- Co-manage with endocrinologist
- For use of thyroid drugs during pregnancy, please refer to Chapter 20 on "Medications in Pregnancy and Lactation"

e. Epilepsy

- Co-manage with neurologist and optimise *antiepileptic drug* regime (AED)
- Use monotherapy at the lowest possible dose
- Attend counselling on congenital malformations, e.g. cleft lip/palate
- Take the required amount of folic acid (high dose — 5 mg per day)

- For patients who are seizure-free for two or more years, stop AED six months prior to conception
- Get referral to a genetic counsellor
- For use of AED in pregnancy, please refer to Chapter 20 on "Medications in Pregnancy and Lactation."

f. Major psychiatric disorders

- Co-manage with a psychiatrist
- Use of benzodiazepines may be associated with anomalies like cleft lip and palate as well as withdrawal syndrome in newborn
- Exposure to tricyclic antidepressants (TCA) and selective serotonin reuptake inhibitors (SSRI) — late in pregnancy — may be associated with withdrawal syndrome in newborns (adaptation syndrome)
- For use of drugs, refer to Chapter 20 on "Medications in Pregnancy and Lactation."

g. Malignant disorders

- Consider storage of semen /cryopreservation of ovarian tissue before cancer treatment

h. Obesity

- Optimise weight control (aim for ideal BMI of 18–23 kg/m^2)
- Aim for a maintenance diet of 1800 calories per day while trying to conceive
- Exercise

i. Venous Thromboembolism (VTE)

All women should undergo a documented assessment of risk factors for venous thromboembolism (VTE) listed below in early pregnancy or before pregnancy.

This assessment should be repeated if the woman is admitted to hospital for any reason or develops other intercurrent problems.

Women at high risk of VTE in pregnancy, such as those with previous VTE, should be offered pre-pregnancy counselling and a prospective management plan for thromboprophylaxis in pregnancy.

Women with a previous non-oestrogen-related VTE provoked by a minor risk factor should undergo testing for thrombophilia, as this will influence management and decisions regarding thromboprophylaxis antenatally.

Risk factors for venous thromboembolism in pregnancy include:

Pre-existing conditions/risk factors

Previous venous thromboembolism

(a) *Thrombophilia*:

Heritable:

Antithrombin deficiency
Protein C deficiency
Protein S deficiency
Factor V Leiden
Prothrombin gene G20210A

(b) *Acquired (antiphospholipid syndrome)*:
Persistent lupus anticoagulant
Persistent moderate/high-titre anticardiolipin antibodies or β2 glycoprotein 1 antibodies

Medical co-morbidities, e.g. heart or lung disease, SLE[a], cancer, inflammatory conditions (such as inflammatory bowel disease or inflammatory polyarthropathy), nephrotic syndrome (proteinuria > 3 g/day), sickle cell disease, intravenous drug user
Age > 35 years

Obesity (BMI[b] > 30 kg/m^2) either pre-pregnancy or in early pregnancy

Parity ≥ 3

Smoking

Gross varicose veins (symptomatic or above knee or with associated phlebitis, oedema/skin changes) paraplegia

Obstetric conditions/risk factors

Multiple pregnancy, assisted reproductive therapy

Pre-eclampsia

Caesarean section

Prolonged labour, mid-cavity rotational operative delivery

PPH[c] (> 1 litre) requiring transfusion

---

[a] SLE = systemic lupus erythematosus
[b] BMI = body mass index;
[c] PPH = postpartum haemorrhage;

New-onset/transient conditions/risk factors

Surgical procedure in pregnancy or puerperium (e.g. ERPC[d], appendicectomy, postpartum sterilisation)

Potentially reversible conditions/risk factors

Hyperemesis, dehydration

Ovarian hyperstimulation syndrome

Admission or immobility (≥ 3 days' bed rest) e.g. symphysis pubis dysfunction restricting mobility

Systemic infection (requiring antibiotics or admission to hospital) e.g. pneumonia, pyelonephritis

Postpartum wound infection

Long-distance travel (> 4 hours)

2. Avoid Teratogenic Drugs (Refer to Chapter 20 on "Medications in Pregnancy and Lactation")

3. Screen for Infections and Genetic Blood Disorders — Treat, Immunise and Counsel

- Full blood count with red cell indices (if MCV is low <80, screen for thalassaemia) — refer to Chapter 25 on "Approach to Prenatal Screening for Thalassaemia"

---

[d] ERPC = evacuation of retained products of conception;

- Syphilis screening
- Hepatitis B surface antigen
- HIV counselling and testing
- Rubella titre
- Varicella (in women with negative history)

Preconception immunisations (rubella/hepatitis B/varicella)
Vaccinate if non-immune. Refrain from getting pregnant within 4 weeks of vaccination.

- Miscellaneous:
  - Toxoplasmosis — avoid cat litter, garden soil, raw meat
  - Cytomegalovirus, parvovirus B19 — frequent hand washing, universal precautions for child care and health care

Cervical screening — PAP Smear

Ultrasound pelvis to exclude pelvic pathologies (e.g. fibroids, ovarian cysts, etc)

Check Dental Hygiene

Gum and dental infections have been shown to increase risk of preterm labour

4. Encourage Appropriate Counselling Sessions

a. Genetic Risk Counselling offered to:

- Older couples
- Couples with neural tube defects (NTD) in previous baby
- Couples with risk of having foetus with haemoglobinopathy
    - Encourage folic acid intake at least 400 μg/day
    - For women with diabetes or epilepsy, higher dose of folic acid 5 mg/day is recommended
    - For mothers with history of babies with neural tube defects, folic acid 5 mg/day is recommended in subsequent pregnancies

b. Avoid High-Risk Activities

- *Alcohol* (associated with risk of miscarriage and foetal malformations): patients should be treated through interventional counselling and referral to treatment programme
- *Smoking* is associated with miscarriage, intrauterine growth restriction, preterm labour, attention deficit disorder in the child

Smoking cessation requires:

- Behavioural techniques/support groups/family help
- Nicotine patches/gum may be helpful before conception but strict supervision by the doctor is recommended

- *Substance abuse* — recreational drugs such as heroin, cocaine, opiates and marijuana are associated with miscarriage, intrauterine growth restriction, preterm labour, abruption and neuro-behavioural abnormalities
- Refer to substance abuse treatment programme
- For women with heroin abuse, referral to a supervised withdrawal programme prior to conception is recommended. An alternative is supervised methadone maintenance programme, i.e. if the patient is unable to complete/tolerate the withdrawal programme

c. Exercise

- Regular moderate exercise is generally beneficial. Pregnant women should limit vigorous exercises to avoid an increase in core body temperature above 38°C (100.4°F) which can increase the risk of neural tube defects

d. Nutrition

- ***Dietary and Vitamin Supplementation***

Using *folic acid* before conception and continuing intake for the first three months of pregnancy is effective in reducing neural tube defects in offspring of women in the general population (at low risk — 400 mcg daily), as well as in offspring of women with previously affected babies. (Recommendation — 5 mg daily)

Strict vegans may have deficiencies in amino acids, zinc, calcium, iron and Vitamins D and B_{12}. Refer to dietician

Women with *milk intolerance* can benefit from consuming lactose reduced milk, lactose tablets or calcium supplements

Avoid overdose of:

— Vitamin A (limit to 3000 IU per day). Teratogenic in dosages of 20,000 to 50,000 IU/day.

— Vitamin D (limit to 400 IU per day). 1600 — 2000 IU/day can cause fetal hypercalcemia and growth retardation

— Caffeine (limit to a maximum of one cup per day; high intake may increase the risk of miscarriage and low birth weight)

Recommended dietary allowence (RDA) for iron during pregnancy — 30 mg of elemental iron per day

RDA for calcium during pregnancy — 1200 mg per day

e. Screen for Domestic Violence and Counselling

f. Lifestyle

- Recommend regular moderate exercise
- Avoid hyperthermia (hot tubs, overheating)

- Caution against obesity and being underweight
- Assess nutritional deficiencies (vegan/pica/milk intolerance/calcium and iron deficiency)
- Avoid environmental toxins such as:-
  - Metals like lead and mercury
  - Pesticides (2, 4, 5T and 2, 4-D organophosphates)
  - Radiation
  - Plastics (vinyl chloride)
  - Solvents like trichloroethylene, benzene, toluene present in paint strippers, dry cleaning fluids)

Chapter 2

ROUTINE ANTENATAL FOLLOW-UP

OBJECTIVES OF ANTENATAL VISITS

1. Assess maternal and foetal well-being.
2. Identify risk factors and consider appropriate interventions.
3. Provide advice, reassurance, education and support for the patient and her family.
4. Offer Down Syndrome screening for all women at any maternal age.
   - First trimester screening at $11–13^{+6}$ weeks of gestation
   - Maternal serum screening at 15–20 weeks of gestation
   - Diagnostic tests (chorionic villous sampling, amniocentesis) if screening test indicates high risk (1 : 300)
5. Review all the investigation results promptly to ensure normality or act appropriately if the results are abnormal.

Recommended Routine Antenatal Follow Up

Trimester	Weeks	Labs/Screening	Procedure/Imaging
First	First antenatal visit 8–12 weeks	– Full blood count – Blood type. Rhesus status and antibody screen – Urine FEME to detect asymptomatic bacteriuria (urinalysis followed by urine culture if results are positive) – Rubella screen for immunity – Syphilis screen – Hepatitis B surface antigen – HIV antibody testing – Pap smear (if appropriate)	Dating ultrasound scan • Expected date of delivery (most accurate from first trimester scan) • Assess location • Assess viability • Confirm singleton or multiple gestations
	$11–13^{+6}$ weeks	Down syndrome screening (first trimester screening) ("Refer to Chapter 27, Screening for Chromosomal Defects")	First trimester screening (nuchal translucency ultrasound scan +/– maternal serum screening).
Second	15–20 weeks	Down syndrome screening (maternal serum screening if not done earlier)	
	18–22 weeks		Screening ultrasound scan to exclude structural abnormalities

(Continued)

(Continued)

Trimester	Weeks	Labs/Screening	Procedure/Imaging
Third	28 weeks	Oral glucose tolerance test if indicated (24–28 weeks)	• Administer anti-D immunoglobulin if needed • Interval growth scan
Subsequent Visits	32–35 weeks	Routine follow up	Administer anti-D immunoglobulin if needed (34 weeks)
	35–37 weeks (weekly follow up)	• Determine foetal presentation/amniotic fluid index/estimated foetal weight • Screen for Group B streptococcus (GBS) usually at 35–37 weeks *Exclusion*: Those with GBS bacteriuria detected earlier in present pregnancy and previous infant with invasive GBS disease (will need intrapartum antibiotics prophylaxis regardless of confirmation status)	Discuss mode and timing of delivery.
	40 weeks onwards		Discuss induction of labour/delivery if post date.

National Institute for Clinical Excellence (NICE) recommends 10 appointments during first pregnancy and seven during subsequent ones (Guideline, October 2003).

Warning Symptoms in Pregnancy

Symptoms	Action
Abdominal contractions	• Exclude labour by assessment of cervical dilatation • **Refer OBGYN** if in labour • Braxton-Hicks contractions are common in the third trimester. Unlike labour pains, they are irregular in intensity, unpredictable, non-rhythmic, usually taper off and then disappear
Vaginal discharge or leaking liquor	• Use amnicator (Nitrazine test) to exclude leaking liquor • Use Actim-PROM[a] (used in KKH) • Perform high vaginal swab for Group B streptococcus (GBS) infection if indicated; if GBS positive, will need intrapartum antibiotics to prevent neonatal GBS sepsis
Reduced foetal movements (after 24 weeks gestation)	• **Refer OBGYN** for assessment of foetal well-being • Instruct the patient on Cardiff "Count-to-ten" foetal movement chart

[a]ActimPROM-rapid dipstick, detects IGFBP-1 (insulin-like growth factor binding protein-1) in vaginal samples.
Sensitivity — 94.75%
Specificity — 93%
No interference from blood, other vaginal secretions or body fluid.

How to Instruct Your Patient on Cardiff "Count-to-Ten" Foetal Movement Chart?

This method uses an 8-to 12-hour period to record 10 of your baby's movements. The time period you choose is preferably your baby's most active period, for example in the evenings.

(*Continued*)

(Continued)

When charting, start your timing at around the same time each day. The first time you feel your baby move, record the time and write it down on your graph. Try to count every movement or kick until your baby has moved ten times. When you feel your tenth movement, note the time.

If your baby has at least 10 movements within this 12-hour period, he/she is thought to be well. If your baby has not moved in 12 hours or you are concerned, you should see your doctor immediately.

Warning signs in pregnancy

General	Action
Blood Pressure	• Repeat if ≥ 140/90. Check for proteinuria • **Refer OBGYN** if still elevated • Start antihypertensives as appropriate
Weight	• Expect a normal weight increase • *Ideal Weight Gain in Pregnancy* — BMI <18.5 kg/m² (underweight)* — weight gain 12.5 to 18.0 kg — BMI 18.5 to 24.9 kg/m² (normal weight)* — weight gain 11.5 to 16.0 kg — BMI 25.0 to 29.9 kg/m² (overweight)* — weight gain 7.0 to 11.5 kg — BMI ≥ 30.0 kg/m² (obese)* — weight gain 5 to 9.0 kg **WHO International classification of BMI*

(Continued)

(Continued)

General	Action
Urinalysis	• Urine albumin +: exclude urinary tract infection, vaginal discharge, pre-eclampsia or renal disease. Also consider false positives due to semen, blood, vaginal secretions • Check blood pressure and perform blood tests to exclude pre-eclampsia • Do 24-hour urinary total protein (abnormal if >0.3g/ day) if persistent proteinuria $\geq$ 2+ • Protein:creatinine ratio may be reasonably used as an alternative to the 24-hr urine collection method The protein creatinine ratio of $\geq$ 0.3 is an indicator of protein excretion $\geq$ 300 mg/24 hr. (Sensitivity, 98.2%; specificity, 98.8%) • Glycosuria: exclude diabetes mellitus if persistent ($\geq$ 2 episodes). Do 75 g oral glucose tolerance test (OGTT) • **Refer OBGYN** if tests are abnormal

Examination	Action
Symphyseal fundal height (smaller than dates)	• **Refer OBGYN** for assessment of small-for-gestation foetus (IUGR) if dating is correct
Malpresentation	• Repeat scan for presentation at 34 weeks • **Refer OBGYN** if non-cephalic presentation
Doptone (after 12 weeks of gestation)	• **Refer OBGYN** if doptone is negative to suggest intrauterine death (IUD)

Chapter 3

VACCINATION IN PREGNANCY

GENERAL PRINCIPLES

- No evidence of risk to foetus from vaccinating pregnant women with inactivated virus, bacterial vaccine or toxoid
- The benefits of vaccinating pregnant women outweigh potential risks when the likelihood of disease exposure is high or when infection would pose a risk to the mother or foetus. Ensure all vaccines administered are fully documented in the patient's medical record
- Live-virus vaccines are contraindicated for pregnant women because of the **theoretical** risk of transmission of the vaccine virus to the foetus
- If a live-virus vaccine is inadvertently given to a pregnant woman, or if a woman becomes pregnant within 4 weeks after vaccination, she should be counselled about the potential effects on the foetus. It is not ordinarily an indication to terminate the pregnancy
- No known risk to the foetus from passive immunisation of pregnant women with immune globulin preparations

- Neither inactivated nor live vaccines administered to a lactating woman affect the safety of breastfeeding for mothers or infants
- Breast-feeding does not adversely affect immunisation and is not a contraindication for any vaccine

The need for certain vaccines like mumps, measles, rubella (MMR), varicella, diphtheria, tetanus and pertussis vaccination (DTap) should be assessed before conception. It is advisable that a woman refrains from getting pregnant within 4 weeks of vaccination of these vaccines.

HepBsAg should also be tested during every pregnancy. If the mother is found to be HepBsAg positive ensure that the infant receives hepatitis B vaccine no later than 12 hours after birth and completes the recommended hepatitis B vaccine series on schedule. Hepatitis B immunoglobulin should also be administered to neonates of hepatitis B positive mothers within 12 hours of birth.

VACCINATIONS CONTRAINDICATED IN PREGNANCY

In general, live vaccines are contraindicated in pregnancy. These include:

- Mumps, measles and rubella (MMR)
- Varicella
- Bacillus Calmette-Guerin (BCG)
- Poliomyelitis
- Smallpox

Vaccinations

Type of Vaccine	Recommendation of Use in Pregnancy	Remarks
Hepatitis B	*Recommended in some circumstances	Not a contraindication. The vaccine contains non-infectious HBsAg particles
Human papillomavirus (HPV)	Not recommended	If pregnant patient inadvertently given 1st dose, complete the three-dose series postpartum. No intervention is needed
Influenza (inactivated)	Recommended	May be given at any trimester. Increased risk of influenza-related complications if not vaccinated
Meningococcal conjugate (MCV4)	Inadequate data for specific recommendation	No safety data in pregnancy
MMR (mumps, measles, rubella)	Contraindicated	Exclude pregnancy before administration. Postpartum women previously unimmunised and seronegative — to be vaccinated a few days after delivery
Pneumococcal polysaccharide	**Recommended in some circumstances	No adverse consequences have been reported among newborns whose mothers were inadvertently vaccinated during pregnancy

(Continued)

(*Continued*)

Type of Vaccine	Recommendation of Use in Pregnancy	Remarks
Bacillus Calmette-Guerin (BCG)	Contraindicated	Live freeze-dried vaccine. No harmful effects of BCG vaccination on the foetus have been observed; however, further studies required to prove its safety
Rabies	Use when benefits outweigh risks	Pregnancy is not considered a contraindication to post-exposure prophylaxis. Some studies have indicated no increased incidence of abortion, premature births or foetal abnormalities
Tetanus and diphtheria (Td)	Recommended	Td toxoid is indicated for pregnant women although it is not routinely given in Singapore **Regime: Primigravida 2 doses — 1 month apart in the 2nd or 3rd trimester. Multigravida — 1 dose if immunised in previous pregnancy** Previously vaccinated pregnant women who have not received a Td vaccination within the last 10 years could receive a booster dose. Although no evidence exists that tetanus and diphtheria toxoids are teratogenic, waiting until the **second** trimester of pregnancy to administer Td is a reasonable precaution for minimising any theoretical concerns

(*Continued*)

(*Continued*)

Type of Vaccine	Recommendation of Use in Pregnancy	Remarks
Tetanus, diphtheria, and pertussis (Tdap)	Recommended	Unvaccinated pregnant women should get one dose of Tdap during the third trimester or late second trimester (after 20 weeks gestation). If not administered during pregnancy, Tdap should be administered immediately postpartum
Typhoid	NA	Insufficient data to recommend use
Varicella	Contraindicated	Pregnant women without immunity who are exposed should be strongly considered for varicella zoster immune globulin (VZIG). There is no evidence of foetal infection, congenital varicella syndrome or neonatal varicella in women administered VZIG.
Yellow Fever	May be used if benefits outweigh risks	Not recommended unless there is a significant risk of exposure. Delay until third trimester, if possible

*Women at risk for hepatitis B infection during pregnancy (e.g. having more than one sex partner during past six months, been evaluated or treated for STI, recent or current injection drug use or having had a HBsAg — positive sex partner).

**Recommendations if at risk of pneumococcal disease during pregnancy.

Chapter 4

APPROACH TO BLEEDING IN EARLY PREGNANCY

Causes

1. Miscarriage (threatened/missed/inevitable/incomplete/complete)
2. Ectopic pregnancy*
3. Local causes — polyps (common), cervical cancer (rare)
4. Molar pregnancy (rare)
5. Implantation bleeding

---

*Note: Important not to miss an ectopic pregnancy as it is potentially life-threatening.

Management of Early Pregnancy Bleeding

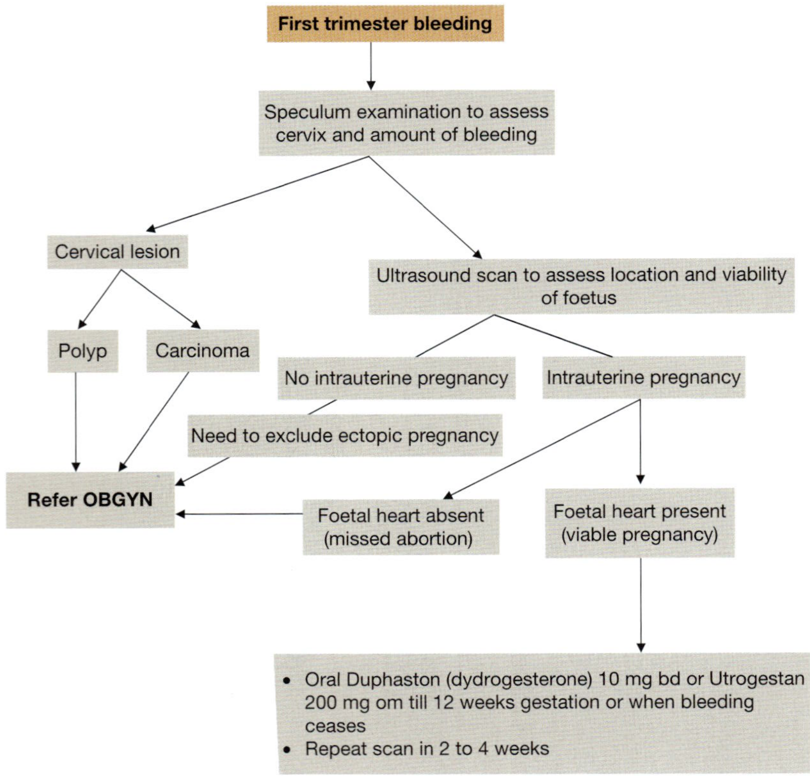

Approach to Bleeding in Early Pregnancy

History

- **Menstrual history**
  - Number of weeks amenorrhoea, regularity of menstrual cycles
- **Vaginal bleeding**
  - Onset, quantity, trigger factors
- **Associated symptoms**
  - Lower abdominal pain, giddiness

↓

Physical Examination

- **Vital parameters**
  - Assess if haemodynamically stable
  - Haemodynamic instability usually associated with ruptured ectopic pregnancy, severe haemorrhage from miscarriage, gestational trophoblastic disease
- **Abdomen**
  - Abdominal tenderness
  - Signs of acute abdomen such as guarding and rebound tenderness usually associated with ruptured ectopic pregnancy
- **Vaginal examination**
  - Amount of ongoing bleeding
  - Cervical or vaginal lesions such as polyps, malignancy
  - Products of conception
  - Cervical os dilatation

↓

INVESTIGATIONS

Ultrasound Scan

— To assess location of pregnancy and foetal viability

— A *gestational sac* may be identified as early as 5 weeks gestation, usually when the serum βhcg is above 1500 IU/L via a *transvaginal* ultrasound of the pelvis (discriminatory level of βhcg)

(*Continued*)

(*Continued*)

— A *double decidual sign* indicates an intrauterine pregnancy
— The *yolk sac* is usually visualised by 5–6 weeks gestation, and disappears by 10 weeks gestation
— A *blighted ovum* is diagnosed when the **IUGS is > 25 mm** but there is no yolk sac
— A *miscarriage* is diagnosed with the **CRL is > 7 mm** without foetal cardiac activity or if the CRL does not increase in size with gestation.
— If a miscarriage is diagnosed, identification of remnant products of conception, and thickness of endometrium should be measured to determine if surgical evacuation of uterus is needed
— If an ectopic pregnancy is suspected in the absence of an intrauterine gestational sac (IUGS), efforts should be made to look for adnexal masses or free fluid within the pouch of douglas
— *Complete* molar pregnancy has the classical image of a cystic snowstorm appearance whereas *partial* molar pregnancies are often diagnosed retrospectively by histology, after evacuation of uterus, as they may often be mistaken as miscarriages on ultrasound scan

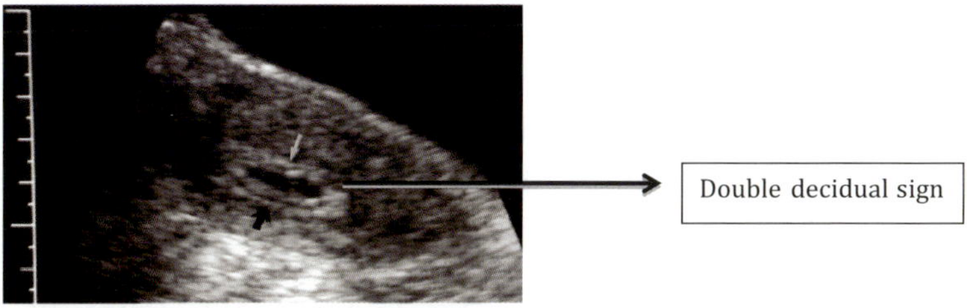

Figure 1. Intrauterine gestational sac (IUGS).

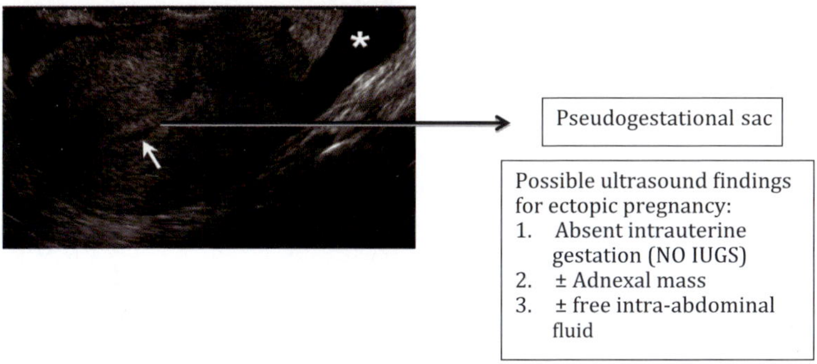

Figure 2. Ectopic pregnancy.

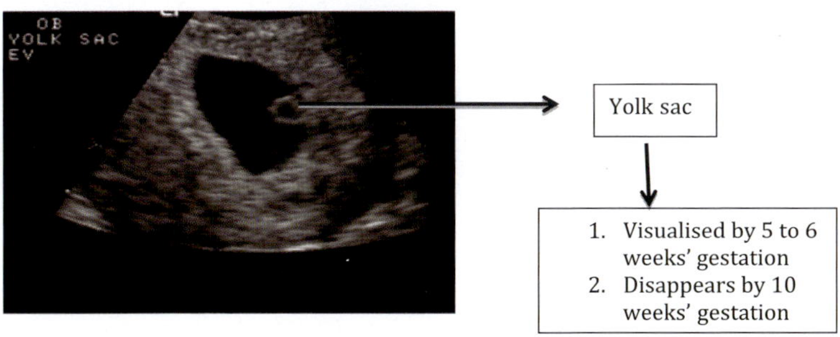

Figure 3. Yolk sac.

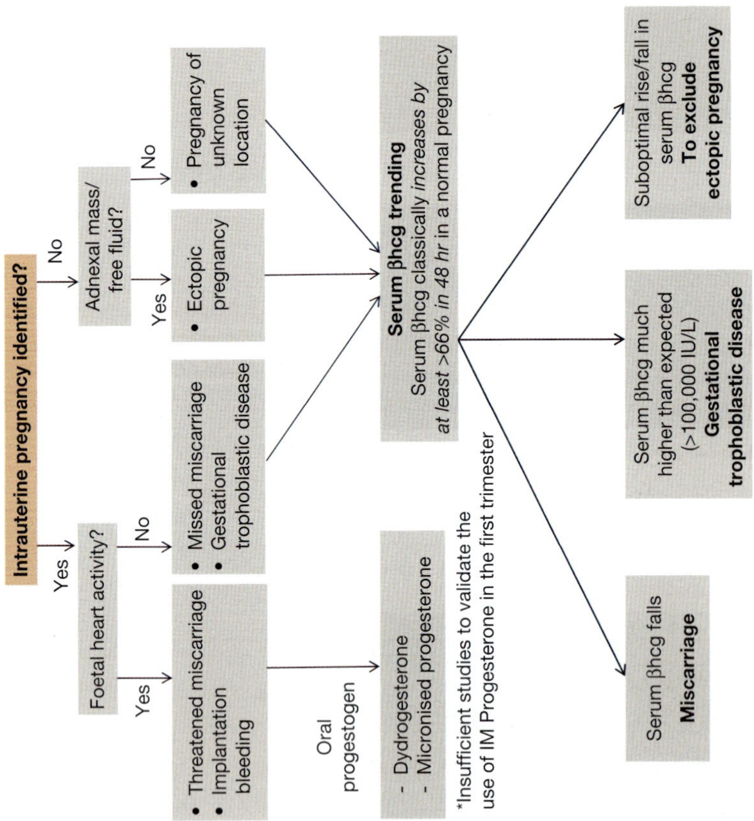
Intrauterine pregnancy identified?
Yes
No
Foetal heart activity?
Yes
No
Adnexal mass/ free fluid?
Yes
No
• Threatened miscarriage
• Implantation bleeding
• Missed miscarriage
• Gestational trophoblastic disease
• Ectopic pregnancy
• Pregnancy of unknown location
Oral progestogen
- Dydrogesterone
- Micronised progesterone
*Insufficient studies to validate the use of IM Progesterone in the first trimester
Serum βhcg trending
Serum βhcg classically increases by at least >66% in 48 hr in a normal pregnancy
Serum βhcg falls
Miscarriage
Serum βhcg much higher than expected (>100,000 IU/L)
Gestational trophoblastic disease
Suboptimal rise/fall in serum βhcg
To exclude ectopic pregnancy

Chapter 5

APPROACH TO SPONTANEOUS MISCARRIAGE

Spontaneous miscarriage is defined as the loss of a clinically recognised pregnancy prior to the 24th week of gestation. The incidence of spontaneous miscarriage averages around 15% in the general population, with a rate of 8–20% in the first trimester, and decreasing to ~3% in the second trimester.

Aetiologies

1. Chromosomal Abnormalities
   - Account for 50% of first trimester miscarriages and 30% of second trimester miscarriages
   - Usually due to aneuploidies, structural abnormalities and mosaicism

2. Congenital Anomalies
    - Caused by genetic, chromosomal abnormalities or from extrinsic factors such as exposure to teratogens
3. Endocrine Disorders
    - Poorly controlled diabetes mellitus
    - Thyroid disorders
    - Polycystic ovarian syndrome (PCOS)
4. Hypercoagulable Disorders
    - *Thrombophilia*: Antithrombin III deficiency, protein C/S deficiency
    - *Autoimmune*: Antiphospholipid syndrome, systemic lupus erythematosus (SLE)
5. Maternal Infections
    - Listeria monocytogenes, toxoplasma gondii, parvovirus B19, rubella, herpes simplex, cytomegalovirus
6. Structural Uterine Abnormalites
    - *Congenital*: Uterine septum, uterine didelphys
    - *Acquired*: Fibroids
7. Unexplained

Spontaneous Miscarriages

	Threatened	Incomplete	Complete	Missed	Septic
History	• PV[a] staining • Occasional abdominal pain	• PV bleeding • Abdominal pain • POC passed	• PV bleeding • Abdominal pain • POC passed	• PV staining • No abdominal pain	• PV bleeding/ discharge • Abdominal pain • Fever
Physical Exam	• Cervical os closed • Minimal PV bleeding	• Cervical os open • PV bleeding • POC seen	• Cervical os closed • +/– PV bleeding	• Cervical os closed	• Cervical os open • PV bleeding • Cervical excitation • Fever
US Pelvis	• FH[b] present	• FH absent • Irregular sac • RPOC[c]	• Empty uterus	• FH absent	• FH absent • RPOC

(Continued)

(*Continued*)

	Threatened	Incomplete	Complete	Missed	Septic
Management	• Expectant treatment — reassure — 97% have normal outcome • Progestogen support • Bed rest • Avoid strenuous activity • Avoid sexual activity • Repeat scan 1–2 weeks later	• Conservative — antibiotics — analgesics • Surgical — evacuation of uterus — postoperative systemic antibiotics	• Conservative — antibiotics	• Surgical — evacuation of uterus — post-operative antibiotics	• Broad spectrum IV antibiotics • Surgical — evacuation of uterus

[a]PV: Per vaginal.
[b]FH: Foetal heart.
[c]RPOC: Retained products of conception.

When to Try Conceiving Again after a Miscarriage?

Women who conceive within six months of an initial miscarriage have the best reproductive outcomes and the lowest complication rates in a subsequent pregnancy.

Chapter 6

APPROACH TO RECURRENT SPONTANEOUS MISCARRIAGE (RSM)

Recurrent spontaneous miscarriage refers to the occurrence of three or more consecutive losses of clinically recognised pregnancies prior to the 24th week of gestation.

2% of women experience two consecutive pregnancy losses, and 0.5–1% have three consecutive pregnancy losses.

Common Aetiologies

- **Genetic**
- **Anatomic**
  - Septate uterus, submucosal fibroids, endometrial polyps, intrauterine synechiae

- **Endocrine**
    - Poorly controlled diabetes mellitus, thyroid disease, polycystic ovarian syndrome, hyperprolactinaemia

- **Autoimmune**
    - Presence of lupus anticoagulant or anticardiolipin antibodies

- **Thrombophilia**

The evaluation of patients with RSM is often a challenging task as these patients often seek definitive reasons for their condition, and hope for curative measures.

However, the aetiology of RSM may not always be identifiable and there are few evidence-based treatment strategies.

Detailed History

- **Number** of spontaneous miscarriages
- **Features** of prior miscarriages
    - — Gestational age of miscarriage
    - — RSM typically occurs at a similar gestation in consecutive pregnancies

  - Miscarriages at earlier gestations reflect an underlying chromosomal abnormality
  - Miscarriages at later gestations tend to be related to anatomical factors
- **Social history**
  - Emotional trauma couple is experiencing

Investigations

- **Karyotyping**
  - Balanced reciprocal, Robertsonian translocations or mosaicism which may be passed to the foetus in the unbalanced form
  - Karyotypic assessment should be performed on both the parents, and if possible, of the abortus
- **Uterine assessment**
  - US pelvis, hysterosonography or hysterosalpingogram
  - Hysteroscopic evaluation may be considered as well, as it is both diagnostic and therapeutic
- **Endocrine screening**
  - Diabetes mellitus and thyroid disease
- **Autoimmune screening**
  - Antiphospholipid syndrome should be screened for anticardiolipin antibodies and lupus anticoagulant.

Management of RSM should be aimed at the Underlying Aetiology

- Emotional support plays a crucial role
- Parental karyotype anomalies
  - Refer to geneticist for genetic counselling
  - May choose to undergo prenatal genetic studies to determine foetal karyotype
- Uterine anomalies
  - Surgery if the defect is potentially correctable
- Poorly controlled or previously undiagnosed endocrine diseases
  - Refer to a dedicated endocrinologist
- Antiphospholipid syndrome
  - May benefit from aspirin +/– heparin (Refer to Chapter 20 on "Medications in Pregnancy and Lactation")

*Almost 50% of RSM remains unexplained

Nonetheless, the chance of a live birth is >50% without intervention

Chapter 7

APPROACH TO ABDOMINAL PAIN IN PREGNANCY

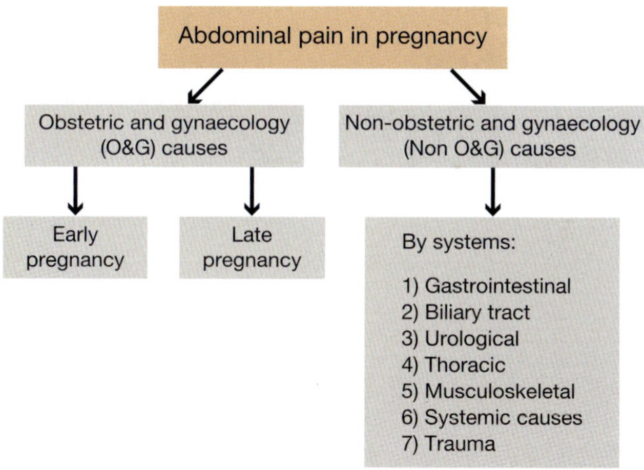

O&G causes of abdominal pain in pregnancy: Simple approach by site of pain

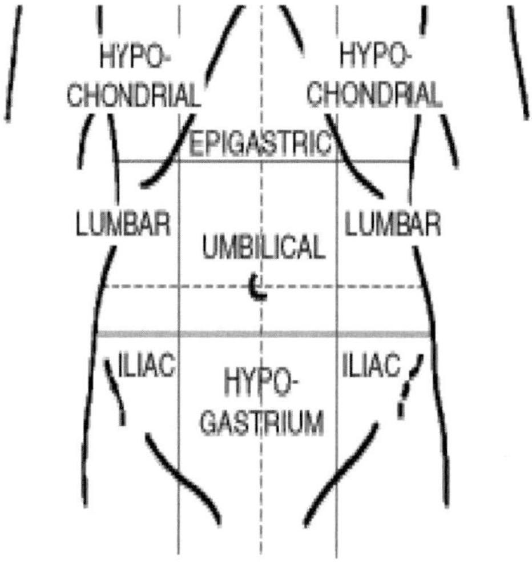

O&G Causes of Abdominal Pain in Pregnancy: Simple Approach by Site of Pain

Right hypochondrium Late pregnancy — Acute fatty liver of pregnancy	**Epigastrium** Late pregnancy — Acute fatty liver of pregnancy — Pre-eclampsia	**Left hypochondrium** Musculoskeletal (e.g. costochondritis)
Right lumbar Ureteric colic	**Umbilical** **Late pregnancy** — Polyhydramnios — Ligamental strain	**Left lumbar** Ureteric colic
Right iliac fossa **Early pregnancy** — Right ectopic pregnancy — Right adnexal torsion — Right ovarian cyst rupture — Fibroid degeneration — Ovarian hyperstimulation syndrome (OHSS) **Late pregnancy** — Right adnexal torsion	**Hypogastrium/suprapubic** **Early pregnancy** — Miscarriage: threatened, inevitable, incomplete, complete, septic — Fibroid degeneration — Acute urinary retention **Late pregnancy** — Labour — Placental abruption — Uterine rupture — Chorioamnionitis — Braxton Hicks contractions — Symphysis pubis dysfunction — Rectus abdominis rupture — Fibroid degeneration	**Left iliac fossa** **Early pregnancy** — Left ectopic pregnancy — Left adnexal torsion — Left ovarian cyst rupture — Fibroid degeneration — Ovarian hyperstimulation syndrome (OHSS) **Late pregnancy** — Left adnexal torsion

Chapter 8

OBSTETRIC & GYNAECOLOGICAL (O&G) CAUSES OF ABDOMINAL PAIN IN EARLY PREGNANCY

- Exclude *Miscarriage*: Refer to Chapter 5 on "Approach to Spontaneous Miscarriage."
- Exclude *Ectopic pregnancy*: Refer to Chapter 12 on "Approach to Ectopic Pregnancy."

Condition	Symptoms	Signs	Investigations	Management
Ruptured ovarian cyst *Risk factors* • Known history of ovarian cysts • Pain may be preceded by strenuous physical activity	• Acute onset of lower abdominal pain • Pain is usually unilateral	• Low grade fever • May have signs of shock: hypotension, tachycardia • Acute abdomen • Cervical examination: adnexal tenderness	• U/S of pelvis: adnexal mass, free fluid in pelvis • FBC, U/E/Cr, GXM • Ovarian tumour markers are not useful in pregnancy	• Advise conservative management for uncomplicated cyst rupture: give analgesia, antibiotics, correct electrolyte imbalance • Monitor clinical symptoms • Surgical management only if patient is haemodynamically unstable or suspected acute abdomen
Adnexal torsion *Risk factors* • Known history of ovarian cysts • Most common in the first trimester	• Twisting abdominal pain which may wax and wane • Nausea, vomiting	• Low grade fever • Acute abdomen with signs of peritonism	• U/S of pelvis: adnexal mass with absent or impaired ovarian venous flow on Doppler ultrasound scan • FBC, U/E/Cr, GXM • Ovarian tumour markers are *not* useful in pregnancy	• Surgical evaluation of ovarian viability, detorsion with/without cystectomy with/without salpingo-oophorectomy • Give analgesia, anti-emetics • Antibiotics • Correct electrolyte imbalance

(*Continued*)

(Continued)

Condition	Symptoms	Signs	Investigations	Management
Fibroid degeneration *Risk factors* • Known history of fibroids • Higher risk if fibroid is >5 cm in size	• Constant localised pain over fibroid • Nausea, vomiting	• Low grade fever • Tenderness over fibroid	• U/S of pelvis: fibroid with degenerative cystic changes may be present • FBC, U/E/Cr, GXM	• Conservative management: • Give analgesia, anti-emetics, correct any electrolyte imbalance
Acute urinary retention • Usually between 10th and 14th week of gestation (especially with retroverted uterus)	• Abrupt inability to pass urine • Lower abdominal/ suprapubic discomfort	• Palpable bladder • Suprapubic tenderness	• FBC, U/E/Cr • UFEME, urine culture • U/S of pelvis to exclude pelvic mass e.g. fibroid	• Insertion of indwelling catheter • Antibiotics if infection is present • Correct any electrolyte imbalance

(Continued)

(*Continued*)

Condition	Symptoms	Signs	Investigations	Management
Ovarian hyper-stimulation syndrome (OHSS) *Risk factors* • Recent treatment with gonadotrophin stimulation to induce ovulation • Recent treatment with assisted reproductive technology e.g. *in vitro* fertilisation (IVF)	• Abdominal pain, distension • Nausea, vomiting, diarrhoea • Shortness of breath • Rapid weight gain • Oliguria • Lower limb swelling	• Tachypnoea • Pleural effusion • Right or left iliac fossa tenderness • Ascites • Peripheral oedema		
Grade 1 (mild OHSS) • Affects 33% of IVF cycles • Bilateral ovarian enlargement, corpus luteum cyst (5 cm–8 cm)	• Abdominal pain and bloating			*Mild* OHSS: — Outpatient monitoring — Increase oral fluids — Bedrest — Analgesia (Paracetamol/ Codeine) — No contraindication to progesterone luteal support

(*Continued*)

(Continued)

Condition	Symptoms	Signs	Investigations	Management
Grade 2 (moderate OHSS) • Ovarian size 8–12 cm^3	• Moderate abdominal pain. Nausea, vomiting, ultrasound scan shows evidence of ascites		*Moderate* OHSS: — FBC (twice weekly) — U/E/Cr (twice weekly) — LFT (weekly) — PT/PTT (weekly) — U/S of pelvis	*Moderate* OHSS — Inpatient monitoring — Daily measurement of abdominal girth and weight — Intake/output monitoring and fluid management — Correct electrolyte imbalance — Consider i/v 20% albumin 100ml, 6–12 hourly — Antiemetics

(Continued)

(Continued)

Condition	Symptoms	Signs	Investigations	Management
Grade 3 (severe OHSS) • Affects 3–8% of IVF cycles. Corpus luteum cyst (> 12 cm³) *Critical* OHSS	• Clinical ascites, oliguria, haemo-concentration • haematocrit >45% • hypo proteinaemia. • Tense ascites, • large hydrothorax, haematocrit > 55%. • white cell count > 25 000/mL • oliguria/anuria • thrombo-embolism. • acute respiratory distress syndrome.		*Severe* OHSS: — FBC (daily) — U/E/Cr (daily) — LFT (twice weekly) — PT/PTT (twice weekly) — ABG — U/S of pelvis — Consider judicious use of CT pulmonary angiogram (if pulmonary embolism is suspected). — ECG and echo-cardiogram (if pericardial effusion suspected).	*Severe* OHSS/critical OHSS — Inpatient monitoring — Admission to ICU if necessary — Refer to Anaesthetist — Consider central monitoring lines — Daily measurement of abdominal girth and weight — Intake/output monitoring and fluid management — Correct electrolyte imbalance — Consider intravenous 20% albumin 100 mL, 6–12 hourly — Subcutaneous enoxaprine (Clexane® 0.4 mL OM) — Paracentesis under ultrasound guidance

Chapter 9

OBSTETRIC & GYNAECOLOGICAL (O&G) CAUSES OF ABDOMINAL PAIN IN LATE PREGNANCY

Condition	Symptoms	Signs	Investigations	Management
Labour	• Regular painful contractions (increasing in frequency and intensity) +/– Leaking liquor +/– Show	• Dilated cervix • Ruptured membranes • Show	• Cardiotocography (CTG)	• Term labour: admit for delivery • Preterm labour: admit to inhibit labour • Corticosteroids • Consider Tocolysis
Placental abruption	• Constant periumbilical or suprapubic pain +/– Per vaginal bleeding	• May have signs of hypovolaemic shock: tachycardia, hypotension • Woody hard uterus on abdominal palpation • Per vaginal bleeding on speculum examination	• CTG • FBC, PT/PTT, GXM • U/E/Cr	• Resuscitation and stabilisation • Expedite delivery • Neonatal standby at delivery • Active management of third stage of labour • Correct DIVC if present

(Continued)

(Continued)

Condition	Symptoms	Signs	Investigations	Management
Uterine rupture *Risk factors* • Previous caesarean section • Previous uterine surgery, e.g. myomectomy • Grand multiparity	• Sudden onset severe constant pain +/– Per vaginal bleeding	• May have signs of hypovolaemic shock: tachycardia, hypotension • Tender uterus on abdominal palpation • Foetal parts may be palpated per abdomen • Per vaginal bleeding on speculum examination	• CTG • FBC, PT/PTT, GXM	• Resuscitation and stabilisation • Expedite delivery: caesarean section — consent for hysterectomy • Neonatal standby at delivery

(Continued)

(*Continued*)

Condition	Symptoms	Signs	Investigations	Management
Chorioamnionitis *Risk factors* • History of leaking liquor	• Abdominal pain • Foul smelling vaginal discharge • Fever	• May have signs of septic shock: tachycardia, hypotension • Fever • Tender uterus on abdominal palpation • Foul smelling vaginal discharge on speculum examination	• CTG • FBC, CRP • Vaginal swab culture • Blood culture • UFEME, urine culture	• Resuscitation and stabilisation if required • IV antibiotics • Expedite delivery • Neonatal standby at delivery

(*Continued*)

(Continued)

Condition	Symptoms	Signs	Investigations	Management
Severe pre-eclampsia (PE)/ Impending eclampsia	• Epigastric / right hypochondrial pain +/– Headache +/– Vomiting +/– Blurring of vision	• Raised blood pressure • Epigastric/right hypochondrial tenderness +/– Brisk reflexes +/– Clonus +/– Papilloedema	• CTG • *PE bloods:* FBC U/E/Cr/Uric acid LFT PT/PTT T&S • Urine dipstick for albumin • 24-hr UTP or Urine protein: creatinine ratio *HELLP syndrome:* • Haemolysis • Elevated liver enzymes • Low platelet count	• Resuscitation and stabilisation if required • BP and SaO_2 monitoring • Involvement of high dependency/ intensive care unit and multidisciplinary team • Start anti-hypertensives • Indwelling catheter • Intake/output monitoring and fluid management • Intravenous magnesium sulphate ($MgSO_4$) • Expedite delivery

(Continued)

(*Continued*)

Condition	Symptoms	Signs	Investigations	Management
Acute fatty liver of pregnancy • Typically presents in third trimester *Differential diagnosis* • Pre-eclampsia • Acute viral hepatitis • Obstetric cholestasis	• Epigastric / hypochondrial pain +/– Nausea, vomiting +/– Malaise, anorexia +/– Jaundice +/– Polyuria, polydipsia	• Epigastric / right hypochondrial tenderness +/– Jaundice +/– Hypertension	• CTG • FBC, U/E/Cr, LFT, PT/PTT, Uric acid • Hypocount • *Viral hepatitis screen:* ○ Hepatitis A: • Hep A IgM ○ Hepatitis B: • HepBsAg • HepBeAg, Anti • HepBc IgM • Anti HepBc IgG ○ Hepatitis C: • Anti HCV antibodies • Ultrasound scan of liver	• Resuscitation and stabilization if required • Involve high dependency / intensive care unit and multidisciplinary team • Correction of hypoglycemia or coagulopathy • Expedite delivery • Postnatal liver function monitoring

(*Continued*)

(Continued)

Condition	Symptoms	Signs	Investigations	Management
Rectus abdominis rupture	• Sudden onset abdominal pain • Usually precipitated by coughing or vomiting	• Hematoma over rectus abdominis on abdominal palpation	• CTG • FBC, PT/PTT, GXM	• Analgesia • Conservative management • Consider referral to general surgeon for surgical exploration and drainage (if the haematoma is expanding in size)
Braxton Hicks Contraction	• Irregular painful/ painless tightenings • No leaking liquor or show	• No progressive cervical dilatation/ effacement	• CTG	• Reassurance • Outpatient follow up
Symphysis pubis dysfunction	• Suprapubic pain, which is worse with movement	• Suprapubic tenderness • Closed cervix	• CTG	• Physiotherapy • Analgesia • Reassurance • Outpatient follow up

Chapter 10

NON OBSTETRIC & GYNAECOLOGICAL (NON O&G) CAUSES OF ABDOMINAL PAIN IN PREGNANCY: SIMPLE APPROACH BY SITE OF PAIN

1) Right hypochondrium **Thoracic** — Right lower lobe pneumonia — Right pleural effusion **Biliary** — Cholecystitis — Biliary colic — Cholangitis	**Hepatic** — Hepatitis — Hepatic abscess **Gastrointestinal** — Peptic ulcer **Musculoskeletal** — Costochondritis	**2) Epigastrium** **Gastrointestinal** — Oesophagitis — Gastritis — Peptic ulcer disease — Gastro-Oesophageal reflux — Pancreatitis		**3) Left hypochondrium** **Thoracic** — Left lower lobe pneumonia — Left pleural effusion **Gastrointestinal** — Peptic ulcer disease — Pancreatitis — Diverticulitis	**Musculoskeletal** — Costochondritis
4) Right lumbar **Biliary** — Cholecystitis — Cholelithiasis — Cholangitis **Urological** — Pyelonephritis — Hydronephrosis — Renal calculi	**Gastrointestinal** — Appendicitis	**5) Umbilical** **Gastrointestinal** — Early appendicitis — Bowel obstruction — Gastroenteritis — Inflammatory bowel disease — Colitis **Trauma**	**Systemic** — Diabetic ketoacidosis — Sickle cell crisis **Musculoskeletal** — Umbilical hernia	**6) Left lumbar** **Urological** — Pyelonephritis — Hydronephrosis — Renal calculi	

(Continued)

(*Continued*)

7) Right iliac fossa **Gastrointestinal** — Appendicitis — Mesenteric adenitis — Colitis — Hernia — Inflammatory bowel disease		**8) Hypo-gastrium/suprapubic** **Urological** — Cystitis — Urinary tract infection — Acute retention of urine — Bladder calculi		**9) Left iliac fossa** **Gastrointestinal** — Constipation — Diverticulitis — Colitis — Hernia — Inflammatory bowel disease	

Chapter 11

NON OBSTETRIC & GYNAECOLOGICAL (NON O&G) CAUSES OF ABDOMINAL PAIN IN PREGNANCY

Condition	Symptoms	Signs	Specific Investigations	Management
1) Urological				
Lower urinary tract infection/cystitis	• Suprapubic pain +/– Urinary frequency +/– Urgency, dysuria +/– Haematuria +/– Fever	• Fever • Suprapubic tenderness • Haematuria	• Urine dipstick • UFEME, urine culture	• Oral antibiotics (e.g. PO Cephalexin 500 mg TDS) • Increase fluid intake • Encourage post-coital voiding and perineal hygiene
Pyelonephritis	• Loin pain radiating to abdomen +/– Fever, chills, rigors +/– Urinary frequency +/– Urgency, dysuria +/– Haematuria	• Fever • Loin tenderness • Renal punch positive	• Urine dipstick • UFEME, urine culture • FBC (note: total white count may be mildly elevated in pregnancy) • CRP, U/E/Cr • Blood culture • Ultrasound kidneys • Screen for diabetes	• Inpatient treatment • IV antibiotics • IV fluids • Analgesia

(Continued)

(*Continued*)

Condition	Symptoms	Signs	Specific Investigations	Management
Renal calculi (nephrolithiasis)	• Loin to groin pain, colicky +/– Nausea, vomiting +/– Haematuria +/– Stones passed in urine • May present with cystitis or pyelonephritis	• Renal angle tenderness • Suprapubic tenderness • Renal punch positive • Haematuria	• Urine dipstick • UFEME, urine culture • Ultrasound KUB • X-ray KUB **not** routinely done; consider only if benefits outweigh risks	• Consider inpatient treatment • IV fluids • Analgesia • Refer to urologist urgently if evidence of obstruction is present
2) Gastrointestinal				
• Gastritis • Peptic ulcer disease • Gastro-oesophageal reflux disease (GERD)	• Epigastric pain • Burning sensation related to meals +/– Nausea, vomiting +/– Bloatedness	• Epigastric tenderness		• Antacids/H_2 receptor antagonists (e.g. PO antacid, PO Ranitidine) • Advise regular meals • Refer to general surgeon or gastroenterologist (if severe and persistent symptoms)

(*Continued*)

(*Continued*)

Condition	Symptoms	Signs	Specific Investigations	Management
Appendicitis • Location of the appendix migrates cephalad with the enlarging uterus, hence location of pain may be atypical	• Central umbilical pain with subsequent radiation to right iliac fossa. +/– Loss of appetite +/– Nausea, vomiting +/– Fever	• Tachycardia • Fever • RIF tenderness +/– rebound/ guarding	• FBC (note: total white count may be mildly elevated in pregnancy) • C-reactive protein (CRP) • Ultrasound abdomen and pelvis • Serial abdominal examinations	• Inpatient treatment • Refer to general surgeon • Keep nil by mouth • IV fluids • IV Antibiotics
Intestinal obstruction *Risk factors* • Previous abdominal surgery • Hernia	• Colicky abdominal pain with nausea and vomiting • Constipation	• Abdominal tenderness +/– rebound/ guarding • Tinkling or absent bowel sounds • Fever	• FBC, U/E/Cr • ABG • Judicious use of X-ray (erect/ supine) in pregnancy	• Inpatient treatment • Refer to general surgeon • Keep nil by mouth • IV fluids • NG tube insertion • Correct electrolyte imbalance

(*Continued*)

(Continued)

Condition	Symptoms	Signs	Specific Investigations	Management
Pancreatitis *Risk factors* • Gallstone disease • Hyperlipidaemia • Steroid use • Autoimmune disease • Trauma • Alcohol intake	• Epigastric pain radiating to back +/– Nausea, vomiting +/– Loss of appetite	• Tachycardia, low grade fever • Epigastric tenderness	• Amylase, lipase (note: levels may be mildly elevated in pregnancy) • FBC, U/E/Cr, LFT, lactate dehydrogenase, Ca/Mg/PO_4 • ABG • Ultrasound abdomen	• Inpatient treatment • Refer to general surgeon • Keep nil by mouth • IV fluids • Analgesia • Monitor intake/ output • Correct electrolyte imbalance • Anticipate and manage complications of renal failure, acute respiratory distress syndrome, infection

(Continued)

(Continued)

Condition	Symptoms	Signs	Specific Investigations	Management
Gastroenteritis *Risk factors* • Recent travel history • Contact history	• Colicky abdominal pain +/– Nausea, vomiting +/– Diarrhoea +/– Fever	• Fever • Mild abdominal tenderness	• Consider stool sample for cysts, ova, parasites, culture in cases of positive travel history or prolonged diarrhoea	• Symptomatic treatment • Intake/output chart • Increase oral fluids • Advise hand hygiene • Consider antibiotics if systemically unwell
Diverticulitis	• LIF pain +/– Nausea, vomiting +/– Fever +/– Constipation or diarrhoea	• Fever • LIF tenderness • Palpable LIF mass	• FBC, CRP, U/E/Cr	• Inpatient treatment • Refer to general surgeon • Keep nil by mouth • IV fluids • IV antibiotics • Analgesia

(Continued)

(*Continued*)

Condition	Symptoms	Signs	Specific Investigations	Management
5) Thoracic				
Pneumonia *Risk factors* • Recent travel history • Positive contact history	• Fever • Cough, shortness of breath • Hypochondrial pain if lower lobe pneumonia	• Fever • Tachypnoea, tachycardia • Confusion if severe • Inspiratory crepitations	• FBC, CRP, U/E/Cr • ABG • H1N1 swab • Sputum for gram stain, culture • Sputum for AFB stain, TB culture • Blood culture • CXR (with abdominal shield)	• Inpatient treatment • Refer to infectious disease physician • Isolate patient • SaO_2 monitoring • O_2 support • IV fluids • IV antibiotics

(*Continued*)

(*Continued*)

Condition	Symptoms	Signs	Specific Investigations	Management
6) Systemic				
Diabetic ketoacidosis (DKA) *Risk factors* Known history of diabetes mellitus +/– trigger for DKA e.g. infection, non compliance to medications	• Vomiting, shortness of breath • Confusion, lethargy • Low urine output • Abdominal pain	• Dehydration • Tachycardia, hypotension • Fever • Kussmaul breathing • Decreased consciousness • High hypocount or blood glucose	• Hypocount • FBC, U/E/Cr • ABG • Serum lactate • Serum glucose • ECG +/– CXR (with abdominal shield) +/– Blood, urine or sputum cultures	• Inpatient treatment • Refer to endocrine physician • Intake/output charting • IV fluids • IV insulin bolus followed by IV infusion • Monitor serum K^+ and blood glucose levels • Treat precipitating factors e.g. sepsis, dehydration

(*Continued*)

(*Continued*)

Condition	Symptoms	Signs	Specific Investigations	Management
Sickle cell crisis *Risk factors* Known history of sickle cell disease with trigger for painful crisis, e.g. dehydration, stress, over exertion, infection	• Abdominal pain • Nausea, vomiting • Painful joints/ bones • Chest pain, shortness of breath	• Dehydration • Tachycardia • Fever • Pallor • Abdominal tenderness	• FBC, CRP, U/E/Cr, LFT • GXM • ECG +/– CXR with abdominal shield +/– Blood, urine or sputum cultures	• Inpatient treatment if in severe pain • IV fluids • Oxygen supplementation • Analgesia • Thromboprophylaxis e.g. TED stockings • Treat precipitating cause e.g. infection, dehydration • Early recognition of complications, e.g. acute coronary syndrome, acute stroke +/– Blood transfusion

(*Continued*)

(*Continued*)

Condition	Symptoms	Signs	Specific Investigations	Management
7) Trauma				
History of abdominal trauma, e.g. involvement in road traffic accident	• Abdominal pain +/– Contractions +/– Leaking liquor +/– Per vaginal bleeding	• Activate advanced trauma life support (ATLS) if necessary • Assess and secure airway, breathing, circulation, neurological evaluation • Secondary survey: head to toe assessment • Speculum and vaginal examination	• CTG • FBC, U/E/Cr, PT/PTT • GXM	• Prompt multidisciplinary team input • Resuscitation and stabilisation of patient • Early recognition of penetrating abdominal trauma, uterine rupture, abruptio placentae, preterm prelabour rupture of membranes, preterm labour — prompt management accordingly

(*Continued*)

(Continued)

Key:

ABG = Arterial blood gases
Ca = Calcium
CRP = C-Reactive protein
DIVC = Disseminated intravascular coagulopathy
FBC = Full blood count
GXM = Group crossmatch
KUB = Kidney, ureter, bladder
LFT = Liver function test
Mg = Magnesium
PO_4 = Phosphate
PT/PTT = Prothrombin time/Partial thromboplastin time
T&S = Type and screen
U/E/Cr = Urea, electrolytes, creatinine
UFEME = Urine full examination, microscopic examination
U/S = Ultrasound scan
UTP = Urinary total protein

Chapter 12

APPROACH TO ECTOPIC PREGNANCY (EP)

Ectopic pregnancy is the leading cause of pregnancy related maternal death in the first trimester.

Hence a high clinical index of suspicion should be entertained if a patient presents with per vaginal bleeding and abdominal pain in early pregnancy.

Natural Progession

- Tubal abortion
- Tubal rupture
- Spontaneous resolution

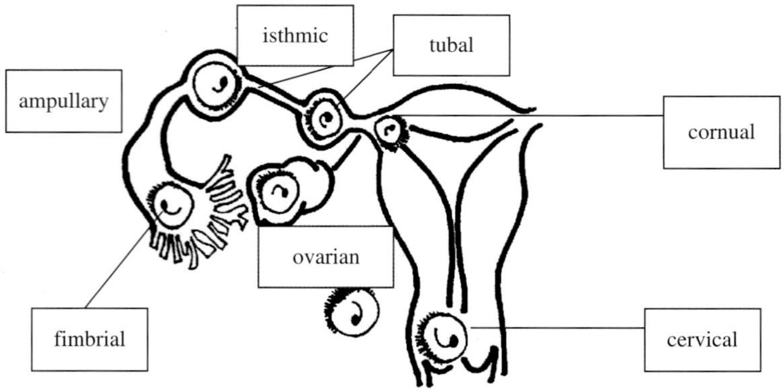

Incidence of Ectopic Pregnancy

- Fallopian tube – 98%
  - Ampulla – 70%
  - Isthmus – 12%
  - Fimbria – 12%
  - Cornu – 2 – 3%
  - Interstitial – 2 – 3%
- Abdominal - 1.3%
- Ovarian – 0.5%
- Cervical – 0.2%
- Caesarean scar ectopic — 1 in 1800 – 2200 pregnancies
- Heterotopic – 1.5 per 1000 Assisted Reproductive Technology (ART) procedures

Figure 1. Possible sites of ectopic pregnancy.

Classical Triad of an Ectopic Pregnancy

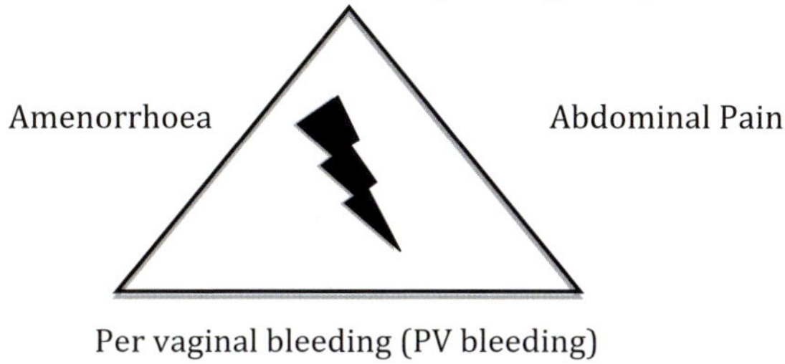

History

- *Presenting complaints*: amenorrhoea, lower abdominal pain, PV bleeding
- *Risk factors*:
  - — Uterine anomalies/Asherman syndrome
  - — Previous tubal surgery (Re-anastomosis/ligation)
  - — Previous pelvic inflammatory disease (chronic salpingitis)
  - — Previous ectopic pregnancies

    Risk of recurrence after 1 prior ectopic pregnancy — 15%

    Risk of recurrence after 2 prior ectopic pregnancies — 30%
  - — Assisted reproductive techniques (ART)
  - — Presence of intrauterine contraceptive devices (IUCD)
    - — women using IUCDs have a lower incidence of ectopic pregnancy than non-contracepting women

because IUCD prevents fertilisation and implantation. (However, IUCD users are at higher risk of having an ectopic pregnancy if a pregnancy occurs)

— Smoking
— Previous caesarean section

Physical Examination

Vital Parameters:
— Assess for haemodynamic instability which may indicate a ruptured ectopic pregnancy

- *Abdominal examination*:
  — Assess for signs of acute abdomen — guarding and rebound tenderness
- *Vaginal examination*:
  — Assess for adnexal tenderness which may indicate free fluid in the cul-de-sac/Pouch of Douglas

↓

Investigations

Transvaginal ultrasound scan (TVUS)

- Absent intrauterine gestation sac (no IUGS)
- +/−Adnexal mass
- +/−Free intra-abdominal fluid

+

Serum βhcg

- Discriminatory zone
  — A gestational sac should be seen when βhcg >1500 IU/L usually via transvaginal ultrasound scan (TVUS)
- Serum βhcg increases at least >66% over 48 hours
- Suboptimal rises in βhcg are commonly seen in ectopic pregnancies

Algorithm For Diagnosis of Ectopic Pregnancy (EP)

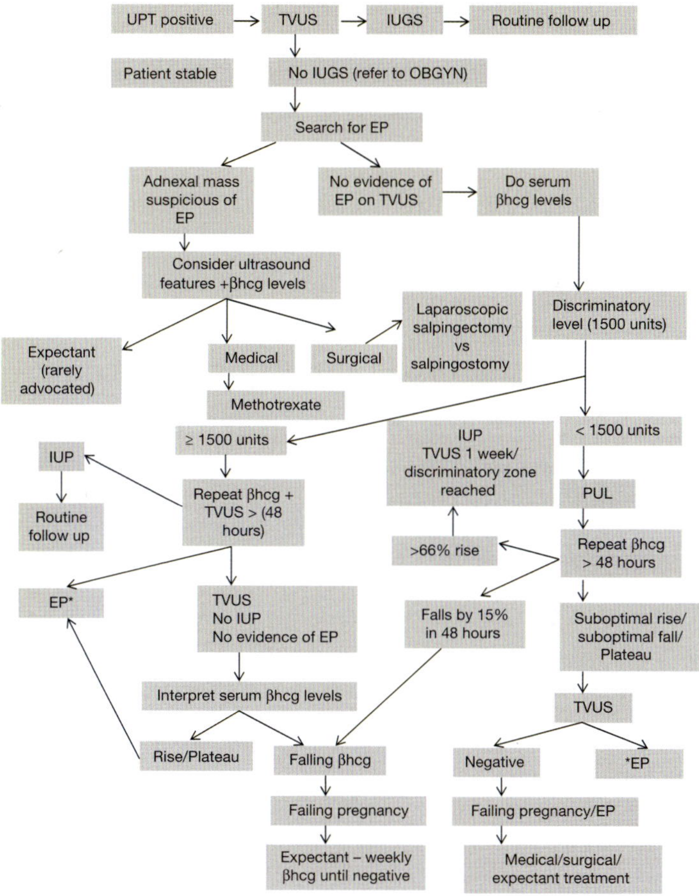

EP	: Ectopic pregnancy	PUL	: Pregnancy unknown location
IUGS	: Intrauterine gestation sac	TVUS	: Transvaginal ultrasound scan
IUP	: Intrauterine pregnancy	UPT	: Urine pregnancy test

Ultrasound Features of Normal Early Gestation

Intradecidual sign: Gestation sac located within the endometrial cavity and deviates from the endometrial lining seen at gestation age of 4 weeks + 5 days, with βhcg ≥ 1500 IU/L and mean sac diameter ≥ 3 mm.

Double decidual sign: two concentric echogenic rings surrounding an IUGS which is visible at gestation age of 4 to 6 weeks. IUGS then contains a yolk sac and a foetal pole.

Ultrasound Features of Tubal Ectopic Gestation

Begels sign: A tubal ring about 5 mm in size that appears at 6 weeks and later becomes a sonolucent sac with or without a yolk sac and/or a live embryo.

Intrauterine pseudosac, centrally located. No echogenic rim.

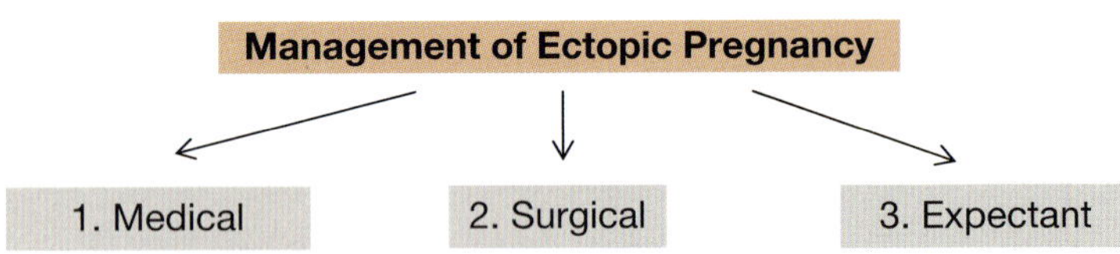

1. Medical Management of Ectopic Pregnancy

Intramuscular Methotrexate (MTX)

- Dose adjusted to body surface area (50 mg/m^2)
- *Criteria*:
  - — Stable vital parameters
  - — No evidence of acute abdomen
  - — Unruptured ectopic
  - — Adnexal mass < 2 cm
  - — Absence of foetal cardiac activity
  - — Serum βhcg < 3000 IU/L
  - — No contraindication to MTX
  - — Presence of reliable follow up
- **Failure rates 15–25%**
- Treatment failure (persistently elevated βhcg levels or symptoms) may still necessitate surgical intervention
- Single dose associated with:

  Risk of rupture — 7%

  Further MTX (2nd dose) — 14%

  Surgical intervention — 10%
- Avoid pregnancy till 3–6 months after MTX due to risk of foetal teratogenicity

Advantage:

Less invasive/cheaper

Risk of recurrent ectopic is the same as with surgery.

Contraindications to Intramuscular Methotrexate

- Haemodynamic instability
- Impending ectopic rupture (evidence of haemoperitoneum)
- Non compliance
- Immunodeficiency, acute peptic ulcer disease
- Abnormalities in FBC/renal function/liver function
- Hypersensitivity to methotrexate
- Heterotopic pregnancy
- Breastfeeding

Side Effects of Intramuscular Methotrexate

Conjunctivitis, stomatitis, dermatitis, xerostomia, alopecia, pneumonitis, impaired liver function, abdominal pain, nausea, diarrhoea, neutropenia.

Follow up after Intramuscular Methotrexate

βhcg on Day 5, Day 12 then weekly until βhcg < 20 IU/L (initial βhcg may rise Day 1 to Day 3, 15% decline between Day 4 and Day 7).

If fall is < 15% within a week, administer second dose of methotrexate. Repeat βhcg on Day 4 and Day 7 after second dose.

2. Surgical Management of Ectopic Pregnancy

Laparoscopy vs Laparotomy (Salpingectomy/Salpingostomy)

Criteria:

1. Haemodynamic instability
2. βhcg > 5000 IU/L
3. Known tubal disease with planned IVF in future
4. Failed medical therapy
5. Size > 3 cm live ectopic

- ***Ensure haemodynamic stability***
- Surgery is the mainstay of treatment
- Laparoscopy is the gold standard
- **Salpingostomy** (tube preserved) or **salpingectomy** (tube removed)
- Salpingostomy is performed when the contralateral fallopian tube is diseased and future fertility is desired
- Salpingectomy is performed when the ectopic pregnancy is too large for tubal preservation or rupture has occurred
- No difference in subsequent fertility rates

- Post-surgical weekly surveillance of βhcg is necessary till zero
  — this is especially necessary when salpingostomy is performed due to 5–15% rate of persistent trophoblastic tissue
- Day 1 postoperative βhcg declines more than 50%
- *Evacuation of uterus is not routinely performed, but may be undertaken to reduce post-surgical per vaginal bleeding which may occur due to decidual reaction*

Management of tubal pregnancy in the presence of haemodynamic instability should be by the most expedient method.

Reproductive outcome of laparoscopic salpingostomy

- Intrauterine pregnancy (IUP) 60%
- Recurrent ectopic risk is 15% if contralateral tube absent/abnormal

Reproductive outcome of laparoscopic salpingectomy

- Intrauterine pregnancy (IUP) 40%
- Recurrent ectopic risk 10%

Recommendations for salpingectomy

- Uncontrolled bleeding
- Severely damaged tube

- Large ectopic (> 5 cm) pregnancy
- Recurrent ipsilateral ectopic pregnancy
- Women who require IVF in future/who do not desire fertility

3. Expectant Management of Ectopic Pregnancy

Spontaneous resolution expected if
- βhcg low < 200 IU/L
- Declining βhcg levels

TVUS:

- Absence of extrauterine gestation sac
- Absence of adnexal mass/small adnexal mass < 3 to 4 cm
- Absence of free fluid

Criteria

- Haemodynamically stable
- Asymptomatic women

Success rate 90% (200 IU/L cut-off βhcg)

Follow up

βhcg levels 2 times a week and TVUS weekly
Expect βhcg levels to decrease to less than 50% within 7 days
Expect adnexal mass to reduce in size in 7 days

Other Types of Ectopic Pregnancies (EP)

1. *Isthmic EP*:

- Narrow compact portion of tube
- EP invades quickly into muscularis of tube
- Ruptures early (as in ampullary which is the commonest site of EP)

2. *Interstitial EP*:

- Tortuous portion of the tube
- Difficult to diagnose
- Late rupture — higher rate of catastrophic haemorrhage
- Higher mortality rate

  Diagnosis: interstitial "line" sign — echogenic line between sac and cavity. Thin myometrium — less than 5 mm around the sac. The term is interchangeable with cornual EP which traditionally refers to pregnancy within the horn of a bicornuate uterus.

  Treatment: surgical (cornual resection). The risk of uterine rupture in subsequent pregnancy is unknown.

3. *Angular EP*:

- Implantation medial to round ligament
- Medial to uterotubal junction
- Uterine rupture rare
- 30% present with miscarriage

4. ***Ovarian EP***:

Random occurrence

Diagnosis: Speigelberg criteria

- Tube intact and distinct from ovary
- Gestation sac connected to uterus by utero-ovarian ligament
- Ovarian tissue in wall of gestation sac

Treatment: cystectomy/oophorectomy

5. ***Abdominal EP***:

Sites — posterior cul de sac; mesosalpinx; omentum; bowel; mesentery; liver and spleen

Late diagnosis: "Studdiford" criteria

- Normal fallopian tube — no evidence of recent or remote trauma
- Absent uteroperitoneal fistula

Treatment:

- Early — MTX/surgery
- Advanced gestation — laparotomy and delivery of neonate. Placenta unless easily separated, is left *in situ*

6. ***Cervical EP***:

Implantation within cervical canal beneath the internal os of cervix.

Presentation — painless vaginal bleeding

Diagnosis: enlargement of cervix (barrel shaped)

- Empty uterine cavity
- Gestation sac beneath internal os

Treatment:

- MTX
- Uterine artery embolisation (UAE) followed by curettage
- Cervical artery ligation (descending branches) followed by cervical suction curettage and post-curettage cervical canal balloon tamponade

7. ***Caesarean scar EP***:

   Ultrasound criteria

- Empty uterine cavity and cervical canal
- Gestation sac in anterior part of uterine isthmus
- Absent/thin myometrium between bladder and gestation sac

Treatment:

- MTX (local or systemic) +/− UAE
- Hysteroscopic resection with laparoscopic guidance
- Resection of scar ectopic with repair of defect
- Post-treatment monitoring for declining βhcg level

8. ***Heterotopic EP***:

Simultaneous intrauterine and extrauterine pregnancy

Rising incidence due to assisted reproductive technology (ART)

Treatment:

- MTX — contraindicated
- Surgical — *salpingectomy* is mainstay
  — salpingostomy contraindicated

(as βhcg cannot be monitored postoperatively and MTX is contraindicated if required).

Chapter 13

APPROACH TO GESTATIONAL TROPHOBLASTIC DISEASE (GTD)

Gestational trophoblastic disease is a type of tumour of trophoblastic cells.
It is caused by abnormalities in the fertilisation process. Risk factors include previous gestational trophoblastic disease, or pregnancies at extremes of reproductive life.

Risk of recurrence after 1 prior gestational trophoblastic disease is 2%.
Risk of recurrence after 2 prior gestational trophoblastic disease is 20%.

Types of GTD:

- Complete hydatidiform mole
- Partial hydatidiform mole
- Choriocarcinoma

	Complete Mole	Partial Mole	Choriocarcinoma
Karyotype	Diploid — 46XX — 46XY	Triploid — 69 XXY — 69 XXX — 69 XYY	Aneuploid — X — Y
Histology	• Hydropic villi • No foetal vessels • Hyperplasia of trophoblastic tissue	• Less hydropic villi • Some foetal vessels • Less hyperplasia of trophoblastic tissue	• Malignant cytotrophoblasts, syncytiotrophoblasts without villi
Presenting symptoms	• PV bleeding • Abdominal pain • Nausea and vomiting	• PV bleeding • Abdominal pain • Nausea and vomiting	• +/– Symptoms of distant metastases e.g. *respiratory symptoms*
Examination findings	• Uterus *larger* than dates • Abdominal tenderness • PV bleeding • Products of conception or grape-like vesicles at the introitus	• Uterus *smaller* than dates • Abdominal tenderness • PV bleeding • Products of conception or grape-like vesicles at the introitus	• Uterus *larger* than dates • +/– Signs of distant metastases
Investigations	• Serum βHCG >100,000 IU/L • Pelvic scan — classical snowstorm cystic appearance	• Serum βHCG >100,000 IU/L • Pelvic scan — snowstorm cystic appearance — but features may resemble a missed miscarriage	• Serum βHCG >100,000 IU/L • Pelvic scan • + CXR to rule out distant metastases
Management	• Evacuation of uterus • Serial trending of serum Bhcg till undetectable by 12–16 weeks		• Chemotherapy • +/– Radiotherapy

When to Try Conceiving Again After a Molar Pregnancy?

Women should be advised not to conceive until serum βhcg levels revert to normal levels, usually by 56 days. Women who undergo chemotherapy for choriocarcinoma should be advised not to conceive for a year after completion. Barrier methods of contraception should be used until βhcg levels revert to normal. Once βhcg levels have normalised, the combined oral contraceptive pill may be used. Intrauterine contraceptive devices (IUCD) should be avoided till βhcg levels normalise to reduce the risk of uterine perforation.

Chapter 14

TERMINATION OF PREGNANCY (TOP)

Criteria under the Termination of Pregnancy (TOP) Act in Singapore

- Citizen of Singapore or wife of citizen of Singapore; OR
- Holder or wife of holder of work permit or employment pass; OR
- Person who has resided in Singapore for at least 4 months

unless it is immediately necessary to save the life of the pregnant woman.

Legal limits of Termination of Pregnancy Act in Singapore

- 24 weeks of gestation based on last menstrual period
- May be ascertained by clinical examination/ultrasound scan dating

Mandatory Counselling in Singapore

Criteria for Pre-abortion Counselling

- Singaporeans or permanent residents
- Have 2 or fewer children
- Passed PSLE and has at least some secondary education
- Wife of a holder of an employment pass or work permit pass issued under the Immigration Act
- Person who has resided in Singapore for at least 4 months

Criteria for Ministry of Community Development, Youth & Sports (MCYS) Counselling

- Similar to pre-abortion counselling, **exclude** single women and pregnant women with >20 weeks gestation

Criteria for Referral to Medical Social Worker

- Midtrimester Termination of Pregnancy (MTPT) >20 weeks
- Single
- >2 abortions
- Other social or financial problems

(*Continued*)

Pre-abortion Counselling for Girls Below 16 Years of Age (exception — rape victims)

Refer to Health Promotion Board Counselling Centre

Ensure issuance of Certificate of Attendance (COA)

At least 48 hours must elapse *after counselling* before TOP

Additional considerations:

Comprehensive history

Physical examination

Ultrasound to confirm intrauterine pregnancy and estimate gestation

Discuss methods-risks/benefits/contraception

Consent

Investigations — full blood count, blood group and rhesus status

Refer to Anaesthetist if high risk case

Note : First trimester TOP is safer than second trimester MTPT

Management of TOP

↓

Fulfils TOP criteria in Singapore

↓

Foetal viability scan to date and locate pregnancy

<12 weeks gestation

↓

Vacuum aspiration

↓

Exclusion criteria (**relative contraindications)**
Severe and/or uncontrolled maternal diseases, e.g. unstable angina, valvular heart disease on anticoagulation, cardiomyopathy, myasthenia gravis.

↓

- Done under sedation/general anaesthesia
- Risks of bleeding, infection, uterine perforation, retained products of conception, cervical stenosis or incompetence

Pre-TOP cervical preparation with cervagem/misoprostol is recommended to reduce the risk of uterine perforation and cervical laceration.

≥12–24 weeks gestation

↓

Mid-trimester termination of pregnancy (MTPT)

↓

Exclusion criteria **(relative contraindications)**
Active asthma, decompensated heart disease, severe hypertension.

↓

- Requires hospital admission
- Insertion of 5 cervagem (prostaglandin E1) vaginal pessaries 4 hourly in each course
- Alternative is 5 oral/vaginal misoprostol 400 μg 4 hourly in each course. (for patients with an intact uterus)
- May need repeated course(s) if necessary
- May need evacuation of uterus after abortion of foetus
- Risks of bleeding, infection, uterine perforation, cervical incompetence
- Hysterotomy maybe necessary for failed MTPT (cervagem or misoprostol protocol)
- Counselling must be done regarding increased risk of uterine rupture in patients with previous scar (previous caesarean or myomectomy)

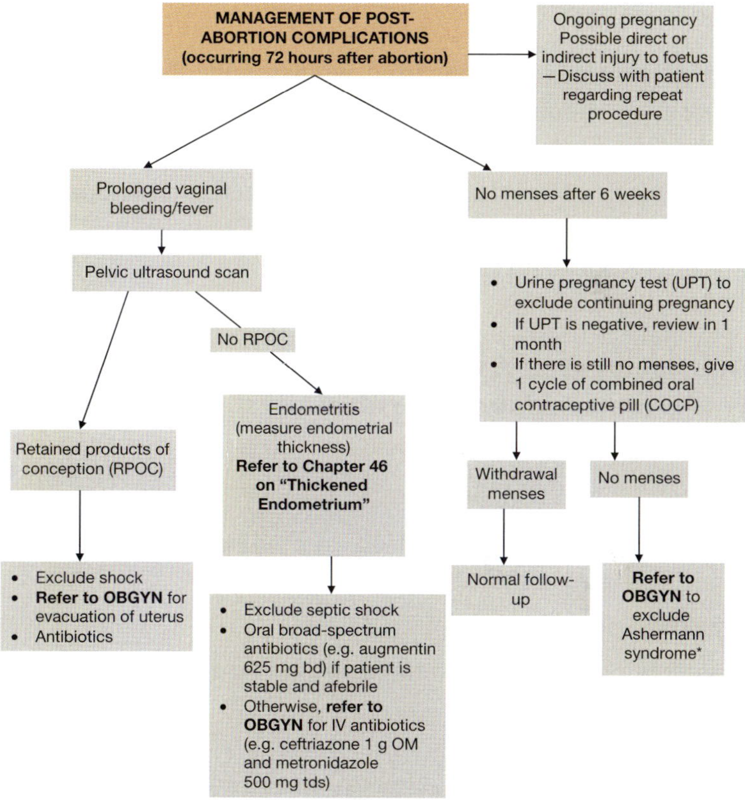
MANAGEMENT OF POST-ABORTION COMPLICATIONS (occurring 72 hours after abortion)
Ongoing pregnancy Possible direct or indirect injury to foetus —Discuss with patient regarding repeat procedure
Prolonged vaginal bleeding/fever
Pelvic ultrasound scan
No RPOC
Retained products of conception (RPOC)
Exclude shock
Refer to OBGYN for evacuation of uterus
Antibiotics
Endometritis (measure endometrial thickness) Refer to Chapter 46 on "Thickened Endometrium"
Exclude septic shock
Oral broad-spectrum antibiotics (e.g. augmentin 625 mg bd) if patient is stable and afebrile
Otherwise, refer to OBGYN for IV antibiotics (e.g. ceftriazone 1 g OM and metronidazole 500 mg tds)
No menses after 6 weeks
Urine pregnancy test (UPT) to exclude continuing pregnancy
If UPT is negative, review in 1 month
If there is still no menses, give 1 cycle of combined oral contraceptive pill (COCP)
Withdrawal menses
No menses
Normal follow-up
Refer to OBGYN to exclude Ashermann syndrome*

Post Top Care

- Rh(D) negative unsensitised women with Rh(D) positive partners should receive Anti-D Immunoglobulin 300 μg (1st trimester: 50 μg)
- Antibiotic prophylaxis to prevent post-abortal endometritis is recommended. (Augmentin/Doxycycline/Flagyl/Ceftriaxone/Ofloxacin)

Management of Asherman Syndrome (Adhesions or Fibrosis within the Uterine Cavity)

Causes:

- Occurs following dilatation and curettage (D&C) on recently pregnant uterus
- After repeated D&C
- Following pelvic infection e.g. pelvic tuberculosis

Investigations:

- Hysteroscopy is the gold standard
- Transvaginal pelvic ultrasound scan
- Hysterosonography

Management:

- Hysteroscopic resection of adhesions (with or without laparoscopic or ultrasound guidance)
- To prevent recurrence after the procedure, some recommend:
  - IUCD
  - Oestrogen (conjugated oestrogen 5 mg or oestradiol 8 mg in divided doses for one month with progestins for the last 10 days with withdrawal bleed)

Chapter 15

MEDICAL DISORDERS AND POTENTIAL RISK FACTORS IN PREGNANCY

1. Anaemia
2. Asthma
3. Antiphospholipid Syndrome (APS)
4. Cardiac Disease
5. Cardiomyopathy
6. Gestational Diabetes Mellitus (GDM)
7. Hyperthyroidism
8. Hypothyroidism
9. Liver Disease
10. Lower Urinary Tract Infection (UTI)
11. Acute Pyelonephritis
12. Acute Renal Failure (ARF)
13. Preeclampsia (PE)

14. Previous Severe Pre-eclampsia (SPE)
15. Pre-existing Hypertension
16. Previous Gestational Diabetes Mellitus (GDM)
17. Pre-existing Diabetes Mellitus (DM)
18. Previous 2nd Trimester Loss
19. Previous One Preterm Birth (PTB)
20. Preterm Prelabour Rupture of Membranes (PPROM)
21. Previous Preterm Prelabour Rupture of Membranes
22. Previous Intrauterine Growth Restriction (IUGR)
23. Systemic Lupus Erythematosus (SLE)
24. Thrombocytopaenia
25. Gestational Thrombocytopaenia
26. Immune Thrombocytopaenia
27. Teenage Pregnancy
28. Advanced Maternal Age (≥ 35 years old)
29. Alcohol Consumption
30. Cigarette Smoking
31. Maternal Underweight (Body Mass Index < 18.5 kg/m^2)
32. Maternal Obesity (Body Mass Index > 30 kg/m^2)
33. Previous Caesarean Sections (2 or more)
34. Grand Multiparity (Parity ≥ 5)
35. Venous Thromboembolism (VTE)

Medical Disorders and Potential Risk Factors in Pregnancy

Risk Factors	Implications	Action
1. Anaemia CDC — Centers for Disease Control and Prevention — US *First/Third Trimester* • Hb < 11 g/dL • Hematocrit < 33% *Second Trimester* • Hb < 10.5 g/dL • Haematocrit < 32%	*Symptoms of Anaemia* Fatigue, Dyspnoea, Palpitations, Dysphagia, Anorexia, Sore Mouth, Headache, Fainting *Signs*: Pallor, tachycardia, systolic flow murmur *Maternal Risks of Anaemia*:- Increased risk of PTL, PTB, prolonged labour, obstructed labour, postpartum haemorrhage, infections, subinvolution of uterus *Foetal Risks of Anaemia*: IUGR/PTB/IUD	*Prevention* *Primary prevention* • Start low dose oral elemental iron supplements (30 mg/day) at first prenatal visit • Diet rich in iron and foods that enhance iron absorption *Secondary prevention* Screen for anaemia at first antenatal visit *Investigations* • FBC: Hb, MCV, MCH, PBF (peripheral blood film) If PBF shows microcytic, hypochromic red blood cells - Do Hb electrophoresis and serum ferritin to differentiate between thalassaemia trait and iron deficiency anaemia. • Reduced serum ferritin (<30 ng/ml) – indicates reduced storage iron • Serum iron and TIBC saturation have lower diagnostic accuracy

(*Continued*)

(*Continued*)

Risk Factors	Implications	Action
		Management • Start oral elemental iron 60–120 mg/day. Once haemoglobin is normal, decrease to 30 mg/day. • Common supplements (Refer to Chapter 20 — Medications in Pregnancy). • *Side effects of iron supplementation* — nausea, heartburn, constipation, black stools. • Indications for Parenteral Iron — iron malabsorption, extreme deficiency, intolerance to oral iron and non-compliance.
2. Asthma • 7% require emergency treatment and 1.5% hospitalisation in pregnancy	• Preterm birth (PTB) • Pregnancy-induced Hypertension (PIH)/ Pre-eclampsia Toxaemia (PET) • Asthma in child (6–30%) • Intrauterine Growth Restriction (IUGR)/ Low Birth Weight Infant (LBW)	• Aim to maintain asthma control • Use inhalational rather than oral route • In active asthma cases — increased foetal growth monitoring • Avoid use of prostaglandin F2, ergot derivatives • IV steroids intrapartum if on chronic oral therapy or >3 weeks of systemic steroids.

(*Continued*)

(*Continued*)

Risk Factors	Implications	Action
3. Antiphospholipid Syndrome (APS) Diagnostic criteria: at least one clinical and one laboratory criteria. *Clinical Criteria* 1) Vascular thrombosis • At least one episode of arterial, venous, or small-vessel thrombosis in any tissue or organ • Confirmed by imaging or biopsy 2) Pregnancy morbidity (≥1 of the following) • At least one unexplained death of morphologically normal foetus ≥10 weeks gestation • At least one premature birth (<34 weeks) of morphologically normal neonate due to eclampsia, severe pre-eclampsia, or placental insufficiency • At least three consecutive spontaneous miscarriages prior to 10 weeks gestation, otherwise unexplained	• Thrombotic — Venous thromboembolism, including deep vein thrombosis (DVT) and pulmonary embolism — 5% — Transient ischaemic attack — Cerebrovascular accident — 12% • Obstetric — PIH/ PET — 30% — IUGR — Preterm birth 32–65% — Pregnancy loss — Catastrophic APS — rare	• Low dose aspirin + low molecular weight heparin (LMWH), e.g. Enoxaparin (Clexane) 40 mg OM • Visits 2–4 weekly until 24 weeks and then 1–2 weekly • Ultrasound scan 2 weekly from 24 weeks • Deliver at term • Postpartum thromboprophylaxis for 6 weeks

(*Continued*)

(*Continued*)

Risk Factors	Implications	Action
Laboratory Criteria • Positive lupus anticoagulant on at least two occasions, at least 12 weeks apart • Medium or high titer IgG or IgM anti-cardiolipin antibody on at least two occasions, at least 12 weeks apart • Medium or high titer IgG or IgM anti-B2 glycoprotein I antibody on at least two occasions, at least 12 weeks apart		
4. Cardiac disease Poor outcome predictors: • New York Heart Association (NYHA) >2 or cyanosis • Left ventricular (LV) outflow tract obstruction • Severe pulmonary hypertension • Cardiac dysfunction • Left ventricular ejection fraction (LVEF) < 40% • Previous arrhythmia requiring treatment • Previous cardiac complication	**Maternal risks** • Pulmonary oedema • Symptomatic arrhythmia • Stroke • Cardiac arrest • Venous thromboembolism • Death	• Manage in collaboration with cardiologist,maternal-foetal specialist,obstetric anaesthesiologist • Treat coexisting anaemia, arrhythmia, hypertension • Termination of Pregnancy (TOP) option in some conditions (Eisenmenger syndrome, pulmonary hypertension, Marfan syndrome with aortic root dilatation, severe left ventricular outflow tract obstruction, severe left ventricular dysfunction)

(*Continued*)

(*Continued*)

Risk Factors	Implications	Action
	Foetal risks • Increased risk of congenital heart disease (CHD) if mother has CHD (2–5% increase in risk) — risk of recurrence varies with specific parental defect. • Frequent recurrent lesions include: Ventricular septal defect,coarctation of aorta, hypoplastic left heart syndrome. • Preterm labour • Foetal acidosis • IUGR • Foetal death	• Avoid or minimise aggravating factors • Foetal echocardiogram • Growth and foetal surveillance especially in left-to-right shunt • Intrapartum prophylactic antibiotics till 6 hr post delivery (IV ampicillin, gentamicin) in certain situations (e.g. artificial heart valves, previous endocarditis, Mitral Valve Prolapse (MVP) with regurgitation, previous rheumatic fever) • Await spontaneous labour. If need to induce, do so in controlled environment. Avoid prolonged inductions. • Caesarean section is usually reserved only for obstetric indications. Caesarean is associated with twice as much blood loss

(*Continued*)

(Continued)

Risk Factors	Implications	Action
		• Encourage left lateral position in labour • Oxygen administration • Haemodynamic monitoring • Appropriate fluid management • Use epidural cautiously • Foetal monitoring in labour • Shorten second stage by assisted vaginal delivery (e.g. in cardiac disease, NYHA class 3 or 4) • Avoid ergotamines, IV bolus oxytocin • Prophylaxis for venous thromboembolism • Contraceptive advice

(Continued)

(*Continued*)

Risk Factors	Implications	Action
• Patients with prosthetic valves	• Structural failure of valve • Heart failure • Thromboembolism • Bleeding due to anticoagulations • Risk of Warfarin embryopathy/ haemorrhage in foetus	• Collaborate with remaining team, including haematologist • Ensure continuous monitoring and therapeutic anticoagulation • Warfarin use is limited to 13–36 weeks • Use unfractionated Heparin/low molecular weight Heparin(LMWH) in first and third trimester. Use Anti-Xa levels to monitor anticoagulation appropriateness (higher risk of valve thrombosis compared with Warfarin, require twice a day injections). Protamine sulphate as antidote • Resume Warfarin on same day as vaginal delivery or a day or two after caesarean section

(*Continued*)

(Continued)

Risk Factors	Implications	Action
5. Cardiomyopathy a. Development of heart failure (HF) in the last month of pregnancy or within 5 months of delivery. b. Absence of determinable cause of HF. c. Absence of demonstrable heart disease before last month of pregnancy. d. Left Ventricular (LV) systolic dysfunction demonstrated by echocardiography with Left Ventricular Ejection Fraction (LVEF) <45%.	• Pulmonary oedema • Cardiogenic shock • Arrhythmia • Thromboembolic disease (TED)/(VTE) • Mortality	• Assisted vaginal delivery preferred in stable patients • Caesarean section should be performed for obstetric reasons or maternal instability

(Continued)

(*Continued*)

Risk Factors	Implications	Action
6. Gestational Diabetes Mellitus (GDM) • Age ≥ 35 years • Race • Family history (first degree relative) • Obesity • Previous GDM • Previous stillbirth • Previous macrosomia • ≥ 2 episodes of glycosuria *Criteria*: • GDM – FBG > 5.1 but < 7 mmol/L • 75 g 2 hr OGTT has at least one abnormal result • FBG > 5.1 but < 7 mmol/L • 1st hr ≥ 10 mmol/L • 2nd hr ≥ 8.5 mmol/L **FBG = fasting blood glucose** *Overt diabetes if at first prenatal visit*: Fasting blood glucose ≥ 7.0 mmol/L HbA1C ≥ 6.5% Random blood glucose ≥ 11.1 mmol/L	*Risk of* : • Pre-eclampsia • Foetal macrosomia • Polyhydramnios • Operative delivery • Birth trauma • Stillbirth • Neonatal hypoglycaemia/ hyperbilirubinaemia/ hypocalcaemia/ respiratory distress/ long term risk to infant — obesity	• Nutrition (diet control) • Insulin (if the following glucose targets are exceeded). FBG >5.5 mmol/L 2 hr post-prandial >6.6 mmol/L • Moderate exercise • Glucose monitoring • Interval growth scans • Induction of labour (IOL) at term • Postpartum low dose OC pill • Recurrence next pregnancy • Risk of cardiovascular disease • Risk of DM after pregnancy (check OGTT 75 g 6 weeks postpartum) 40% risk of developing DM within 20 years of delivery • Recommend lifestyle interventions

(*Continued*)

(Continued)

Risk Factors	Implications	Action
7. Hyperthyroidism If autoimmune, disease may improve as pregnancy advances and antibody levels fall Anti-thyroid drugs: 1. Carbimazole 2. Proplythiouracil (PTU) (Refer Chapter 20 on "Medications in Pregnancy and Lactation")	• Miscarriage • Intrauterine Growth Restriction (IUGR) • Preterm labour • Placental abruption • PIH/Pre-eclampsia • Infection • Foetal/neonatal thyrotoxicosis • Increased perinatal mortality	• Avoid conception 3–6 months after radioiodine treatment. • Advise euthyroid state 3 months before conception • TFT — 3 monthly or within two weeks of switching drugs • Screen for agranulocytosis and hepatitis if on thionamides (e.g. Carbimazole) • Serial growth scans 28, 32, 36 weeks, scan for foetal goiter • Assess infants for hyperthyroidism after birth • Role of surgery — indicated for obstructive symptoms/failure of medical treatment/non-compliance • Measure thyroid-stimulating hormone receptor antibody (TRAb) at 28 weeks — if high, risk of foetal thyroid dysfunction and neonatal thyrotoxicosis

(Continued)

(*Continued*)

Risk Factors	Implications	Action
8. Hypothyroidism Trimester Specific TSH First Trimester 0.1 to 2.5 mµ/L Second Trimester 0.2 to 3 mµ/L Third Trimester 0.3 to 3 mµ/L	• Miscarriage • Increase in pregnancy-induced hypertension (PIH) • Neurodevelopmental delay especially if treatment is delayed in first trimester	• Do Thyroid Function Tests (TFT) (free T_4) at booking and once in each trimester • Adjust levothyroxine dosage accordingly • Do not use other thyroid preparations, such as T3 or natural desiccated thyroid drugs • Avoid taking iron and calcium supplements at same time as levothyroxine as they decrease its absorption • Repeat TFT 4–6 weeks after adjusting dose • Watch for postnatal depression

(*Continued*)

(Continued)

Risk Factors	Implications	Action
Role of Thyroid Antibodies 1) Thyroid peroxidase antibody –TPOAb. Elevated in Hashimoto thyroiditis; Graves disease. Patients at increased risk for postpartum thyroiditis 2) Thyroid stimulating hormone receptor antibody — TRAb Elevated in Graves disease	**TPOAb** *Ordered when* a) symptoms suggesting thyroid disease; b) before starting a patient on a drug therapy that has associated risks of developing hypothyroidism when thyroid peroxidase antibodies are present, such as lithium, amiodarone, interferon alpha or interleukin-2 **TRAb** *Ordered when* a) symptoms of hyperthyroidism; b) monitor the effectiveness of anti-thyroid therapy	*Other facts on TPOAb:* TPOAb has been associated with reproductive difficulties, such as miscarriage, preeclampsia, premature delivery, and in-vitro fertilization failure

(Continued)

(*Continued*)

Risk Factors	Implications	Action
Postpartum thyroiditis (PPT) Thyroiditis induced by an autoimmune mechanism within one year after parturition. *Risk Factors* • type 1 diabetes mellitus • prior history of PPT • positive TPOAb • women on thyroid hormone replacement	Presentation Postpartum • Transient hyperthyroidism alone • Transient hypothyroidism alone • Transient hyperthyroidism followed by hypothyroidism and then recovery	• High or high-normal serum free T4 and T3 concentrations and low serum TSH concentrations during the hyperthyroid phase.Most require no treatment.If symptomatic ,treat with with 40 to 120 mg *propranolol* or 25 to 50 mg *atenolol* daily • During the hypothyroid phase, serum free T4 concentrations are low or low-normal, and serum TSH concentrations are high.Treat if symptomatic with *levothyroxine* (T4) (typically about 50 to 100 mcg/day) • Serum TPOAb – high • 30 percent of women have permanent hypothyroidism. Women with reversible hypothyroidism are also at increased risk for developing permanent hypothyroidism in the future and, therefore, require yearly monitoring of TSH. • Recurrence is likely in future pregnancies

(*Continued*)

(*Continued*)

<table>
<tr><th>Risk Factors</th><th colspan="2">Implications</th><th colspan="2">Action</th></tr>
<tr><td colspan="5">9. Liver Disease
Disease presentation and the timing of onset during pregnancy
Disease Categories</td></tr>
<tr><td>a) Preexisting Liver Disease</td><td colspan="4">Chronic hepatitis B or C, autoimmune hepatitis, primary sclerosing cholangitis, Wilson disease, primary biliary cirrhosis, cirrhosis</td></tr>
<tr><td>b) Newly Acquired Liver Disease in Pregnancy</td><td colspan="4">Viral hepatitis, gallstones, drugs, sepsis, Budd-Chiari syndrome (usually postpartum)</td></tr>
<tr><td></td><td colspan="2">1st Trimester</td><td>2nd Trimester</td><td>3rd Trimester</td></tr>
<tr><td>c) Disease Related to Pregnancy</td><td>Hyperemesis gravidarum</td><td>Obstetric cholestasis</td><td colspan="2">Obstetric cholestasis, preeclampsia, HELLP syndrome, Acute Fatty Liver of Pregnancy (AFLP)</td></tr>
<tr><td>Obstetric cholestasis</td><td colspan="2">• Increased risk of preterm labour, fetal distress, intra-uterine death
• ↑ transaminases, ↑bilirubin, ↑bile acids
• Recurrence up to 40–60%
• Avoid oestrogen containing oral contraceptives</td><td colspan="2">• Ursodeoxycholic acid 500 mg BD – QDS
• Oral Vitamin K
• Serial ultrasound scan for foetal growth
• Consider delivery at term</td></tr>
</table>

(*Continued*)

(Continued)

Risk Factors	Implications	Action
10. Lower Urinary Tract Infection (UTI) Most common: E coli, Klebsiella, Proteus, Enterobacter	• 25–30% acute pyelonephritis • Preterm delivery • Low birth weight	• Do urine culture for diagnosis and 2 weeks later for test of cure • Do not use single dose regime • Ultrasound scan of urinary tract to exclude calculi, structural anomaly of renal tract for relapse/persistence
11. Acute Pyelonephritis	• 25% mild haemolytic anaemia, thrombocytopaenia, • 2% Acute Respiratory distress Syndrome (ARDS) • 15% bacteraemia • Septic shock • Recurrent cystitis 33%	• Admit • IV fluids and IV empirical antibiotics till culture results are available • 14 day antibiotic treatment • Ultrasound scan to exclude calculi, structural anomaly of renal tract for relapse/persistence • If reinfection, continued low dose antibiotic suppression till 4 weeks postpartum • Do urine culture for diagnosis and 2 weeks later for test of cure

(Continued)

(Continued)

Risk Factors	Implications	Action
12. Acute Renal Failure *More common causes*: Haemorrhage, severe pre-eclampsia *Rare*: Septic shock, hyperemesis, Haemolytic uraemic syndrome (HUS)/thrombotic thrombocytopaenic purpura (TTP), acute fatty liver of pregnancy, amniotic fluid embolism		• Identify and correct precipitating insult • Optimal fluid resuscitation • Suspect bilateral renal cortical necrosis if oliguria > 1 week — consider dialysis
13. Preeclampsia (PE) *Risk factors:* • Primigravida • Age ≥40 years old • Pregnancy interval ≥10 years • BMI ≥30 kg/m^2 • Family history of pre-eclampsia • Multiple pregnancy • New sexual partner *Criteria* • BP ≥140/90 mmHg • Proteinuria ≥0.3g/24-hr urine specimen	*Complications secondary to PE*: • Increased blood pressure — eclampsia — stroke • Capillary leak — pulmonary oedema/pleural effusion • Fibrinolysis and Haemolysis — HELLP – Haemolysis elevated liver enzymes, low platelets	• Urine albumin • 24-hr urine total protein or spot urinary protein: creatinine ratio • PE bloods (FBC/U/E/Cr/uric acid/LFT/PT/PTT) • Anti-Hypertensives (Methyldopa/Nifedipine/Labetalol) • Steroide, e.g. Dexamethasone for foetal lung maturity • Ultrasound growth scan and Doppler if indicated • Induction of labour (IOL) at term/caesarean section if suspicious of impending eclampsia (IE)

(Continued)

(*Continued*)

Risk Factors	Implications	Action
	– Renal failure – Ascites – DIVC (Disseminated intravascular coagulopathy) *Placenta associated*: • Abruption • Foetal growth restriction • Preterm birth • Stillbirth	• Magnesium sulphate (if suspicious of IE or severe pre-eclampsia) • Immediate delivery if severe pre-eclampsia • Postnatal surveillance of blood pressure
Severe PE criteria: • Symptoms of impending eclampsia (IE): • Headache/visual disturbances • Nausea/vomiting • Right hypochondrial/epigastric pain • BP ≥160/110 mmHg on 2 occasions 6 hr apart • Proteinuria ≥5 g in 24-hr • Oliguria <500 ml/24-hr		

(*Continued*)

(Continued)

Risk Factors	Implications	Action
14. Previous Severe Pre-eclampsia (SPE)	• Rule out pre-existing renal, thyroid, cardiac pathology • Recurrence 20%	• Pre-pregnancy weight loss if BMI > 30 • Low dose Aspirin from booking till 36 weeks • Monitor BP/urine albumin at each visit.
15. Pre-existing Hypertension a. *Low risk group*	• Maternal and perinatal morbidity and mortality *similar* to general population	• Use antihypertensives like Methyldopa, Labetalol, Hydrallazine, Nifedipine • Stop ACE (angiotensin-converting-enzyme) inhibitors, ARBs (angiotensin II receptor blockers); risk of congenital abnormalites such as hypocalvaria, decreased skull ossification, renal tubular dysgenesis) and diuretics
b. *High risk group* • BP >180/110 mmHg • Hypertension lasting >15 years • Early pregnancy BP >160/110 mmHg • Maternal age >40 years old • Diabetes Class B to F • Renal Disease • Cardiomyopathy • Connective Tissue Disease • Coarctation of aorta	• Abruptio Placenta ***Maternal Risk*** • Exacerbation of hypertension • Superimposed pre-eclampsia toxaemia (PET)	• Consider low dose Aspirin (i.e. 100mg OM) • Serial Ultrasonography for foetal growth 2–3 weekly from 26 weeks depending on maternal and foetal condition • Consider steroids if preterm

(Continued)

(*Continued*)

Risk Factors	Implications	Action
	• Congestive cardiac failure • Intracerebral haemorrhage • Acute renal failure • Maternal mortality ***Foetal Risk*** • Intrauterine growth restriction (IUGR) • Spontaneous / iatrogenic prematurity • Increased perinatal mortality	• Timing and mode of delivery dependent on maternal and/or foetal well being • Postnatal monitoring of BP. Refer to physician if suboptimal control
16. Previous Gestational Diabetes Mellitus (GDM)	• Onset of type 2 diabetes mellitus (DM) later in life	• Pre-pregnancy weight reduction if BMI >25 • OGTT 16–18 weeks, if normal, repeat at 24–28 weeks • Foetal monitoring for growth and AFI (amniotic fluid index)

(*Continued*)

(*Continued*)

Risk Factors	Implications	Action
17. Pre-existing Diabetes Mellitus (DM)	• Increased perinatal morbidity and mortality • Increased risk of miscarriage • Increased congenital malformations (e.g. congenital heart defects, sacral agenesis, neural tube defects, skeletal abnormalities, urogenital, gastrointestinal and facial malformations) • Increased risk of preterm birth • Macrosomia which increases the risk of birth injury • Pregnancy-induced hypertension, pre-eclampsia in mother • Polyhydramnios	• Maintain HbA1c < 6% throughout pregnancy (monitor every 4 weeks) • Booking Thyroid function test, Renal panel, Liver function test, ECG • Fundoscopy • MSU at booking • Growth scan at 28, 32, 36 weeks • Insulin therapy maintain FBG<5.5 mmol/L • 2 hr post prandial BG<6.6 mmol/L • Monitor HbA1c every 4–6 weeks and home self glucose monitoring (7 point BSP) • During night, glucose level should not decrease < 3.3 mmol/L • Induction at term for insulin-dependent diabetes mellitus/ uncontrolled diabetes mellitus

(*Continued*)

(Continued)

Risk Factors	Implications	Action
	• Risk of worsening of Diabetic Nephropathy • Risk of Cardiovascular disease • Risk of Thyroid dysfunction • Risk of infection (e.g. UTI) • Risk of Diabetic ketoacidosis • Risk of hypoglyaecemia • Operative Intervention (LSCS/ shoulder dystocia) • Risk of neonatal complications (hypoglycaemia, respiratory distress syndrome, erythrocytosis, hyperbilirubiinaemia, hypocalcaemia).	

(Continued)

(Continued)

Risk Factors	Implications	Action
18. Previous 2nd Trimester loss • History of cone biopsy • History of large loop excision of transformation zone • Diethylstilbestrol exposure in-utero	• High recurrence (up to 30%)	• 2 weekly scans for cervical length from 12–24 weeks. • Consider cervical cerclage after first trimester (14–16 weeks)
19. Previous one Preterm Birth (PTB)	• 22.5% recurrence	• Pre-pregnancy — lose weight if BMI > 30 — gain weight if BMI < 18 • Mid-Stream Urine for culture (MSU) at booking to rule out asymptomatic bacteriuria • 2 weekly scans for cervical length from 16–24 weeks • Start IM/vaginal progesterone from 16 weeks

(Continued)

(*Continued*)

Risk Factors	Implications	Action
20. Preterm Prelabour Rupture of Membranes (PPROM)	• Chorioamnionitis • Preterm birth • Increased neonatal morbidity • Maternal morbidity	• High vaginal swab • Urine culture • FBC/CRP twice weekly • Ultrasound scan for AFI/Placental location and estimated foetal weight • Antibiotics • Intramuscular Dexamethasone • Deliver if symptoms/signs of chorioamnionitis or gestation >34 weeks
21. Previous Preterm Prelabour Rupture of Membranes (<36 weeks)	• 17–30% recurrence	• High vaginal swab (HVS) to rule out bacterial vaginosis (BV) • Mid-stream urine (MSU) for culture at booking to rule out asymptomatic bacteriuria
22. Previous Intrauterine Growth Restriction (IUGR)	• Detailed history of previous affected pregnancy	• Early dating scan • Serial growth scans from 26/28 weeks 2–3 weekly • Doppler scan if Intrauterine growth restriction is detected.

(*Continued*)

(Continued)

Risk Factors	Implications	Action
23. Systemic Lupus Erythematosus (SLE) • Establish good control • Adjust maintenance medications • Discontinue azathioprine and cyclophosphamide if possible • Worsened outcome if presence of chronic hypertension, Anti-Phospholipid Syndrome (APS), active disease	• Exacerbation • PIH/PET — 20–30% • Pregnancy loss • Preterm birth • IUGR • Neonatal lupus 5% • Complete congenital heart block	• Early dating scan • If renal involvement, perform 24 hr urine collection for creatinine clearance, protein • Visits 2–4 weeks until 24 weeks and then 1–2 weekly • Ultrasound scan 2 weekly from 24 weeks • *Drugs of choice*: antimalarials, steroids, azathioprine (last resort) • Deliver at term
24. Thrombocytopaenia *Pregnancy-related Thrombocytopaenia* • Gestational (or incidental, 75%) • Pre-eclampsia toxaemia (PET) • Haemolysis, elevated liver enzymes and low platelet (HELLP syndrome) • Disseminated intravascular coagulation (DIVC) • Acute fatty liver of pregnancy (AFLP) • Acute folate deficiency		

(Continued)

(*Continued*)

Risk Factors	Implications	Action
Non-Pregnancy-related Thrombocytopaenia • Spurious (EDTA-induced platelet aggregation). Send a citrate sample to exclude this • Autoimmune — immune thrombocytopaenia purpura, drug-induced (e.g. Frusemide, NSAIDS, Penicillin, Qunidine, Sulphonamides, Ranitidine), systemic lupus erythematosus, antiphospholipid syndrome • Viral, e.g. HIV, EBV, CMV, Dengue fever • Von Willebrand type IIB disease • Haemolytic uraemic syndrome (HUS)/thrombotic thrombocytopaenic purpura (TTP) • Congenital/marrow disease/hypersplenism/liver disease • Drugs — e.g. Heparin-induced thrombocytopaenia (*not* low molecular weight heparin)		
25. Gestational thrombocytopaenia • Mild and asymptomatic • No past non-pregnant history of thrombocytopaenia in the mother • Resolves spontaneously after delivery (within 7 days to 6 weeks postpartum) • Bleeding times are normal, unless platelet count falls below 100×10^9/L.	• No neonatal thrombocytopaenia • Occurs late in pregnancy (second trimester) • No association with maternal or neonatal haemorrhage	• Ensure that the thrombocytopaenia resolves spontaneously after delivery

(*Continued*)

(Continued)

Risk Factors	Implications	Action
26. Immune thrombocytopaenia • 1–5 cases per 10000 pregnancies. • 100 times less common than gestational thrombocytopaenia. • majority of cases occur alone • rarely it can be associated with systemic lupus erythematosus, human immunodeficiency virus (HIV), or is secondary to drugs	• Rarely causes thrombocytopaenia in the foetus	• Monitor platelet count 1–2 weekly • Treat if symptomatic (platelet $<20 \times 10^9$/L) • Treat if platelet $< 50 \times 10^9$/L in late pregnancy even if asymptomatic • Prednisolone 10–20 mg/day • High dose intravenous immunoglobulins (IVIG) • Avoid traumatic vaginal delivery, foetal scalp electrode, foetal blood sampling, ventouse • Caesarean section offers *no* benefit over vaginal delivery
27. Teenage Pregnancy	*Increased risk of:-* • Anaemia • Premature rupture of membranes (PROM) • Preterm labour (PTL) • Pre-eclampsia (PE) • Sexually transmitted infection (STI)	• Monitor BP • Iron supplementation for anaemia • Refer to social worker • Screen for sexually transmitted infection (STI) • Postnatal support

(Continued)

(Continued)

Risk Factors	Implications	Action
28. Advanced Maternal Age (≥35 years at EDD)	*Increased risk of:-* • Miscarriage • Down syndrome • Pre-eclampsia, gestational diabetes mellitus • Heart disease, ischaemic heart disease • Caesarean section and operative delivery • Breastfeeding problems • Postnatal depression	• Screen for Down Syndrome/ congenital malformations • Monitor BP • Screen for diabetes mellitus (OGTT) • Postnatal support

(Continued)

(Continued)

Risk Factors	Implications	Action
29. Alcohol Consumption	*Increased risk of:-* • Miscarriage • Stillbirth • Poor growth development • Preterm labour (PTL) • *Foetal alcohol syndrome disorder (FASD)* is a pattern of intellectual and physical defects (e.g. microcephaly, cardiac, skeletal and facial abnormalities) that can develop in a foetus in association with high levels of alcohol • Learning difficulties and behavioural problems in children after birth	• Avoid alcohol consumption in pregnancy

(Continued)

(*Continued*)

Risk Factors	Implications	Action
30. Cigarette Smoking	*Increased risk of:-* • Preterm labour (PTL) • Preterm rupture of membranes (PROM) • Intrauterine growth restriction (IUGR) • Placental abruption • Placenta praevia • Sudden infant death syndrome (SIDS) • Withdrawal symptoms in baby after birth • Other birth defects	• Advise to stop smoking
31. Maternal Under-weight (BMI < 18.5 kg/m²)	*Increased risk of:-* • Small-for-gestational age baby • Preterm delivery • Stillbirth/Neonatal death	• Refer dietician • Good antenatal care • Antenatal supplements

(*Continued*)

(*Continued*)

Risk Factors	Implications	Action
32. Maternal Obesity (BMI >30 kg/m²)	*Increased risk of:-* • Miscarriage • Pre-eclampsia (PE) • Pregnancy induced hypertension (PIH) • Gestational diabetes mellitus (GDM) • Thromboembolism • Vitamin D deficiency • Birth defects in baby • Macrosomia • Difficulty in clinical assessment of presentation and foetal growth • Intrapartum complications (difficult venous access, anaesthetic difficulty, slow progress of labour, operative vaginal delivery, shoulder dystocia)	• Dietary advice • 5 mg folic acid supplementation • Vitamin D supplementation • Low molecular weight Heparin (LMWH) • Compression stockings • Screen for diabetes (OGTT) • Monitor BP • Difficult ultrasound scans because of habitus • Postnatal: diet advice, encourage breastfeeding, contraception (Long acting reversible contraceptives — LARC)

(*Continued*)

(Continued)

Risk Factors	Implications	Action
	• Risks of LSCS • Stillbirth • Neonatal death • Postpartum haemorrhage (PPH) • Breastfeeding problems • Wound infection	
33. Previous Caesarean Sections (2 or more) Contraindication for vaginal birth.	***Maternal risks:*** • Uterine dehiscence/rupture • Morbidly adherent placenta • Postpartum haemorrhage • Blood transfusion • Hysterectomy • Maternal morbidity • Difficult caesarean due to adhesions and high risk of bladder and bowel injury	• Early booking visit, consultant-led care. • Placental localisation at 20 week scan. • If lower anterior placenta, high index of suspicion for placenta accreta/percreta. • Repeat ultrasound scan at 32–34 weeks • Consider MRI scan if accreta suspected • Plan for elective delivery at term. • Consider antenatal steroids before delivery if contemplating early delivery.

(Continued)

(*Continued*)

Risk Factors	Implications	Action
	Foetal risks: If uterine dehiscence/ rupture:- • Risk of prematurity • Birth asphyxia • Foetal death	• Discuss postpartum sterilisation • Senior O&G doctor present at Caesarean section • If accreta/percreta, consider hysterectomy/embolisation
34. Grand Multiparity (Parity ≥ 5)	*Increased risk of:* • Placental abnormalities such as placenta praevia and abruption • Postpartum haemorrhage • Foetal risk — macrosomia (these data are inconsistent)	• Close monitoring of labour • Postpartum haemorrhage prophylaxis

(*Continued*)

(Continued)

Risk Factors	Implications	Action
35. Venous Thromboembolism (VTE) All women should undergo a documented assessment of risk factors for venous thromboembolism (VTE) listed below in early pregnancy or before pregnancy. This assessment should be repeated if the woman is admitted to hospital for any reason or develops other intercurrent problems. Risk factors in pregnancy include: Refer to Chapter 1 on "Preconception Preparation"	• Increased risk of thromboembolic events • Increased risk of haemorrhage in patients on anticoagulants	• Antenatal thromboprophylaxis should begin as early in pregnancy as practical. • Low molecular weight heparins (LMWH) are the agents of choice for antenatal thromboprophylaxis. These are at least as effective as and safer than unfractionated heparin. • Any woman with three or more current or persisting risk factors should be considered for prophylactic LMWH antenatally. • Women with a previous single provoked (excluding oestrogen-related) VTE and no other risk factors require close surveillance; antenatal LMWH is not routinely recommended.

(Continued)

(Continued)

Risk Factors	Implications	Action
		• Women with previous recurrent VTE or a previous unprovoked or oestrogen or pregnancy-related VTE or a previous VTE and a history of VTE in a first-degree relative or a documented thrombophilia or other risk factors should be offered antenatal thromboprophylaxis with LMWH. • Women with asymptomatic inherited or acquired thrombophilia may be managed with close surveillance antenatally. Exceptions are women with antithrombin deficiency, those with more than one thrombophilic defect (including homozygosity for factor V Leiden) or those with additional risk factors, where advice of a local expert should be sought and antenatal prophylaxis considered.

Chapter 16

MULTIPLE PREGNANCY

TWINS

- 3% of all live births
- Monozygotic (MC) twin frequency rates worldwide at 3–5/1000 maternities
- Dizygotic (DC) twin frequency rates are varied, depending on:
    1. geographical location
    2. assisted reproductive techniques
    3. increasing maternal age

Table 1. Frequency of Foetal Complications in Twins

	Singleton	Dichorionic	Monochorionic
2nd trimester miscarriage risk	1%	2%	10%
Perinatal death	0.5%	1.5%	3%
Intrauterine growth restriction (IUGR)	5%	20%	30%
Preterm delivery <32 weeks	1%	5%	10%
Major defects	0.5%	1%	4%

Antenatal Care

First trimester ultrasound provides:

- Accurate dating
- Determination of foetal number
- Chorionicity (accuracy of first trimester ultrasound~100%) — allows for risk stratification and the initiation of more intensive surveillance
- Amnionicity

Monochorionic, Monoamniotic Twins

- Monoamniotic twinning occurs in 1–2% of MC gestations (1 in 3000–6000 pregnancies)
- Occurs as a result of zygotic separation beyond 8 days of conception
- Associated with the highest perinatal loss rate ~30–60% due to prematurity or cord accidents
- Higher rates of congenital abnormalities (20–25%) and growth restriction.

Complications of Multiple Pregnancy — Foetal Causes

1) Chromosomal abnormalities
2) Structural abnormalities

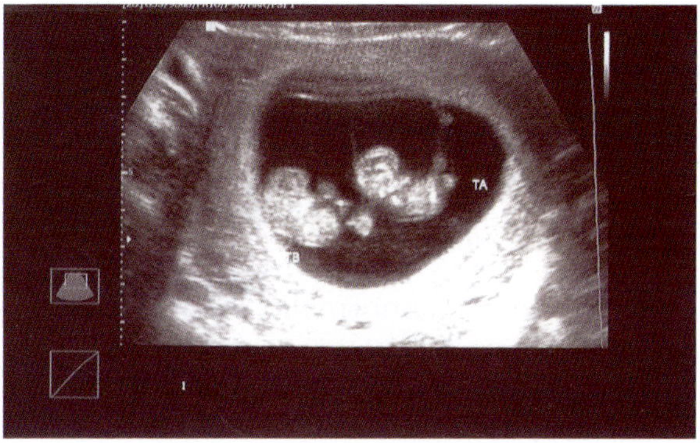

Figure 1. Ultrasound scan image of monochorionic (MC) twins.

3) Intrauterine growth restriction (IUGR)
4) Twin to twin transfusion syndrome (TTTS)
5) Twin reversed arterial perfusion (TRAP)
6) Single twin demise
7) Preterm delivery

1. *Chromosomal abnormalities*

- Risk of Down syndrome for MC twins is the same as for singleton pregnancy, but for DC twins, this risk is doubled as each twin has its own individual risk.
- Screening test of choice — nuchal translucency (NT).

- Rate of miscarriage associated with invasive testing in multiple pregnancies is increased (3% for CVS and 2% for amniocentesis).

2. ***Structural abnormalities***

- Frequency of foetal abnormality in dizygotic twins is comparable to that of singleton pregnancies (2–3%).
- Increased frequency of anomalies seen in monozygotic pregnancies (10%)
- Neural tube defects and congenital heart disease
- In monozygotic twinning, abnormal vascular connections predispose to limb reduction defects and bowel atresia.

3. ***Intrauterine growth restriction*** **(IUGR)**

- Increased risk of intrauterine growth restriction, with 20% in DC twins and 30% in MC twins
- Foetal weight discordance is estimated using two or more biometric parameters at each scan from 20 weeks
- Referral to a tertiary centre should be made if there is > 25% difference in size. Surveillance of growth-restricted twins will include monitoring of foetal Dopplers (umbilical artery, middle cerebral artery and ductus venosus), liquor volume and biophysical profile.

4. *Twin to twin transfusion syndrome* (TTTS)

- Complicates 10–20% of MC twin pregnancies
- Occurs via unidirectional arteriovenous (AV) connections between the circulations of both twins, such that there is a net flow of blood from one twin (the "donor") to the other (the "recipient")
- Results in hypovolaemia and oligohydramnios in donor twin, and overload and polyhydramnios in recipient twin
- Quintero introduced ultrasound staging of TTTS to describe a progression from early (stage I) to late (stage IV) disease (Table 2).

Table 2. The Quintero Classification System

Stage	Classification
I	Discrepancy in amniotic fluid volume with oligohydramnios of a maximum vertical pocket (MVP 2 cm) in one sac and polyhydramnios in the other sac (MVP 8 cm) The bladder of the donor twin is visible and Doppler studies are normal
II	The bladder of the donor twin is not visible, but Doppler studies are normal
III	Abnormal Doppler studies in either twin characterised by reversed end diastolic flow (EDF) in the umbilical artery, reversed in the ductus venosus or pulsatile umbilical venous flow
IV	The presence of hydrops in the recipient
V	Death of one or both twins

TTTS Staging (Quintero)

Stage	Oligohydramnios/ Polyhydramnios	Absent Urine in Donor Bladder	Abnormal Doppler Blood Flow	Hydrops Foetalis	Foetal Demise
I	+	–	–	–	–
II	+	+	–	–	–
III	+	+	+	–	–
IV	+	+	+	+	–
V	+	+	+	+	+

- Treatment of choice before 26 weeks of gestation is laser ablation of the intercommunicating vessels (dependent on availability of this treatment technique at respective tertiary centre). Other management options include:
  - serial amnioreduction with or without septostomy
  - occlusive foetocide
- It may be appropriate to consider conservative or expectant management, or to offer a termination of pregnancy if the foetuses are extremely premature or severely compromised.

5. *Twin reversed arterial perfusion* (TRAP)

- Rare complication unique to MC placentation
- Occurs when (because of an apparent lack of well-formed cardiac structure) an acardiac twin is abnormally perfused by a structurally normal co-twin (pump twin) via a single superficial artery-to-artery anastomosis
- Overall,with conservative management
  - intrauterine death of the pump twin occurs in 25%
  - polyhydramnios in 50%
  - preterm birth in 80% of cases
- Overall pump twin survival rate with no intervention is 60%
- Conservative management should be contemplated in cases of TRAP sequence where there is an abdominal circumference ratio of <50% with no evidence of compromise of the pump twin
- *In utero* interventions considered are:
  - cord occlusion
  - intrafoetal ablation
- Both procedures can be performed under ultrasound or foetoscopy guidance.

6. *Single twin demise*

- Following the death of one twin, the risk of MC and DC co-twin demise is 15% and 5%, respectively.

- Risk of neurological abnormality of surviving co-twin is 20% for MC and 1% for DC twins, respectively.

7. *Preterm delivery*

- Higher risk of spontaneous or iatrogenic preterm delivery
- Incidence of preterm delivery prior to 37 weeks can be up to 40%
- Delivery at less than 32 weeks vary with the type of twinning, ranging from 5% for DC and 10% for MC twins as compared with 1% for singleton pregnancies

Maternal complications of multiple pregnancy

- Mothers with multiple pregnancies are at higher risk of obstetric complications such as:
  - Hyperemesis
  - Increased mechanical symptoms of pregnancy
  - Gastro-oesophageal reflux
  - Pre-eclampsia
  - Gestational diabetes mellitus
  - Anaemia
  - Operative delivery
  - Postpartum haemorrhage
  - Perinatal mental health disorders
- Close surveillance is required

Summary of Management of Twins	
Dichorionic (DC) twins	**Monochorionic (MC) twins**
• Multidisciplinary team • Scan at 10–13 weeks: (a) viability, (b) chorionicity, (c) nuchal translucency (NT): aneuploidy • Structural abnormality scan — 19–22 weeks • Serial foetal growth scans, e.g. at 24, 28, 32 weeks and then every 2 weeks • Blood pressure and urinalysis at 20, 24 and 28 weeks and then every 2 weeks • Discussion of woman's/family's needs relating to twins • 34–38 weeks: discussion of mode of delivery and intrapartum care • Elective delivery at 37–38 completed weeks • Postnatal advice and support to include breastfeeding and contraceptive advice	• Multidisciplinary team • Scan at 10–13 weeks: (a) viability, (b) chorionicity, (c) nuchal translucency: aneuploidy/Twin-Twin Transfusion syndrome (TTTS) • Scan surveillance for TTTS and discordant growth: at 16 weeks and then every 2 weeks • Structural abnormality scan at 19–22 weeks (including foetal echocardiography) • Serial foetal growth scans every 2 weeks until delivery • Blood pressure and urinalysis at 20, 24, 28 weeks and then every 2 weeks • Discussion of woman's/family needs relating to twins • 32–34 weeks: discussion of mode of delivery, caesarean section and intrapartum care • Elective delivery at 34–36 completed weeks (if uncomplicated) • Postnatal advice and support to include breastfeeding and contraceptive advice

Triplets

- Incidence: approximately 1 in 6000 to 8000 births for spontaneous triplet pregnancy

Types of Triplets	Monozygotic	Dizygotic	Trizygotic
Fertilisation	• Single fertilised egg splits into three • One placenta and amniotic sac	• Two sperms fertilising two eggs and one of the two fertilised eggs split into two	• Three sperms fertilising three eggs • Three different placenta and amniotic sacs

Significant complications of triplets

	Singleton	Triplets
Spontaneous reduction	20%	50%
Aneuploidy	Age-related risk	3 times age-related risk
Hyperemesis gravidarum	Common	More common
Premature rupture of membranes	2%	15–30%
Mean delivery gestation	38 weeks	32 weeks
Birth weight	<2500g : 5% <1500g :1.1%	<2500 g : 95% <1500 g : 35%
Pre-eclampsia	5%	20–50%
Anaemia	25%	50%
Postpartum haemorrhage	0.5%	10–35%

Delivery (as suggested by NICE Guideline)

Information about timing of birth:

- Discuss with the woman timing of birth and possible mode of delivery early in the third trimester
- Inform woman that spontaneous preterm birth and elective preterm birth are associated with an increased risk of admission to a special care baby unit

Uncomplicated twin pregnancy

Inform woman that:

- ~60% of twin pregnancies result in spontaneous birth before 37 weeks **and**
- Elective birth from 36 week for MC twins and 37 weeks 0 days for DC twins does not appear to be associated with increased risk of serious adverse outcomes **and**
- Continuing twin pregnancies beyond 38 weeks increases the risk of foetal death

Offer elective delivery:

- 36 weeks for MC twin pregnancies after a course of corticosteroids has been offered
- 37 weeks for DC twin pregnancies

Uncomplicated triplet pregnancy

Inform woman that:

- ~75% of triplet pregnancies result in spontaneous birth before 35 weeks **and**
- Continuing triplet pregnancies beyond 36 weeks increases the risk of foetal death

Offer elective delivery from 35 weeks, after a course of corticosteroids given

- If elective delivery is declined, offer weekly appointments with specialist obstetrician
- Offer fortnightly foetal growth scans and weekly biophysical profile assessments

Chapter 17

INFECTIONS IN PREGNANCY

Antenatal Screening for Infection

Do	Don't
Hepatitis B (HbsAg) HIV (HIV antibody) Rubella (Rubella IgG) Syphilis (VDRL) Asymptomatic bacteriuria (urine culture) GBS	Asymptomatic bacterial vaginosis Chlamydia CMV Toxoplasmosis Hepatitis C

Management of Infection in Pregnancy

History	• Date and time of exposure • Time of onset of symptoms • History of previous vaccination or infection • Current gestation of pregnancy
Examination	• Temperature, pulse and blood pressure • Maternal well-being • Stigmata of infection
Investigations	• Confirm maternal infection by testing for pathogen-specific IgG and IgM

(*Continued*)

(*Continued*)

Management	• Refer to infectious disease specialist and foetal medicine specialist • Diagnose foetal infection — in most cases by PCR testing via amniocentesis • Ultrasound surveillance of foetus • Therapeutic options — depending on type of infection
Limitations	• An infected foetus does not always mean the foetus will be damaged by the infection • Risks of transmission and foetal damage depend on pathogen and gestation at infection • Invasive techniques may cause maternal-foetal transmission and infect a non-infected foetus

Infections associated with perinatal infections	Infections associated with *in utero* infections
Hepatitis B Hepatitis C HIV Herpes simplex type 1 and 2 GBS	Rubella Parvovirus Toxoplasmosis CMV Varicella Syphilis Listeriosis

List of Infections in Pregnancy

1. Bacterial Vaginosis
2. Candidiasis
3. *Chlamydia trachomatis*

(1–3:) Refer to Chapter 53 on "Vaginal Discharge and Recurrent Vulvo-Vaginal Candidiasis"

4. Cytomegalovirus (CMV) Infection
5. Dengue Infection

6. Genital Warts Infection
7. Gonorrhoea — Refer to Chapter 55 on "Sexually Transmitted Infections"
8. Group B Streptococcus (GBS) Infection
9. Hand Foot Mouth Disease (HFMD) Infection
10. Hepatitis B Infection
11. Hepatitis C Infection
12. Hepatitis E Infection
13. Herpes Simplex Virus (HSV) Infection
14. H1N1 Influenza Infection
15. HIV Infection
16. Listeriosis Infection
17. Malaria Infection
18. Parvovirus B19 Infection
19. Rubella Infection
20. Shingles (Herpes/Varicella-Zoster Virus) Infection
21. Syphilis (*Treponema Pallidum*) Infection
22. Toxoplasmosis Infection
23. Trichomoniasis Infection — Refer to Chapter 53 on "Vaginal Discharge and Recurrent Vulvo-Vaginal Candidiasis"
24. Tuberculosis Infection
25. Varicella Zoster (Chicken Pox)

4. Cytomegalovirus (CMV) Infection

Incidence	• 2% seroconvert during pregnancy • 40% vertical transmission • 3–4 per 1000 livebirths, commonest cause of congenital infection • Second commonest cause of mental retardation after Down syndrome • 50–60% of women of childbearing age have antibodies to CMV
Maternal symptoms	• Asymptomatic • Flu-like illness
Risks to foetus	• Commonest cause of congenital sensorineural deafness • Miscarriage, stillbirth • IUGR • Microcephaly, learning disability, seizures • Hepatosplenomegaly, thrombocytopaenia, jaundice, haemolytic anaemia • Chorioretinitis, micro-opthalmia, cataract, optic atrophy
Diagnosis	• Usually investigated after findings of an abnormal scan • Maternal CMV-specific IgG and IgM antibodies but IgM persist for 4–7 months • CMV IgG Avidity test can help distinguish primary CMV infection from reactivated infection Low Avidity — Primary CMV (may last up to 17 weeks) High Avidity — Reactivation • Amniocentesis to detect CMV in amniotic fluid but should be delayed for 6 weeks after maternal seropositivity to allow for accumulation of CMV in foetal urine

(Continued)

(*Continued*)

Management	• If CMV is detected in amniotic fluid, assume infected foetus • Consider termination of pregnancy (TOP) if primary infection diagnosed in first trimester • Serial foetal ultrasound scan for sonographic features: cerebral atrophy, ventriculomegaly, calcifications, periventricular cyst formation, leukomalacia, IUGR, echogenic bowel • No therapy to protect at risk foetus • Neonatal treatment with ganciclovir for neonates with congenital CMV and central nervous system signs at birth
Prevention	• Hygiene: wash hands • Avoid finger/mouth contact

5. Dengue Infection

Maternal risks	• Acute fever, headache, retro-orbital pain, severe muscle and joint pains • Fine petechial rash • Dengue haemorrhagic fever • Dengue shock syndrome • Clinical confusion can occur with HELLP syndrome as they have similar clinical presentation • Pregnancy does not predispose to more severe disease
Foetal risks	• No specific threat of foetal malformation or disease-specific foetal harm • Increased incidence of neural tube defects, also associated with other febrile illnesses • If maternal infection occurs near delivery, infants might develop congenital dengue infection — fever, thrombocytopaenia and enlarged liver
Management	• Supportive treatment with fever reduction measures • Careful maintenance of fluid and electrolyte balance
Prevention	• Avoid travel to dengue endemic areas • Mosquito bite-preventive measures should be advised, including the use of an effective insect repellent

6. Genital Warts Infection

Maternal risks	• Genital warts can proliferate and become friable during pregnancy • Complete resolution of warts during pregnancy is seldom achieved
Foetal risks	• Very small risk of warts on the larynx (respiratory papillomatosis) in infants and children. The route of transmission, whether it is transplacental, perinatal or postnatal, has not been established. • Caesarean section is indicated only if the pelvic outlet is obstructed by genital warts or if vaginal delivery would result in excessive bleeding • Trichloroacetic acid can be used
Management	• Imiquimod, sinecatechins, podophyllin, and podofilox should NOT be used during pregnancy • Cryotherapy with liquid nitrogen, electrocautery and laser treatment can be considered • Trichloroacetic acid can be used

7. Gonorrhoea (Refer to Chapter 55 on "Sexually Transmitted Infections")

8. Group B Streptococcus (GBS) Infection

Incidence	• Most common infective cause of mortality in the newborn • 10% overall mortality in early-onset GBS disease
Treatment	• No evidence that antepartum antibiotics reduces GBS carriage rate or affects outcome • Offer treatment to women identified to be at risk of having an infected infant with intrapartum antibiotic prophylaxis
High risk group	• GBS disease in previous baby • Maternal chorioamnionitis • GBS incidentally found in vagina or urine at any time of pregnancy • Preterm labour • Prolonged rupture of membranes 18 hours or more • Maternal pyrexia in labour of more than 38°C
Intrapartum management	• Intrapartum antibiotics to high risk groups • Intravenous 5 Mu Pen G stat and intravenous 2.5 Mu Pen G 4 hourly (in KKH) • If allergic to penicillin, give intravenous clindamycin 900 mg 8 hourly until delivery
Neonatal management	• Neonatologist to review at delivery • Consider treatment if mother did not receive intrapartum antibiotics or if the first dose is less than 4 hours prior to delivery • Observe for at least 12 hours in high risk groups • Treat if baby develops signs and symptoms of infection

9. Hand-Foot-Mouth Disease (HFMD) Infection

Symptoms	• Blister-like or pimple-like rash on hands, feet, buttocks, mouth ulcers and fever • Some may get sore throat, runny nose, vomiting and diarrhoea
Risk to foetus	• Normally no risk to foetus but there have been reported cases of miscarriage and stillbirth in infected pregnant women • Infection in the newborn can occur if pregnant women acquired infection close to delivery
Prevention	• Ensure good hygiene • Wash hands immediately after contact with infected child or handling diaper changes, and before handling food • Wear mask when in close contact with children suffering from runny nose and cough

10. Hepatitis B Infection

Incidence	• 1 in 35 people in Singapore are carriers				
Risk to foetus	• No congenital syndrome • Neonatal hepatitis — high mortality • 90% become chronic carriers if vertically infected • Risk of developing cirrhosis and hepatocellular carcinoma (incubation period 20 to 30 years) • 5% occur due to transplacental transmission • 95% occur during delivery				
Management	• Counsel, screen and vaccinate partner • Record in notes and notify carers • Infection control measures during invasive procedures • Consider hepatitis B immune globulin administered to neonate within 12 hours of delivery • First dose of HBV vaccine within 12 hours of birth • Second dose at 1 month, third dose at 6 months • Test for HbsAg at 12–15 months				
Prevention of neonatal infection				HBV vaccine	HBVIg
	HbsAg +	HBeAg +	AntiHBe –	+	+
	HBsAg +	HBeAg –	AntiHBe –	+	+
	HBsAg +	HBeAg –	AntiHBe +	+	–

11. Hepatitis C Infection

High risk groups	• IV drug users
Diagnosis	• Anti HCV positive — a positive hepatitis C antibody test implies a persistent infection
Risk to foetus	• Vertical transmission 5% unless mother is in acute phase of illness or co-infected with HIV • HCV RNA status negative, no reported transmission • Babies of infected mothers need testing for HCV RNA at 6 and 12 months of age • Breastfeeding not contraindicated
Vaccine	• Not available

12. Hepatitis E Infection

Transmission	• Water-borne infection with faeco-oral transmission
Maternal risks	• Usually a self-limiting infection but pregnancy is associated with a 6-fold increase in maternal mortality • Especially in third trimester with 15% fulminant hepatic failure and 5% mortality
Treatment	• No specific treatment

13. Herpes Simplex Virus (HSV) Infection

Incidence	• Genital herpes lesions are usually caused by HSV type 2 virus • Increasing incidence of HSV type 1 amongst young adults • HSV1 not protective against HSV2
Transmission risk	• 40% if vaginal delivery occurs with active primary infection • Less than 3% if the infection is recurrent
Risk of recurrence during pregnancy	• 75% will have 1 or more recurrent infection • Infection not more severe in pregnancy • Risk of neonatal herpes is low
Risk to foetus	• Neonatal herpes (rare) • Causes meningitis, encephalitis, hepatitis, disseminated skin lesions • 70–90% mortality in disseminated disease • Requires early recognition and treatment with acyclovir
Current practice	• Treatment with acyclovir is associated with reduced duration, severity of symptoms and duration of viral shedding • Acyclovir should be used with caution before 20 weeks gestation • All women presenting with 1st episode genital herpes at time of labour or within 6 weeks of the expected date of delivery, caesarean section is recommended • Routine caesarean section is not recommended for women with recurrent genital herpes

14. H1N1 Influenza Infection

Maternal risks	• Pregnant women are at increased risk of developing complications • 4-fold increase in risk of being hospitalised for complications as compared to non-pregnant population • Risk is highest in the third trimester • Women with asthma, morbid obesity, COPD, diabetes, and heart disease appear to have a higher risk of severe disease
Effect on pregnancy	• Associated with preterm delivery, especially in women admitted to the intensive care unit (ICU) • Vertical transmission has not been reported
Criteria for hospital referral	• Signs of respiratory distress, oxygen saturation less than 94% in room air, dehydration, shock, any sign of sepsis, altered conscious level or seizures
Risk factors for ICU admission	• Dyspnoea, tachypnoea (respiratory rate >30/min) • Supplementary oxygen requirement • Pneumonia • Tachycardia • Altered conscious level
Antiviral therapy	• Most effective if given within 48 hours of symptom onset • Zanamivir recommended as first line in pregnancy as no systemic absorption
Vaccination	• Inactivated H1N1 virus • Antibody response in pregnant women as effective as in non-pregnant women • *Side effects*: pain at injection site, myalgia, Guillain-Barre syndrome (rare) • Recommended after first trimester • Influenza vaccines are safe to administer in all trimesters of pregnancy

15. HIV Infection

Incidence	• Very low in Singapore
Transmission risk	• Can be reduced to less than 2% with anti-retroviral therapy (mother and neonate) • Mode of delivery dependent on viral load • Breastfeeding is contraindicated
Risk to foetus	• Risk of miscarriage, preterm delivery, low birthweight in advanced maternal disease
Management	• Multidisciplinary team including consultant obstetricians, infectious disease specialist and neonatologists • At booking, check hepatitis B, C, CMV, toxoplasmosis, VZV, syphilis, CD 4 count, viral load and viral resistance test • Screen for genitourinary infection • Prophylaxis against *Pneumocystis carinii* pneumonia depends on CD 4 count • Advise all women to take antiviral therapy, to start at 20–28 weeks if not needed for their own health, the aim being to achieve undetectable viral load of <50 copies/mL prior to delivery • Planned vaginal delivery is possible in women taking highly active antiretroviral therapy (HAART) with viral load <50 copies/mL • Delivery by elective caesarean section at 38 weeks in (a) women taking HAART with a viral load >50 copies/mL (b) women taking zidovudine monotherapy (c) women with HIV and hepatitis C co-infection
Neonatal management	• Early cord clamping • Early bathing • Anti-retroviral therapy within 4 hours of birth (for 4 weeks) • Avoidance of breastfeeding • HIV PCR test should be performed at day 1, 6 weeks and 12 weeks. A confirmatory HIV antibody test should be performed at 18 months of age

16. Listeriosis Infection

Prevention	• Do not eat unpasteurised dairy products, soft cheese and pate • Food-borne transmission
Maternal symptoms	• Asymptomatic • Flu-like symptoms • Usually a mild illness but can get severe ARDS • More common in third trimester
Diagnosis	• Need a high index of clinical suspicion • Gram stain from blood culture • Meconium stained liquor
Risks	• Miscarriage, premature labour • Congenital listeriosis is a cause of foetal hydrops • Perinatal listeriosis
Treatment	• High dose ampicillin and gentamicin • Early aggressive treatment may allow continuation of pregnancy with good outcome

17. Malaria Infection

Risk to mother in pregnancy	• Pregnant women are twice as likely to be bitten by mosquitoes (Anopheles mosquito), to contract and to die from malaria than non-pregnant women
Risk to foetus	• Miscarriage, premature birth, stillbirth, intrauterine growth restriction
Prevention in pregnancy	• Do not travel to a malaria endemic country unless essential • If travel is unavoidable, advise women to seek guidance from centre with expertise on risk and avoidance strategies • Flu-like illness when travelling or upon returning home for up to 1 year or more may be malaria • *"ABCD" of malaria prevention* • **A**wareness of risk — transmission risk, rainy or dry season, drug resistant strains, rural or urban travel, length of stay • **B**ite prevention — risk period dawn to dusk, skin repellents containing 50% DEET, knock-down mosquito sprays, insecticide treated bed nets, clothing and room protection • **C**hemoprophylaxis — no malaria prophylaxis is 100% protective. *Mefloquine* is the only drug considered safe for prophylaxis in pregnancy • **D**iagnosis and treatment must be prompt — suspect if flu-like illness and temperature more than 38°C

(Continued)

(*Continued*)

Safety of drugs in pregnancy	• Mefloquine — safe in the second and third trimester; its use in first trimester may be justified if risk of acquiring *Plasmodium falciparum* is high. Contraindicated in depression, epilepsy, hypersensitivity to quinine or mefloquine • Atovaquone and proguanil — use if mefloquine or chloroquine resistance • Doxycycline — contraindicated as it affects foetal bone growth and teeth discolouration • Primaquine — contraindicated as it causes haemolysis • Chloroquine — contraindicated due to widespread drug resistance
Symptoms	• Fever, headache, myalgia, nausea, vomiting, diarrhoea, cough, jaundice, pyrexia, splenomegaly, respiratory distress
Diagnosis	• Blood film and malaria rapid antigen test
Management	• Start antimalarials immediately according to species and severity of disease • Multidisciplinary team approach • Notify

18. Parvovirus B19 Infection

Incidence	• 1% of susceptible adults are infected each year • 1 in 400 pregnancies • Annual seroconversion rate among susceptible primary school employees is 5%, hospital staff, 2%
Maternal presentation	• Asymptomatic (30–40%) • Flu-like illness, arthralgia, erythematous rash, slapped cheek appearance • Once rash appears, patient is no longer infectious • More than 50% adults are immune
Foetal risk	• Transplacental transmission rate 30% • No evidence of increased risk of congenital malformations • Spontaneous miscarriage risk 10% • Foetal anaemia, cardiac failure • Foetal hydrops 3% with 50% mortality • Foetal infection occurs 2–12 weeks after maternal infection • No congential syndrome
Diagnosis	• Maternal B19 specific IgM — detectable 3 days after the onset of symptoms and may persist for up to 6 months • B19 IgG is detectable by the 7th day of illness and persists for life. Conveys lasting immunity to infection • Elevated maternal serum αFP may be a marker for foetal parvovirus B19 infection • Invasive testing only when there are signs of foetal anaemia or hydrops. Foetal parvovirus B19 IgM and DNA by PCR required via amniocentesis or foetal cord blood

(Continued)

(*Continued*)

Management	• If patient is IgG positive, reassure • If IgG negative, check serum IgM and IgG 21 days after contact • If IgG negative and IgM negative, patient is susceptible but not infected. Reassure patient and follow-up any future contacts • If IgM positive, refer to tertiary centre • Serial ultrasound scans 1–2 weekly for up to 12 weeks (signs of foetal anaemia like ascites, hydrops, measure MCA-PSV) • Foetal blood sampling and *in utero* blood transfusion • Deliver foetus if gestation age permits

19. Rubella Infection

Incidence	• 1–2% women of childbearing age are thought to be susceptible
Maternal symptoms and signs	• Asymptomatic • Mild symptoms • Maculopapular rash • Arthralgia • Infectious from 7 days before until 7 days after onset of rash • Incubation period 14–21 days
Risk to foetus	• The earlier the maternal infection, the worse the foetal abnormalities • *First 12 weeks*: 90% risk of foetal infection, most severely infected • *12–16 weeks*: 55% risk of foetal infection, 20% risk of foetal anomaly • *16–20 weeks*: 45% risk of infection, slight risk of sensorineural deafness • *After 20 weeks*: Almost no risk to foetus • *Congenital rubella syndrome* o *Eyes*: cataract, retinopathy, glaucoma, micro-opthalmia o *Heart*: PDA, PA stenosis, coarctation of aorta, VSD, ASD o *Ear*: bilateral and progressive hearing loss o *IUGR, oligohydramnios* • Neonatal hepatosplenomegaly, purpura, jaundice, meningoencephalitis, thrombocytopaenia

(*Continued*)

(*Continued*)

Diagnosis	• Rubella specific IgM antibodies, peak at 10 days, present for 4–8 weeks • IgG is present 1 week after onset of rash, use avidity test if indicated to distinguish recent and distant infection
Management	• If infected in first trimester, offer termination of pregnancy • Ultrasound growth surveillance • Foetal echocardiography
Prevention	• Vaccination programme (15 year protection 98%) • Check status before becoming pregnant; 2% vaccinees non-immune • If seronegative, advice vaccination before pregnancy or after delivery • Maternal re-infection in immune women has been reported but foetal risk is less than 5%
Vaccine	• Live attenuated vaccine, contraindicated in pregnancy • Risk of rubella-induced foetal malformations with inadvertent immunisation is 1% • Avoid pregnancy for 1 month after vaccination

20. Shingles (Herpes/Varicella-Zoster Virus) Infection

Mode of transmission	• Shingles only occur if a person previously had chicken pox because both are caused by the same virus: herpes varicella-zoster virus (VZV) • If a person is not immune to chicken pox, it is possible to be infected by someone who has shingles • However, the risk is low, particularly if the person's rash is covered, e.g. by clothing or a dressing • In shingles, the virus is passed by direct contact with the rash. The risk is higher if the rash is widespread or situated on an exposed part of their body such as the face
Foetal risks	• Does not appear to have foetal sequelae
Management	• Symptomatic treatment for pain • Avoid contact with other pregnant women in case they are not immune to VZV • Keep the rash covered until the last blister has scabbed

21. Syphilis (*Treponema pallidum*) Infection

Incidence	• Active syphilis usually detected by routine screening • 5 in 10,000 pregnancies • Increasing incidence
Maternal symptoms	• Asymptomatic • Positive serology at antenatal screening
Risks	• Transplacental infection occurs at all stages • Congenital syphilis — 40% risk if primary/secondary syphilis; 10% risk if later stages • Preterm labour 25% • Foetal loss 25%
Management	• Treat with penicillin G — cures maternal infection and foetal infection but will not reverse established foetal damage • Screen for other sexually transmitted infections (STIs) • Refer to Department of STI Control, contact tracing

22. Toxoplasmosis Infection

Incidence	• 2 per 1000 pregnancies • 90% of women of childbearing age are susceptible
Presentation	• Asymptomatic • Non-specific febrile illness
Transmission to foetus	• Risk of infection increases with gestation age 15% first trimester, 30% second trimester, 60% third trimester • Risk of affection decreases with gestation age • Risk of severely affected infants — 65% first trimester, 0% third trimester • Highest risk of having affected foetus between 15–30 weeks
Risk to foetus	• Classic triad of intracerebral calcification, hydrocephalus, chorioretinitis (uncommon) • Spontaneous first trimester miscarriage • IUGR, microcephaly, learning disability • Hepatosplenomegaly • 10% of infected neonates will be symptomatic at birth but if infected, nearly all will develop neurological or ophthalmic problems later • All infected babies must be treated at birth
Maternal diagnosis	• Toxoplasmosis specific IgG/ IgM antibodies • IgM appears within 2 weeks of exposure; can persist for 18 months • IgG appears 2 weeks after exposure and is lifelong. Immunity is lifelong unless the individual becomes immunocompromised • Biopsy of lymph node

(*Continued*)

(*Continued*)

Foetal diagnosis	• Amniocentesis from 16 weeks to detect presence of *Toxoplasma gondii* DNA in amniotic fluid • May need to repeat amniocentesis as presence of toxoplasmosis in amniotic fluid may take up to 6 weeks after maternal seroconversion and foetal diuresis is only fully established from 18–20 weeks • No accurate method to predict severity of foetal disease
Treatment	• Spiramycin therapy to infected mothers result in 60% reduction in the risk of foetal infection • Treat foetal infection with pyrimethamine, sulphadiazine and folinic acid • Infected neonates require treatment for the first year of life
Prevention	• Source: undercooked or cured meat with toxoplasma tissue cysts, cat is host • Wash hands before handling food • Thorough washing of fruits and vegetables, including ready-prepared salads, before eating • Thorough cooking of raw meats and ready-prepared chilled meats • Wear gloves and thoroughly washing hands after handling soil and gardening • Avoid cat faeces in cat litter or in soil

23. Trichromoniasis (Refer to Chapter 53 on "Vaginal Discharge and Recurrent Vulvovaginal Candidiasis.")

24. Tuberculosis Infection

Incidence	• More likely in areas with a higher incidence of tuberculosis • Tuberculosis infection should be suspected in women who come from endemic areas and ethnic minority with non-specific symptoms
Maternal risks	• Outcome of tuberculosis infection is not affected by pregnancy • Delayed or untreated infection can result in increased maternal morbidity
Foetal risks	• Increased risk of preterm labour and intrauterine growth restriction • Congenital tuberculosis is very rare — primary hepatic complex and caseating granulomas in infants
Management	• Tuberculin skin testing (Mantoux test) is safe in pregnancy and the result is not affected by pregnancy • Chest X-ray (radiation <0.01 mGy) with abdominal shield is safe in pregnancy • Chemotherapy should be started in consultation with an infectious disease specialist • Isoniazid, rifampicin, pyridoxine and ethambutol can be used • Patients are non-infectious 2 weeks after initiation of treatment • Breastfeeding can be continued

25. Varicella Zoster (Chickenpox) Infection

Incidence	• Primary chicken pox infection occurs in 3 in 1000 pregnancies • 90% of adult population are immune
Maternal risks	• Severe disease in adults, particularly in pregnancy • Severity increases with increasing gestation • Complications include pneumonia, hepatitis and encephalitis • Women at greater risk of pneumonia are those who smoke, have COPD, immunocompromised, extensive or haemorrhagic rash or who are in the latter half of pregnancy
Risk to foetus	• Foetal varicella syndrome — 1% risk at less than 28 weeks, very rare between 20–28 weeks and does not occur after 28 weeks • Risk lowest in early pregnancy (0.5% in first trimester); highest at 13–20 weeks • Defects do not occur at time of initial infection but are secondary to a herpes zoster type re-activation *in utero* • Skin loss and scarring, usually unilateral and segmented • Hypoplasia of limb bud development, rudimentary digits • Mental retardation with cortical and cerebellar atrophy, microcephaly • Micro-opthalmia, chorioretinitis, cataracts • Bladder and bowel sphincter dysfunction
Diagnosis	• Clinical diagnosis if rash present • If history of past infection, reassure • If significant contact (face to face for 5 minutes or in the same room for 15 minutes or more), test IgG status • Amniocentesis and detection of VZ virus DNA does not imply foetal varicella syndrome, and thus not recommended

(*Continued*)

(Continued)

Management of suspected exposure to varicella in pregnancy	• If IgG positive, reassure • If IgG negative, recommend VZV immune globulin (VZIG) as soon as possible. Effective within 10 days of contact • Patient is potentially infectious from 8–28 days after VZIG • Patient should be advised to notify a doctor if rash develops even after administration of VZIG • Check for seroconversion VZ IgM 3 weeks after exposure
Management of chickenpox in pregnancy	• Avoid contact with susceptible individuals (other pregnant women and neonates), until the lesions have crusted over • Symptomatic treatment and hygiene to prevent secondary bacterial infection • Oral acyclovir if present within 24 hours of the onset of the rash and if more than 20 weeks gestation (800 mg 5 times per day for 7 days) • Oral acyclovir reduces the duration of fever and symptoms. It is not associated with foetal anomalies although there is a theoretical risk of teratogenesis in the first trimester • Refer to hospital if the patient develops: chest or neurological symptoms, haemorrhagic rash or bleeding, a dense rash with or without mucosal lesions

(Continued)

(*Continued*)

Neonatal chickenpox	• The severity of the infection depends on the timing of the maternal infection. It is greatest if maternal infection occurs 4 days prior to delivery and up to 2 days postpartum • Mortality up to 30% of cases • VZIG recommended if the mother develops chicken pox within 7 days before or after delivery • Neonatal infection should be treated with acyclovir following discussion with neonatologist
Vaccination	• Live attenuated vaccine • Should be considered pre-pregnancy or postpartum in women who are found to be seronegative • Avoid pregnancy for at least 4 weeks to 3 months ideally and to avoid contact with other susceptible pregnant women should a post-vaccination rash occur • Inadvertent exposures to vaccine in pregnancy have been reported with no cases of foetal varicella syndrome or increase in foetal abnormalities

Chapter 18

SKIN DISORDERS IN PREGNANCY

There are three categories of common skin conditions in pregnancy:

1. Hormone-related Skin Disorders

Striae gravidarum (stretch marks), hyper-pigmentation (e.g. melasma), hair, nail and vascular changes.

2. Pre-existing Skin Disorders

Atopic dermatitis, psoriasis, fungal infections, cutaneous tumours.

3. Pregnancy-specific Skin Disorders

Pruritic urticarial papules and plaques of pregnancy (PUPPP — most common), prurigo of pregnancy, intrahepatic cholestasis, pemphigoid (herpes) gestationis, impetigo herpetiformis and pruritic folliculitis of pregnancy.

- Most skin conditions resolve postpartum and only require symptomatic treatment.
- Specific treatments needed for melasma, intrahepatic cholestasis of pregnancy, impetigo herpetiformis, and pruritic folliculitis of pregnancy.
- Antepartum surveillance recommended for intrahepatic cholestasis of pregnancy, impetigo herpetiformis and pemphigoid (herpes) gestationis.

Pregnancy-specific Skin Disorders

Condition	Rash Presentation	Pregnancy Risk	Treatment
1. Pruritic urticarial papules and plaques of pregnancy (PUPPP) • mainly occurs in first pregnancy • usually present from 36 weeks' gestation to one week postpartum (Figure 1)	Intensely pruritic urticarial plaques and papules with or without erythematous patches of papules and vesicles; rash first appears on abdomen, often along striae and occasionally involves extremities; face, scalp, palms and soles are usually not affected	No identified maternal or foetal adverse effects	Oral antihistamines (chlorpheniramine 4 mg ON) and topical corticosteroids (betamethasone valerate cream 0.1%) for pruritus; systemic corticosteroids for extreme symptoms

(*Continued*)

(*Continued*)

Condition	Rash Presentation	Pregnancy Risk	Treatment
2. **Prurigo of pregnancy/ papular dermatitis of pregnancy** • presents at 25–30 weeks' gestation	Erythematous papules and nodules on the extensor surfaces of the extremities, no urticarial lesions or vesicles	No identified maternal or foetal adverse effects	Mid potency topical corticosteroids and oral antihistamines
3. **Pruritic folliculitis of pregnancy**	Erythematous follicular papules and sterile pustules on the abdomen, arms, chest and back	No identified maternal or foetal adverse effects	Topical cortiocosteroids, topical benzoyl peroxide (Benzac) or ultraviolet B light therapy
4. **Pemphigoid (herpes) gestationis** (rare) • auto-immune • usually onset in 2nd/3rd trimester • postpartum onset (20%) (Figure 2)	Pruritic papules, plaques, and vesicles evolving into generalised vesicles or bullae; initial periumbilical lesions (90%) may generalise, although the face, scalp, and mucous membranes are usually not affected. Palms and soles are commonly involved.	Newborns may have urticarial, vesicular, or bullous lesions; risk of premature deliveries and newborns who are small for gestational age	Skin biopsy shows sub-epidermal blistering, oedematous upper dermis with peri-vascular inflammation. Direct immuno-fluorescence test is positive. Oral antihistamines and topical corticosteroids for mild cases; systemic oral corticosteroids for severe cases. Monitor foetal growth. Avoid COC pills postpartum (may cause flare ups).

(*Continued*)

(Continued)

Condition	Rash Presentation	Pregnancy Risk	Treatment
5. Impetigo herpetiformis (rare) • usually begins in 3rd trimester. (Figure 3)	Round, arched, or polycyclic patches covered with small painful pustules in a herpetiform pattern; most commonly appears on thighs and groin in major flexures, but rash may coalesce and spread to trunk and extremities; face, hands, and feet are not affected; mucous membranes may be involved	Reports of increased foetal morbidity. Patients can be toxic/ febrile, may result in renal or cardiac failure	Systemic corticosteroids; antibiotics for secondarily infected lesions. Delivery is curative. Monitor foetal growth

(Continued)

(*Continued*)

Condition	Rash Presentation	Pregnancy Risk	Treatment
6. Obstetric cholestasis/ intrahepatic cholestasis of pregnancy • genetically linked. • usually present in 3rd trimester. • Pruritus involving palms and soles	Pruritus without primary skin lesions. Excoriations from scratching; distribution is nonspecific. Can have tea-coloured urine with light-coloured stools. Increase in liver transaminases (3-fold increase) consistent with cholestasis. Alkaline phosphatase levels are normally elevated in pregnancy, thus not useful.	Risk of premature delivery, meconium-stained amniotic fluid, intrauterine foetal death. Postpartum haemorrhage.	Exclude viral or auto-immune hepatitis or gall-stone disease. Foetal surveillance for growth. Oral antihistamines for mild pruritus Ursodeoxycholic acid (ursodiol [Actigall]) for more severe cases (15 mg/kg/day) Oral vitamin K 10 mg/day given to mother to reduce risk of maternal and foetal bleeding. Induction of labour at 37 weeks of gestation. Resolves 4–6 weeks after delivery. Tends to recur in subsequent pregnancies up to 40–60%.

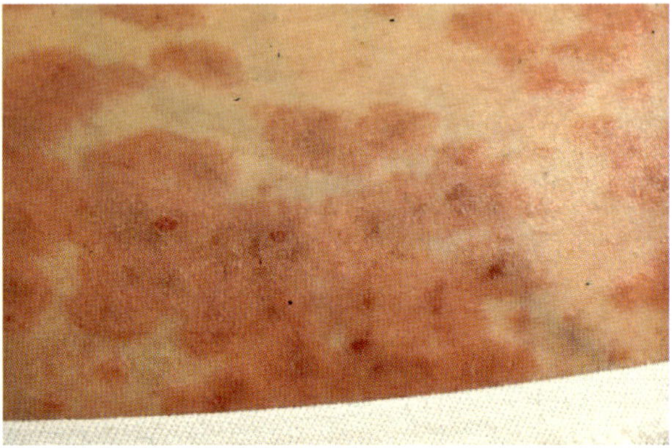

Figure 1. Pruritic and urticarial papules and plaques of pregnancy (PUPPP).

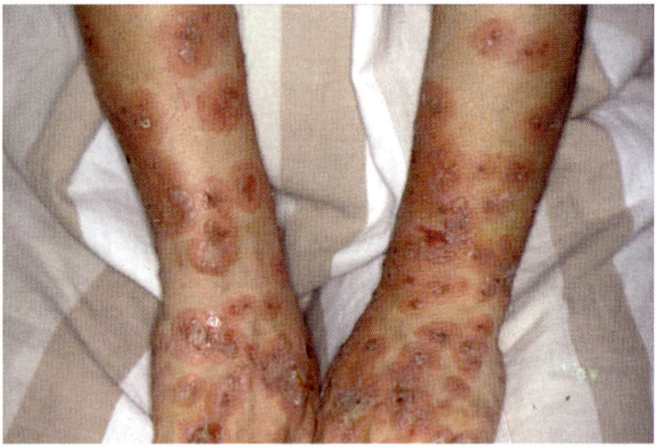

Figure 2. Pemphigoid (herpes) gestationis.

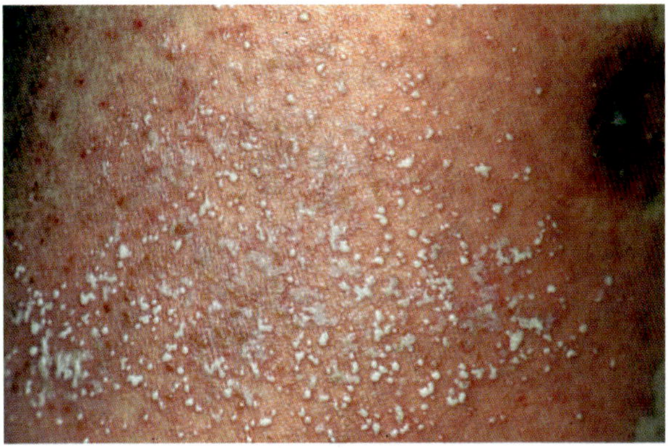

Figure 3. Impetigo herpetiformis.

Chapter 19

APPROACH TO DEPRESSION IN PREGNANCY

Depression affects 12% of pregnant women and 7% of post-partum women.

Antenatal Depression is associated with:

(a) Substance abuse

(b) Poor antenatal compliance/nutrition

(c) Increased risk of preterm labour (PTL)

If untreated, depression progresses into postpartum period in up to 50% of cases.

Postnatal Depression is associated with:

(a) Impaired mother-infant bonding

(b) Poor parenting practices

These are known to affect the intellectual and emotional development of the infant.

(c) Maternal suicide (most serious adverse outcome)

(d) Infanticide

Among women with major depression who discontinue anti-depressants, 70% relapse during pregnancy, typically during the first trimester.

Recognition of symptoms is important:

Emotional liability
Poor sleep
Poor appetite
Loss of energy or interest
Negative thinking
Feelings of hopelessness
Suicidal/infanticidal impulses
Comorbid anxiety symptoms — excessive worrying, palpitations, giddiness, breathlessness, muscle cramps and tremors
Panic attacks

In severe depression-associated psychotic symptoms (hallucinations/delusions).

Screening for Depression:

Edinburgh Postnatal Depression Scale (EPDS)
Antenatal Depression — cut off score of 15
Postnatal Depression — cut off score of 13
Two questions can be effectively used to identify possible depression:

1. "During the past month, have you often been bothered by feeling down, depressed or hopeless?"
2. "During the past month, have you often been bothered by having little interest or pleasure in doing things?"

A "yes" answer to either one or both questions is suggestive of depression, and the patient can be offered help with the question: "Is this something you feel you need or want help with?"

Screening also includes identifying those at greater risk of adverse outcomes especially maternal suicide. It is strongly recommended that specialist psychiatric care be arranged for pregnant or postpartum women with:

- past or present severe mental illness including schizophrenia, bipolar disorder, psychosis in the postnatal period and severe depression
- previous treatment by a psychiatrist/specialist mental health team including inpatient care
- a family history of perinatal mental illness.

Treatment

Refer to Chapter 20 on "Medications in Pregnancy and Lactation."

Chapter 20

MEDICATIONS IN PREGNANCY AND LACTATION

Food Drug Administration (FDA) Classification for Drugs in Pregnancy:

United States FDA Pharmaceutical Pregnancy Categories	
Pregnancy Category A	Adequate and well-controlled human studies have failed to demonstrate a risk to the foetus in the first trimester of pregnancy (and there is no evidence of risk in later trimesters).
Pregnancy Category B	Animal reproduction studies have failed to demonstrate a risk to the foetus and there are no adequate and well-controlled studies in pregnant women OR Animal studies have shown an adverse effect, but adequate and well-controlled studies in pregnant women have failed to demonstrate a risk to the foetus in any trimester.
Pregnancy Category C	Animal reproduction studies have shown an adverse effect on the foetus and there are no adequate and well-controlled studies in humans, but potential benefits may warrant use of the drug in pregnant women despite potential risks.
Pregnancy Category D	There is positive evidence of human foetal risk based on adverse reaction data from investigational or marketing experience or studies in humans, but potential benefits may warrant use of the drug in pregnant women despite potential risks.
Pregnancy Category X	Studies in animals or humans have demonstrated foetal abnormalities and/or there is positive evidence of human foetal risk based on adverse reaction data from investigational or marketing experience, and the risks involved in use of the drug in pregnant women clearly outweigh potential benefits. The drug is contraindicated in women who are or may become pregnant.
Pregnancy Category N	FDA has not classified this drug

Teratogenic Mechanisms Associated with Medication Use

a) **Folate antagonism,** e.g. antiepileptic drugs, methotrexate, trimethoprim.

This is mainly associated with defects such as neural tube defects.

b) **Endocrine disruption,** e.g. diethylstilbestrol.

Diethylstilbestrol may cause genital anomalies in female and male infants.

c) **Neural crest disruption,** e.g. retinoids.

Retinoids may cause craniofacial, cardiovascular, skeletal defects and disruption in CNS function.

d) **Oxidative stress,** e.g. thalidomide, antiepileptics, class III antiarrhythmics.

May cause skeletal, limb and neural tube defects

e) **Vascular disruptions,** e.g. misoprostol, ergotamine, pseudoephedrine.

May cause structural birth defects resulting from interference with or extrinsic breakdown of an originally normal prenatal development of the arteries, veins and capillaries.

f) **Specific receptor or enzyme mediated teratogenesis,** e.g. angiotensin II receptor blockers, ACE inhibitors, statins, NSAIDS. ACE inhibitors have been shown to cause possible lung and kidney hypoplasia, hypocalvaria, oligohydramnios, neonatal convulsions, etc.

Drugs to Avoid in Pregnancy

The drugs listed in the table below should raise "warning" signs if used during pregnancy. The benefits of these drugs must be weighed against their risks. Use only if necessary. The table below indicates a few examples:

Drugs	Category
Antibiotics	
Ciprofloxacin	C
Nitrofurantoin (avoid in 3rd trimester)	B
Tetracycline,doxycycline,	D
Trimethoprim (avoid particularly in 1st and 3rd trimester)	C
Anticoagulants	
Warfarin	X D in mechanical heart valves
Anticonvulsants	
Phenobarbitone	D
Phenytoin	D
Sodium valproate	D
Carbamazepine	D
Lamotrigine	C

(Continued)

(Continued)

Drugs	Category
Antifungal drugs	
Griseofulvin	C
Ketoconazole	C
Itraconazole	C
Fluconazole	C
Antihelmintic	
Mebendazole	C
Anti-inflammatory drugs	
NSAIDS e.g. mefenamic acid	C
COX-2 inhibitors e.g. etoricoxib	N
Antileprotic	
Dapsone	C
Cardiovascular drugs	
Beta-blockers (atenolol) in 1st trimester	D
Minoxidil	C
ACE inhibitors, e.g. enalapril	D
Angiotensin II receptor antagonists, e.g. losartan	C (Ist trimester), D (2nd and 3rd trimester)
Spironolactone	C
Methotrexate	X
Cyclophosphamide	D
Busulphan	D

(Continued)

(Continued)

Drugs	Category
Endocrine related drugs	
Carbimazole (methimazole)	D
Propylthiouracil	D
Chlorpropamide	C
Glipizide	C
Iodine	Foetal risk has been demonstrated
Sex hormones	Not recommended
Psychotropic drugs	
Lithium	D
Vitamin A analogues	
Acitretin	X
Isotretinoin	X
Other drugs	
Thalidomide	X
Biphosphonates	C
Misoprostol	X
Statins, e.g. simvastatin	X
Fibrates, e.g. fenofibrate	C
Tamoxifen	D

Live vaccines, e.g. MMR should not be administered routinely to women because of the theoretical risk of foetal infection.

**Disclaimer*: The above list is not exhaustive. Please check pregnancy categories when in doubt. Pregnancy categories are subject to change.

Drugs to Avoid in Pregnancy for G6PD Deficient Individuals

Drugs with *Definite* Risk of Haemolysis	Drugs with *Possible* Risk of Haemolysis
Chloramphenicol (topical route acceptable)	Acetanilide
Ciprofloxacin	Aminopyrine
Co-trimoxazole	Aminosalicylic acid
Dapsone	Antazoline eye drop
Dimercaprol	Ascorbic acid
Furazolidone	Aspirin (acceptable up to 1 g daily)
Gatifloxacin	Benzhexol
Levofloxacin	Carbidopa
Mesalazine	Chloroquine
Methylene blue	Colchicine
Moxifloxacin	Diphenhydramine
Nalidixic acid	Dopamine
Niridazole	Glibenclamide
Nitrofurantoin	Glipizide
Norfloxacin	Hydralazine
Ofloxacin	Hydroxychloroquine
Pamaquine	Isoniazid
Phenazopyridine	Levodopa
Primaquine	Menadione and derivatives (vitamin K)
	Methyldopa

(Continued)

(Continued)

Drugs with *Definite* Risk of Haemolysis	Drugs with *Possible* Risk of Haemolysis
Rasburicase	Penicillamine (during therapy of Wilson's disease)
Sulfasalazine	Phenacetin
Sulfisoxazole	Phenazopyridine
Sulpha pyridine	Phenylhydrazine
Sulpha pyrimidine	Phenytoin
Sulphamethoxy pyridine	Procainamide
Sulphanilamide	Proguanil
Sulfisoxazole	Pyrimethamine (Maloprim)
Toluidine blue	Probenecid
	Quinacrine
	Quinidine
	Quinine (acceptable in acute malaria)
	Streptomycin
	Trihexyphenidyl (benzhexol)
	Trimethoprim
Disclaimer: The list above is not exhaustive. Please check if in doubt.	

Commonly Prescribed Medications during Pregnancy

Analgesia

Medication	Dose	Comments
Codeine phosphate *FDA Category C*	30–60 mg tds	Avoid in 1st trimester and 3rd trimester especially near term/ delivery. Consider safer alternatives. If necessary, to use strictly at lowest effective dose and for shortest duration. Max dose: 1. Panadeine 2 tablet qds (64 mg/day) 2. Procodin 10 mL tds (54 mg/day) 3. Codeine phosphate 60 mg/day Max duration: 7 days
Paracetamol *FDA Category B (oral)*	500–1000 mg qds	Painkiller of choice during pregnancy. Do not exceed 8 tabs per day or 2 tablets per dose
Tramadol *FDA Category C*	50–100 mg qds	May be used if paracetamol unable to control pain. Chronic use during pregnancy could result in physical dependence and postpartum withdrawal in the newborn. For short term use only

Antenatal Supplementation

Medication	Dose	Comments
Ascorbic Acid	100–200 mg tds	To increase absorption of iron
Calcium	RDA for pregnancy is 1000–1300 mg/day	Different brands have varying elemental calcium content
Ferrous Fumarate	200 mg bd	Iron supplemention especially for patients with iron deficiency anaemia
Folic acid	5 mg om	For peri-conception and 1st trimester to reduce the risk of neural tube defects
Ganilia®	2 tablet od (contains DHA and EPA)	Contents of 1 capsule : vitamin A 950 IU, vitamin B1 1.05 mg, vitamin B2 1.05 mg, vitamin B5 3 mg, vitamin B6 1.3 mg, vitamin B12 1.56 mcg, vitamin C 63.9 mg, vitamin D 100 IU, vitamin E 2.2 IU, iron 14.25 mg, iodine 57 mcg, folic acid 400 mcg & calcium (elemental) 76 mg, DHA 150 mg, EPA 30 mg, niacinamide 8.35 mg
Magnesium	250 mg (elemental) tablet	Recommended for leg cramps in pregnancy
Natal Care Plus®	1–2 capsule daily	DHA 102 mg, EPA 27 mg, arachidonic acid 18 mg, oleic acid 70 mg, D-alpha-tocopherol 4 mg, help support baby's brain and eye development. Suitable for all trimesters; recommended from 12 weeks onwards

(Continued)

(*Continued*)

Medication	Dose	Comments
Nata Boost™	1–2 softgels daily from the 2nd trimester to lactation	Per capsule: DHA 157.5 mg, EPA 13.5 mg, arachidonic acid 9 mg Plant source essential fatty acid supplement to help support baby's brain and eye development. Suitable for all trimesters; recommended from 12 weeks onwards
NeuroGain S®	1 tablet om	DHA 383 mg, EPA 23 mg. DHA-rich edible with added vitamin E as antioxidant in a soft vegetable capsule Help support baby's brain and eye development. Suitable for all trimesters; recommended from 12 weeks onwards.
New Obimin®	1 tablet om	Antenatal vitamin supplementation Each tablet contains vitamin A 3,000 USP units, vitamin D 400 USP units, vitamin C 100 mg, vitamin B1 10 mg, vitamin B2 2.5 mg, vitamin B6 15 mg, vitamin B12 4 mcg, niacinamide 20 mg, calcium panthotenate 7.5 mg, folic acid 1 mg, iron 30 mg, calcium 35 mg, copper 100 mcg, iodine 100 mcg. To be taken *before* food for better absorption.

(*Continued*)

(*Continued*)

Medication	Dose	Comments
Prenaforte®	1 tablet om	Vitamin A 4000 IU, vitamin B1 1.5 mg, vitamin B2 1.7 mg, vitamin B5 8.33 mg, vitamin B6 2.6 mg, vitamin B12 4 mcg, vitamin C 100 mg, vitamin D 400 IU, vitamin E 11 IU, iron 27 mg, iodine 150 mcg, folic acid 800 mcg, calcium (elemental) 100 mg,copper 2 mg, phosphorus 40 mg, selenium 20 mcg, zinc oxide 25 mg
Sangobion®	1–2 tablet om	Each capsule contains copper sulfate 200 mcg, ferrous gluconate 250 mg, folic acid 1 mg, manganese sulfate 200 mcg, sorbitol 25 mg, vitamin B12 7.5 mcg, vitamin C 50 mg. Stools may darken due to iron content.

Anti-Asthmatics

Asthma should be well controlled during pregnancy. Drugs for asthma should preferably be administered via inhalation to minimise exposure of the foetus. During severe acute exacerbations of asthma, **conventional therapy** can be given to ensure patient's condition is stabilised as soon as possible. Prednisolone is the preferred corticosteroid of choice for oral administration as little of the drug crosses the placenta.

Medication	Dose	Comments
Prednisolone *FDA Category C*	Initially 10–20 mg daily	Maximum — 60 mg daily. Advisable to use lower doses for short period of time

Anti-Diabetics

Medication (Insulin)	Dose	Comments
Actrapid	Subcutaneous (according to titration)	Fast acting, onset half an hour, effect lasts approx. 8 hours
Insulatard	Subcutaneous (according to titration)	Intermediate acting Insulin — onset 1–2 hours, effect lasts 14–24 hours

Oral anti-diabetics are not recommended during pregnancy as they do not regulate blood sugar as effectively as insulin.

Metformin/Glipizide — FDA Category C

Anti-Emetics

Medication	Dose	Comments
Domperidone *FDA Category N*	10–20 mg tds PO	Take when necessary half to one hour before food. Can also be used for lactation to increase milk flow.
Metoclopramide *FDA Category B*	10 mg tds PO/IV/IM	Dose can also be given as IM/IV injection. Take when necessary half to one hour before food.
Ondansetron *FDA Category B*	4 mg–8 mg tds PO/IV	$5HT_3$ antagonist

(Continued)

(Continued)

Medication	Dose	Comments
Promethazine theoclate	25 mg tds PO	Antihistamine. May cause drowsiness
Pyridoxine	50 mg om PO	Vitamin B_6. May be taken regularly. Helps to alleviate/prevent symptoms of hyperemesis gravidarum

Antihypertensives

Medication	Dose	Comments
Hydralazine	IV bolus 5–10 mg, may be administered every 20 minutes up to a maximum dose of 30 mg	Direct peripheral arteriolar vasodilator, slow onset of action. Used in acute hypertensive episodes and management of pre-eclampsia
Labetalol	100–400 mg bd–tds PO. Maximum: 2400 mg/day	May cause tiredness and headache
Methyldopa	125–500 mg bd-qds PO Maximum: 3 g/day	Side effects are dizziness, headaches, nasal congestion and weakness
Nifedipine (short acting)	10 mg when necessary PO	For acute episodes. May cause tachycardia, palpitations and headaches
Nifedipine (long acting)	30–60 mg daily Maximum dose: 90 mg/day	Short acting preparation not suitable for maintenance

Antipyretic

Medication	Dose	Comments
Paracetamol *FDA Category: B*	1 g qds PO	Drug of choice during pregnancy. Do not exceed 8 tabs per day or 2 tablets per dose

Cough and Cold

Dry cough

Medication	Dose	Comments
Dextromethorphan (DMP)	10 mL tds PO	Recommended for pregnant women with dry cough. Does not contain alcohol
Procodin (Codeine/ Promethazine)	10 mL tds PO	To avoid use during 1st and 3rd trimester. If necessary, can be used all three trimesters up to 7 days duration

Productive cough

Medication	Dose	Comments
Diphenhydramine (MBE)	10mL tds PO	Recommended for cough with phlegm

Mucolytic

Medication	Dose	Comments
Acetylcysteine (e.g. Fluimucil)	600 mg daily/200 mg bd or tds PO	Acute and chronic respiratory infections
Bromhexine (e.g. Bisolvon®)	1 tablet tds PO	May cause more cough initially

Sorethroat

Medication	Dose	Comments
Benzydamine lozenges (e.g. Difflam)	1–2 tablet tds (prn)	To suck when necessary
Dequalinum lozenges	1–2 tablet tds (prn)	To suck when necessary

Cold (Antihistamines may also be used for rash/itch)

Medication	Dose	Comments
Cetirizine *FDA Category B*	10 mg om PO	Alternative to be used usually in 2nd and 3rd trimester. May be used during 1st trimester if necessary
Chlorpheniramine *FDA Category B*	4 mg tds PO	Can cause drowsiness. Preferred antihistamine for all three trimesters
Loratidine *FDA Category B*	10 mg om PO	Alternative to be used usually in 2nd and 3rd trimester. May be used during 1st trimester if necessary

Gastrointestinal System

Anti-diarrhoeal medication

Medication	Dose	Comments
Charcoal	2 tablets (500 mg) tds	Absorbs toxins. May blacken stools
Kaolin	10 mL tds	Absorbs toxins
Lacteol Fort	1–2 sachet tds	Helps promote good bacterial flora in the gut
Lomotil (Atropine sulphate 25 mcg, diphenoxylate HCl 2.5 mg)	1–2 tablets tds	Anticholinergic. Reduces intestinal motilty
Loperamide	2–4 mg tds	Reduces intestinal motility

Gastric Medications

Medication	Dose	Comments
Antacids	1–2 tablet tds	Some antacids may contain simethicone. Relatively safe as simethicone is not absorbed
Famotidine *FDA Category B*	20–40 mg od or bd PO	H_2 antagonists are preferred in pregnancy.
Hyoscine butylbromide (e.g. Buscopan) *FDA Category C*	10–20 mg tds PO Can also be given IV or IM	For stomach cramps
Magnesium carbonate	10 mL TDS	Reduces gastric acid
Omeprazole *FDA Category C*	20 mg bd or 40 mg om PO	2nd line in pregnancy. For gastric reflux
Ranitidine *FDA Category B*	150 mg bd PO i.v.: 50 mg 8H	H_2 receptor antagonist. Inhibits gastric acid production

Constipation

Medication	Dose	Comments
Bisacodyl (e.g. Dulcolax®)	5–10 mg once Per rectal/PO	May cause abdominal cramps. Can be given orally if necessary. Rectal route — 30 minutes effect
Fleet enema	Per 118 mL fleet enema PR	For bowel evacuation
Fybogel	1 sachet om	Bulk laxative. Takes up to 48 hours to see effect
Lactulose	10–20 mL bd	Stool softener
Liquid Paraffin (e.g. Agarol)	10 mL bd	Stool softener
Senna/ sennosides	1–2 tablets daily or bd	May cause abdominal cramps

Lactation Suppression

Medication	Dose	Comments
Cabergoline (Dostinex®) 0.5 mg/tab	1 mg stat	If lactation not initiated
Cabergoline (Dostinex®) 0.5 mg/tab	0.25 mg bd × 2 days	If lactation initiated

Lactation Promotion

Medication	Dose	Comments
Fenugreek 610 mg	1–3 capsule bd-tds (up to max. 9 capsules/day)	Excessive intake can cause loose stools in mother
Maxolon	10 mg tds PO, for 7–14 days	Increases prolactin level and milk supply

Infections

Antibiotics

In general, penicillins and cephalosporins are the safest antibiotics during pregnancy.

Medication	Dose	Comments
Amoxycillin *FDA Category B*	500 mg tds	Broad spectrum antibiotic. Considered for urinary tract infections, respiratory tract infections, chlamydia and group B streptococcus infection
Amoxycillin-clavulanate (Augmentin) *FDA Category B*	625 mg bd	For urinary tract infection and respiratory tract infection. *Not recommended for use in PPROM due to reported risk of necrotising enterocolitis in exposed neonates.*

(*Continued*)

(*Continued*)

Medication	Dose	Comments
Azithromycin *FDA Category B*	1g as a single dose	*Chlamydia trachomatis* infection
Cephalexin *FDA Category B*	500 mg tds PO	Broad spectrum antibiotic i.e. urinary tract infection
Clindamycin *FDA Category B*	150–450 mg tds-qds PO	Recommended for staphylococcal bone, joint, skin and soft tissue infections. Can also be used for bacterial vaginosis.
Erythromycin stearate (base) *FDA Category B*	500 mg tds-qds PO	Similar to amoxicillin. For those with penicillin allergy
Metronidazole *FDA Category B*	200 mg tds or 400 mg BD PO	Avoid use in first trimester Indications include parasitic infections/bacterial vaginosis (2nd and 3rd trimester)
Nitrofurantoin *FDA Category B*	50–100 mg qds PO	Contraindicated in 3rd trimester due to possible haemolytic anaemia in neonates
Penicillin G *FDA Category B*	5MU IV stat (loading dose) and 2.5 MU IV q4H (maintenance dose) until delivery	Group B streptococcus infection. *If penicillin allergy: 900 mg IV clindamycin q8H or 500 mg IV erythromycin q6H until delivery*

Vulvo-Vaginal Candidiasis

Medication	Dose	Comments
Clotrimazole pessary	100 mg ON × 6 days	Advise pregnant women NOT to use applicator provided
Nystatin pessary	1/1 ON × 14 days	Each pessary contains 100 000 units nystatin

(*Continued*)

(*Continued*)

Medication	Dose	Comments
Flagystatin® pessary	1/1 ON × 10 days	Each pessary contains 500 mg metronidazole and 100 000 units nystatin Useful in treating bacterial vaginosis
Gynotrosyd® pessary	1/1 ON × 3 days	Each pessary contains 100 mg tioconazole. Use with caution in 1st trimester
Gynotravogen® pessary	1/1 ON × 1 day	Each pessary contains 600 mg isoconazole nitrate
(Avoid oral anti-fungal medication in pregnancy.)		

Herpes Virus Infections

Medication	Dose	Comments
Acyclovir *FDA Category B*	<u>Herpes simplex (HSV):</u> <u>*First infection*</u>: 400 mg tds (7–10 days) or 200 mg 5 times a day (7–10 days) <u>*Recurrent*</u>: 400 mg tds (3–5 days or 800 mg bd (5 days) <u>Varicella zoster (chicken pox)</u>: 800 mg qds for 5 days	No data to indicate an increased risk for major birth defects as compared with the general population during the first trimester

Topical

External medications for topical use or ophthalmic/otic/nasal use are generally quite safe as long as they are used within the licensed indications and dosings. However, preparations containing vitamin A/tretinoin are not advisable to use during pregnancy.

Topicals (Creams/Ointments/Suppositories)

Itch/Rash

Medication	Dose	Comments
Betamethasone cream (0.025%)	Once daily or when necessary	Topical use. Apply thinly
Calamine lotion	When necessary	Topical use
Chlorhexidine 1% cream	Once daily or when necessary	Antiseptic cream
Combiderm/Triderm® (Betamethasone 0.05% / Clotrimazole 1%/ Gentamicin 0.1% cream)	Once daily or when necessary	Allergy & inflammatory dermatitis, dermatomycosis
Hydrocortisone cream 1%	Once daily or when necessary	Topical use. Apply thinly
Miconazole 2% cream	Contains miconazole	Antifungal cream. Apply thinly
Miconazole 2%/ hydrocortisone 1%	Once daily or when necessary	
Neoderm® (neomycin/ hydrocortisone) cream	Once daily or when necessary	Corticosteroid cream with anti-infective agent
Travocort® cream (Isoconazole, diflucortolone valerate)	Once daily or when necessary	Broad-spectrum antifungal with a steroid additive. Apply thinly.

Pain relief

Medication	Dose	Comments
Diclofenac gel	bd or tds prn	Apply sparingly. Caution in 3rd trimester
Lignocaine 1% gel	bd or tds prn	To reduce pain via numbing action
Proctosedyl ointment	bd or tds prn	Haemorrhoids/piles. To reduce pain, inflammation and itchiness

Ear/Eye/Nose Drops

Medication	Dose	Comments
Hypromellose 0.3% eye drops	When necessary	Eye drop — lubricant for dry eyes
Oxymetazoline 0.05% nose drops	1 drop tds/prn	As nasal decongestant. Do not use continuously for more than 5 days.
Sodium chloride 0.9% eye/nose drops	1–2 drops tds /prn	Eye drop — lubricant for dry eyes. Nasal use for blocked nose

Threatened Miscarriage

Medication	Dose	Comments
Dydrogesterone (e.g. Duphaston®)	10–20 mg bd/tds	Till 12 weeks of gestation. Take with or after food
Natural micronized progesterone (e.g. Utrogestan®)	100–200 mg om or bd PO/PV	Till 12 weeks of gestation

Tocolytics (To Prevent Contraction)

Medication	Dose	Comments
Glyceryl trinitrate (GTN) 10 mg patch	Apply 10 mg (GTN) patch to the skin of the abdomen. After 1 hour, if there is no reduction in contraction frequency or intensity, an additional patch can be applied	No more than two patches are to be administered simultaneously. Patches can be left in place for 24 hours
Nifedipine (short acting)	5–20 mg bd, tds or qds PO	May cause flushing, oedema, headache and dizziness.

Other Medications commonly used in Pregnancy

Medication	Dose	Comments
Cinnarizine	25 mg tds PO	For giddiness and motion sickness
Diosmin 450 mg/ Hesperidin 50 mg (Daflon® 500 mg)	Acute: 2 tablets tds for 4 days then 2 tab bd for 3 days then 2 tab od for 1–2 weeks. Chronic: 2 tablets od or 2 tab bd	For haemorrhoids/ piles
Prochlorperazine	5–10 mg bd or tds PO	For giddiness and also to prevent nausea and vomiting
Promethazine Theoclate	25 mg ON PO	For insomnia

Special Conditions in Pregnancy

This section is intended to cover briefly on the medications used during pregnancy for certain conditions where medications are unavoidable and the selection of medication is largely dependent on the risk/benefit ratio. The physician should evaluate both the benefits and risks of the medications and ensure that the patient is fully aware of the risks of the medications in pregnancy.

Hyperthyroidism

The mainstay of the medications used for hyperthyroidism are carbimazole and propylthiouracil. In addition, beta blockers such as atenolol and propranolol are used to treat the symptoms of hyperthyroidism like tachycardia and tremors. However, their use should be limited to a few weeks and long-term treatment should be avoided due to potential effects on intrauterine growth restriction, respiratory depression and hypoglycaemia. Radioiodine is absolutely contraindicated during pregnancy.

The main goal of treatment is to maintain the serum free T4 concentration at a normal range using the lowest possible dose.

Medication	Dose	Comments
Carbimazole (CMZ) *FDA Category D*	*Initial*: 15–40 mg daily PO *Maintenance*: 5–15 mg daily PO	Recommended from 2nd trimester onwards. Teratogenic effects of carbimazole are more severe during organogenesis period
Propranolol *FDA Category C* (1st trimester) *FDA Category D* (2nd/3rd trimester)	20–40 mg tds to qds PO	Short term use only. To be weaned as soon as symptoms are controlled
Propylthiouracil (PTU) *FDA Category D*	*Initial*: 200–400 mg daily PO *Maintenance*: 50–150 mg daily PO	Recommended for 1st trimester use only. Hepatotoxicity may occur at any time during PTU treatment. Monitor liver enzymes during administration of PTU

Thyroidectomy may be necessary in pregnancy for those who cannot tolerate thionamides due to allergy or agranulocytosis.

Lactation. Both carbimazole and propythiouracil have been rated as safe by the American Academy of Pediatrics . However, both are present in breast milk and therefore neonatal development should be closely monitored in mothers on these medications and who breastfeed their infants.

Hypothyroidism

Thyroxine (T4) is the treatment of choice for hypothyroidism in pregnancy. As there may be slight differences in bioavailability in T4 formulations, patients are advised to use the same brand. There is no evidence of increased risk of congenital anomalies following the use of levothyroxine (T4). The aim of T4 replacement is to maintain euthyroidism as soon as possible.

For those with pre-existing hypothyroidism, they may require more T4 during pregnancy up to as much as 50% of their usual dose.

Medication	Dose	Comments
Levothyroxine (T4)	*Initially*: 50–100 mcg daily PO *Maintenance*: 100–200 mcg daily PO	To be taken on an empty stomach in the morning. Usual dose may be increased for some pregnant patients

Epilepsy

Pregnant women with epilepsy are at a greater risk of having a child with a major or minor congenital malformation than women without epilepsy. Most of the antiepileptic drugs (AED) are classified as Category D and have been associated with foetal malformations, especially in the 1st trimester. Therefore, women of childbearing potential should discuss with their doctor the impact of both epilepsy and its treat ment on pregnancy outcome.

However, it is important that the pregnant women continue to take their AEDs throughout pregnancy. Frequent and prolonged maternal fits can increase the risk of miscarriage, intracranial haemorrhage, preterm labour or even restrict blood flow and transfer of oxygen and nutrients to the foetus, resulting in foetal hypoxia with bradycardia and brain damage.

Folic acid supplementation is recommended to reduce the risk or neural tube defects (NTD) before conception and throughout 1st trimester.

Medication	Dose	Comments
Anti-epileptic drugs like phenytoin, lamotrigine. *Do not switch if condition is stabilised in pregnancy*	Lowest effective dose. Monotherapy is recommended	Treatment with more than 1 drug increases risk of teratogenicity. Sodium valproate is associated with a higher risk of major and minor congenital malformations
Folic acid	5 mg–10 mg PO	1st trimester to prevent NTD
Vitamin K	10 mg–20 mg PO	May be given in last trimester after 36 weeks for prevention of haemorrhagic complications, especially for patients on carbamazepine or phenytoin

Lactation. Women who are on monotherapy may breastfeed. However, more advice should be sought if the women are on combination therapy or if there are other risk factors such as premature birth. All infants should be monitored for sedation, feeding difficulties, adequate weight gain and developmental milestones. Withdrawal effects may occur if breast-feeding is stopped abruptly for mothers who are on phenobarbital or lamotrigine.

Depression

The main goal of treatment is to maintain euthymic mood in the mother throughout pregnancy and preventing postpartum depression. Psychotherapy should be considered as an initial treatment for mild to moderate symptoms of anxiety disorders before pharmacotherapy is considered. The potential risks of drugs include major malformation (first-trimester exposure), neonatal toxicity (third trimester exposure), and long-term neurobehavioural effects.

It is important to note that safety in breastfeeding where these medications are involved should be considered as it is not advisable to switch the patient's antidepressant medications if their condition is stable even if the lactation data proves superior.

Tricyclic antidepressants (TCA) have been widely used throughout second trimester pregnancies without apparent detriment to foetuses and are preferred in pregnancy. Management strategy includes using a minimal effective dose in divided doses to minimise peak levels and therefore foetal exposure. Use of the antidepressant should be tailed off in the last trimester to minimise neonatal withdrawal symptoms. In the event that the pregnant mother is severely depressed, and requires continued dosing, neonatal standby should be arranged peripartum.

Selective serotonin re-uptake inhibitor (SSRI) are not major teratogens but have been associated with increased risk of septal defects and omphalocoele with early exposure, spontaneous abortion and decreased birth weight. SSRI, when taken in late pregnancy, may be associated with the increased risk of persistent pulmonary hypertension of the neonate.

Medication	Dose	Comments
Fluoxetine (SSRI)	20 mg om PO (maximum 60 mg)	Best studied SSRI in pregnancy for safety and efficacy due to its presence in market — most evidence regarding adverse pregnancy effects. Has long half-life and active metabolite
Imipramine (TCA)	Up to 25 mg daily PO	More experience with use, but poor side effect profile, e.g. constipation
Paroxetine (SSRI)	20 mg om PO	Controversy with regards to its safety. Not 1st line SSRI in pregnancy
Sertraline (SSRI)	50 mg om (may increase to maximum 200 mg PO)	Can be considered in pregnancy if needed, especially if there is previous efficacy in individual patient. May be used in 2nd trimester. Emerging evidence clear regarding association with septal defects. Low serum level for breastfeeding

(Continued)

(*Continued*)

Medication	Dose	Comments
Amitriptyline (TCA)	10–25 mg daily in divided doses or at bedtime PO	Same as with imipramine
Dothiepin (TCA)	Initial 25 mg on (PO); increase gradually 25 mg bd; preferably not more than 75 mg in pregnant or breastfeeding mother	May be used in 2nd trimester for moderate–severe depression. Should be tailed off in last trimester if depression is not severe.
Haloperidol (Typical antipsychotic)	500 mcg bd PO	For short-term management of severe anxiety. May be used throughout pregnancy
Trifluoroperazine (Phenothiazines)	2–4 mg daily in divided doses PO	For short term management of severe anxiety. May be used throughout pregnancy

Indications of Anti-D Immunoglobulin Administration in Pregnancy

1. All non-sensitised Rh-D negative women at 28 weeks, repeated at 34 weeks and post delivery if baby is Rh-D positive (KKH regime)
2. All non-sensitised Rh-D negative women after potentially sensitising events during pregnancy and labour, such as:

   (a) Invasive prenatal diagnosis (amniocentesis, chorionic villous sampling, cordocentesis, intrauterine transfusion).

(b) Other intrauterine procedures (insertion of shunts, embryo reduction and laser).
(c) Recurrent vaginal bleeding in pregnancy.
(d) Antepartum haemorrhage.
(e) External cephalic version (including attempted).
(f) Any abdominal trauma (direct/indirect, sharp/blunt, open/closed).
(g) Foetal death.

Note: This Anti D-Ig (Anti D-immunoglobulin) should be given in addition to any already received.

Dose and Frequency of Administration of Anti-D Immunoglobulin

- For antepartum prophylaxis, the recommended dose of Rho(D) immunoglobulin is 300 mcg (1500 IU) intramuscularly, given at 28 weeks of gestation. Repeat dose at 34 weeks. An additional dose is recommended post-delivery within 72 hours if the baby is Rh (D) positive (KKH regime).
- If there is large foetomaternal haemorrhage (FMH) or recurrent bleeding, Kleihauer test can be performed. An additional dose of Anti-D Ig can be administered (500 IU or greater) depending upon the size of FMH. Events associated with a large FMH are: caesarean section, manual removal of placenta, intrauterine foetal death, unexplained hydrops foetalis, twins and abdominal trauma during the third trimester with placental abruption.

Indications of Aspirin Use in Pregnancy

Risk of hypertensive disorders in pregnancy	**High Risk Women:** a) PIH during previous pregnancy b) Chronic Kidney disease c) Autoimmune disease — SLE/APS d) Type 1 or 2 Diabetes Mellitus e) Chronic Hypertension **Moderate Risk Women (≥1 risk factor)** a) First pregnancy b) ≥40 years old c) Pregnancy interval ≥10 years d) BMI ≥35 kg/m^2 e) Family history of Pre-eclampsia f) Multiple pregnancy
Abnormal uterine artery Doppler	a) Uterine artery notching (unilateral or bilateral) b) Increased resistance index c) Increased pulsatility index
Early onset IUGR	
Previous placental abruption	
Recurrent miscarriages	a) Antiphospolipid antibody (aPL) positive b) Lupus anticoagulant positive
Previous perinatal death	Pre-eclampsia related
Acute Myocardial Ischaemia in pregnancy	
Cerebrovascular accident in pregnancy	

Dosage of Aspirin

- Recommended dose of aspirin is 100 mg/day
- To be initiated as early as 8–10 weeks and not later than 16–18 weeks
- Discontinue at 35–36 weeks of gestation

Mechanism of Action of Aspirin

- Improves placentation by improvement of the uterine spiral arteries
- Improves uterine artery blood flow in the first and second trimester

  Note: In Antiphospholipid Syndrome (APS), low dose Aspirin can be used with low molecular weight heparin.

Chapter 21

APPROACH TO POSTNATAL PROBLEMS

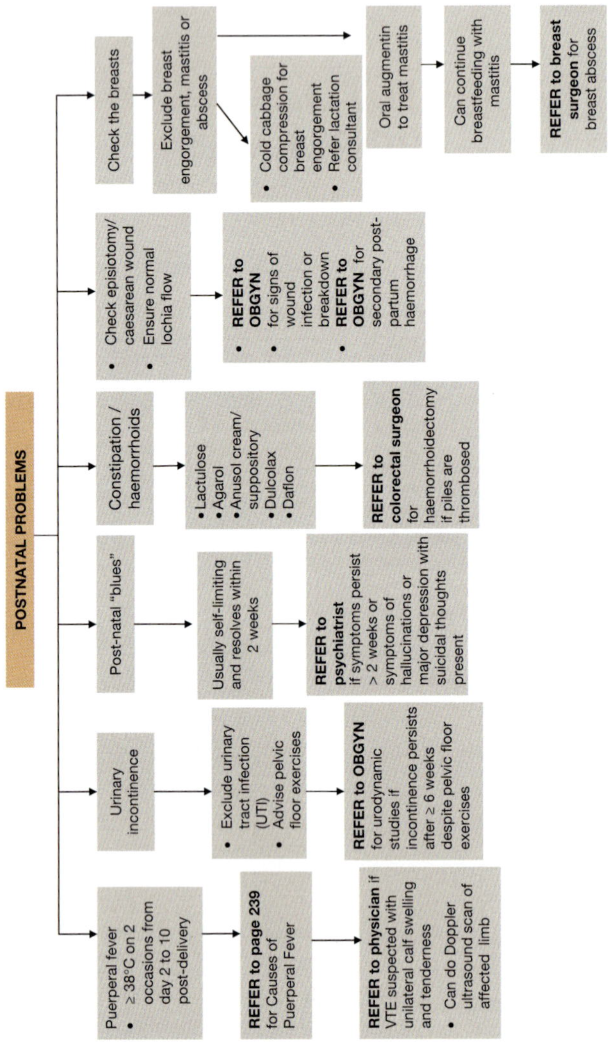
POSTNATAL PROBLEMS
Puerperal fever
• ≥ 38°C on 2 occasions from day 2 to 10 post-delivery
REFER to page 239 for Causes of Puerperal Fever
REFER to physician if VTE suspected with unilateral calf swelling and tenderness
• Can do Doppler ultrasound scan of affected limb
Urinary incontinence
• Exclude urinary tract infection (UTI)
• Advise pelvic floor exercises
REFER to OBGYN for urodynamic studies if incontinence persists after ≥ 6 weeks despite pelvic floor exercises
Post-natal "blues"
Usually self-limiting and resolves within 2 weeks
REFER to psychiatrist if symptoms persist > 2 weeks or symptoms of hallucinations or major depression with suicidal thoughts present
Constipation / haemorrhoids
•Lactulose
•Agarol
•Anusol cream/ suppository
•Dulcolax
•Daflon
REFER to colorectal surgeon for haemorrhoidectomy if piles are thrombosed
• Check episiotomy/ caesarean wound
• Ensure normal lochia flow
• REFER to OBGYN
• for signs of wound infection or breakdown
• REFER to OBGYN for secondary post-partum haemorrhage
Check the breasts
Exclude breast engorgement, mastitis or abscess
• Cold cabbage compression for breast engorgement
• Refer lactation consultant
Oral augmentin to treat mastitis
Can continue breastfeeding with mastitis
REFER to breast surgeon for breast abscess

Bladder Care After Vaginal Delivery

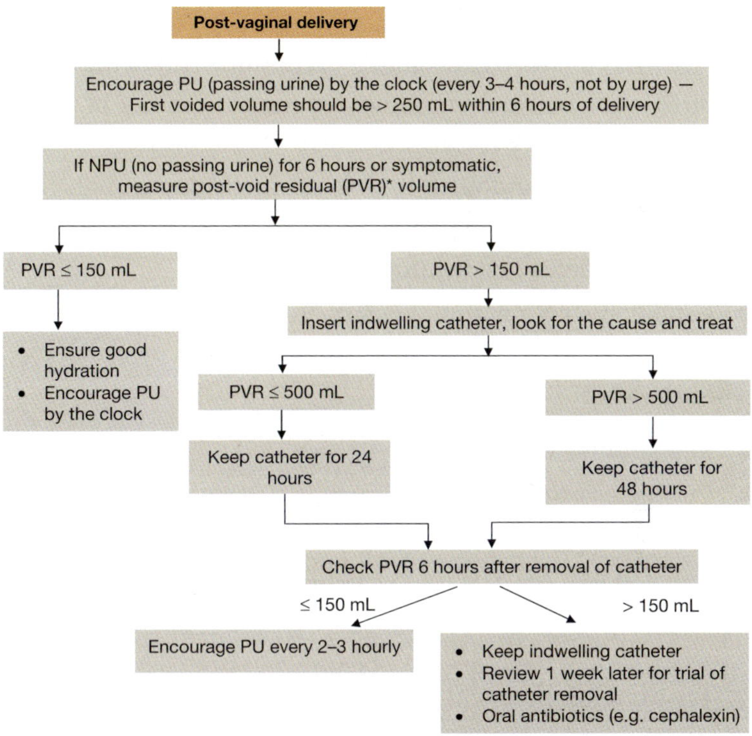

PVR (post void residual)

*The significance of PVR varies with the total volume of urine voided.

* Do not use bladder scan for postnatal patients

Postnatal Problems

1. Postnatal blues

- Postnatal blues ("Baby blues") is common following childbirth, in which new mothers experience lability of mood and tearfulness with the newborn
- Usually peaks on fourth to fifth postnatal day and resolves by the 10th day of delivery
- Postnatal blues is self-limiting and mild
- Usually resolves within 2 weeks after delivery

Management

- Reassurance
- Encourage support from partner, family and friends to cope with the newborn
- **Refer to psychiatrist** for evaluation if symptoms persist for more than 2 weeks

2. Postnatal depression (PND)

- Is a major depressive episode associated with childbirth
- Typically occurs at first month to first year after delivery
- May resolve within several months if woman is not treated but can linger into the second year postpartum
- Common symptoms include depressed mood, insomnia, loss of weight and appetite, apathy and lethargy

- PND is often overlooked in primary care clinics
- Can be treated in primary care settings and is highly treatable

Management

- **Refer to psychiatrist**
- Psychotherapy intervention is highly acceptable and effective
- New mothers need not discontinue breastfeeding if they initiate antidepressants
- Common antidepressants used: fluoxetine (20 mg PO/ day), sertraline (50 mg PO/ day), paroxetine (20 mg PO/ day) and venlafaxine (75 mg PO/ day)
- Fluoxetine is linked to irritability, sleep disturbance and poor feeding in some infants exposed to it in breast milk. Little evidence established with most medications
- No adverse effects are reported with sertraline, paroxetine and venlafaxine in nursing mothers
- Common antidepressants used in non-nursing mothers: fluoxetine (20–40 mg PO/ day), sertraline (50–100 mg PO/ day), escitalopram (10–20 mg PO/day) and venlafaxine (37.5–75 mg PO/ day)
- Good clinical experience with use of dothiepin, a tricyclic antidepressant (25–75mg PO/day in divided dosing) for nursing mothers; no adverse effects in nursing infant.

3. Puerperal psychosis

- Is a medical emergency with risk of self-harm (suicide) and infanticide
- Usually occurs within first month after delivery
- The woman becomes maniac in nature with increased irritability, agitation and insomnia
- Woman may have hallucinations or delusions

Management

- Urgent referral to psychiatrist
- Requires inpatient admission with mood stabilisers, antipsychotic medications and benzodiazepines

Puerperal fever

Puerperal fever is defined as having fever on 2 occasions from the 2nd day up to the 10th day postpartum. *Sepsis* is defined as an infection with systemic manifestations. Although fever is usually a sign of sepsis, it may not always be present. Other clinical signs include tachycardia, hypotension, oliguria, tachypnoea and decreased conscious level.

Causes of Puerperal Fever

Cause	Risk factors	Remarks
1. Endometritis	Caesarean section Prolonged labour Manual removal of placenta Group B streptococcus colonisation	Antibiotic prophylaxis during caesarean section greatly reduces the risk
2. Urinary tract infection (UTI)	Indwelling catheter Epidural anaesthesia Urethral trauma	Catheter should be removed when patient is ambulating to minimise infection
3. Wound infection	Wound haematoma	Usually present on 4th to 7th postoperative day
4. Mastitis	Breast engorgement, cracked nipples and blocked ducts	Important to continue to express milk as stasis of breast milk will predispose to infection
5. Pneumonia	Aspiration pneumonia from general anaesthesia (Mendelson syndrome) Prolonged bed rest	Early ambulation Antibiotics Chest physiotherapy
6. Gastroenteritis	Antibiotic-induced *Clostridium difficile* infection Other pathogens include salmonella and campylobacter	
7. Pharyngitis	Group A streptococcus infection	
8. Spinal abscess	Regional anaesthesia	Rare complication
9. Toxic shock syndrome	Group A streptococcus infection	Causes disseminated rash

(*Continued*)

(*Continued*)

Cause	Risk factors	Remarks
10. Deep vein thrombosis/ pulmonary embolism (VTE)	• Caesarean delivery • Prolonged immobilisation • Advanced maternal age • Obesity • Smoking • Prior or family history of VTE • Thrombophilia	Manage as appropriate • Confirm diagnosis • Refer to physician • Anticoagulation

Risk factors of sepsis

1. Obesity
2. Caesarean section
3. Diabetes — pre-existing or gestational
4. Previous pelvic inflammatory disease
5. Prolonged rupture of membranes
6. Retained products of conception
7. Immunosuppression
8. Group B Streptococcus colonisation

Severe sepsis

Symptoms and signs that warrant urgent referral are:

1. Temperature > 38°C
2. Tachypnoea > 20 breaths/min
3. Tachycardia >120 beats/min
4. Abdominal or chest pain

5. Diarrhoea and/or vomitting
6. Uterine or renal angle pain and tenderness
7. Toxic looking and unwell

Routine Investigations:

1. Blood culture
2. Full blood count
3. Urea, electrolytes, creatinine
4. C-reactive protein
5. Serum lactate

Additional Investigations
to identify the source of sepsis

1. Chest X-ray
2. Urine microscopy and culture
3. Stool cultures
4. Throat swabs
5. Ultrasound scan of pelvis:
   — to exclude retained products of conception
   — to exclude abdominal/pelvic abscess

Treatment is with intravenous broad spectrum antibiotics while awaiting investigations to identify the source of infection. Antibiotics should be continued until the patient is afebrile for at least 24 hours.

Antibiotic	Limitations
1. Amoxycillin-clavulanic acid	Does not cover methicillin resistant *staphylococcus aureus* (MRSA), pseudomonas or extended spectrum beta lactamase (ESBL)-producing organism
2. Metronidazole	Only covers anaerobes
3. Clindamycin	Covers most streptococci and staphylococci, including many MRSA, and switches off exotoxin production which significantly decreases mortality
4. Piperacillin/tazobactam and carbapenems	Covers most organisms except MRSA and are renal sparing (in contrast to amnioglycosides). Piperacillin/tazobactam does not cover ESBL producers
5. Gentamicin	Poses no problem in normal renal function but if doses are to be given regularly; serum levels must be monitored

*Severe sepsis: may need to co-manage with infectious disease specialist.

Chapter 22

LACTATION AND BREASTFEEDING

Introduction

World Health Organization recommends that infants should be breastfed for the first six months for optimal health and development and thereafter with other foods. Breastfeeding can be continued till two years and beyond as desired.

Benefits of Breastfeeding

Benefits for Infant

- Decreases the incidence and severity of infection, diarrhoea, respiratory tract infection, necrotising enterocolitis, otitis media and urinary tract infection
- Decreases the incidence of late-onset sepsis in preterm infants
- Infants with family history of allergy who were exclusively breastfed had significantly lower incidence of atopic disease

Benefits for mother

- Premenopausal breast cancer was lower in women who had previously breastfed
- The protective effect increased with longer duration of breastfeeding
- 20% decrease in the risk of developing ovarian cancer
- More rapid postpartum weight loss

CONTRAINDICATIONS OF BREASTFEEDING

- Maternal human immunodeficiency virus (HIV) infection
- Mother with active and untreated tuberculosis infection
- Mother undergoing treatment for cancer
- Mother who is a recreational drug or alcohol abuse
- Baby with galactosaemia

ANTENATAL PREPARATION

- Breastfeeding education should be initiated as part of the prenatal care during the antenatal period
- Physician recommendation on breastfeeding often makes a positive impact on the woman's decision to breastfeed
- A breast examination should be performed to determine if there is any structural problem or concern
- If a woman's nipples appear to be inverted or non-protractile, reassure and refer to a lactation specialist for further advice

Management of Breastfeeding Related Problems

Latching difficulties

- The newborn should take a large amount of the breast into his or her mouth, with more of the areola and with the nipple pointing towards the soft palate. The mother should hold her breast during the attachment initially and draw the baby to the breast for a good latch
- Different feeding positions such as the football hold or modified cradle hold can be used by those encountering difficulties to facilitate latching onto the breast
- Women with truly inverted nipples often encounter difficulties latching their babies to the breast. The use of niplette as a non-surgical correction of inverted nipples may be recommended from the 2nd trimester.

Sore nipples

- Sore nipples are usually the result of poor positioning or poor latch-on
- Correct positioning and attachment is the key to preventing sore nipples
- Hind milk treatment or purified lanolin cream may be applied to promote healing
- Breast shell may be worn in between feeding to protect the sore nipples from rubbing against the clothing so as to facilitate healing

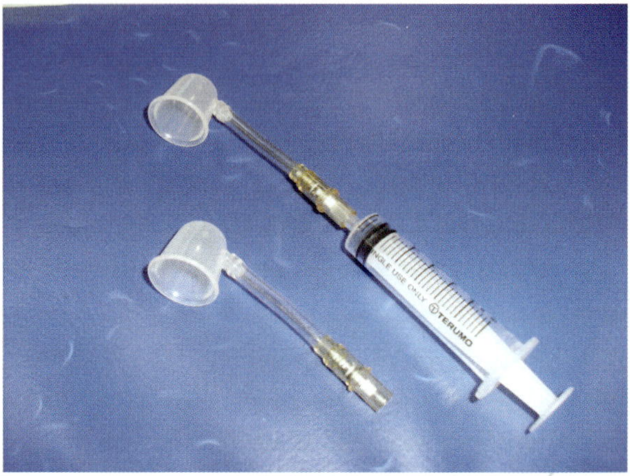

Figure of niplette.

Engorgement of breasts

- Engorgement occurs when there is a decrease in the frequency of feeding causing excessive accumulation of milk in the breast
- Engorgement often occurs during the first week after delivery with the onset of the copious milk and if there is delay in starting breastfeeding or infrequent feeding
- Engorgement usually affects both breasts, involving the areola and the peripheral area of the breast, which becomes full, hard and tender
- Early initiation of breastfeeding, unrestricted feeding day and night and ensuring proper latching for effective

emptying will help to prevent or reduce the severity of engorgement

- If engorgement is not relieved, it may impact on milk production

Treatment of breast engorgement includes:

1. Massaging the breast, nipple and areola area to clear any blockage and enhance milk flow
2. Allowing the baby to breastfeed frequently round the clock as the infant's suckling is the most effective mechanism for removal of milk
3. Apply cold pack or cold cabbage leaves on the breast in between feeding to help reduce swelling, warmth and pain
4. Avoid warm compress as there will be increased vascular heat which may aggravate the swelling if the ducts are blocked
5. Administer analgesia to alleviate the pain

Plugged ducts

- A plugged duct is a localised blockage of milk resulting from milk stasis
- It usually presents as a painful palpable lump with well-defined margins
- It may be caused by inadequate drainage in one area of the breast or by tight or restrictive clothing

- Plugged ducts can develop into mastitis if not treated adequately
- Massage of the breast is an effective way to help dislodge the blocked milk
- Antibiotic is not indicated unless mastitis has developed

Milk Blister

- Milk blister is a whitish, tender area, often found at the tip of the nipple
- It seals a nipple pore preventing the duct system from draining and thus causing milk buildup
- An effective treatment is to break the epithelial tissue using a sterile needle
- Breast massage should be done to clear the milk buildup and breastfeeding continued to clear the blocked milk duct

Candidiasis

- Symptoms often present as sharp shooting pain in the breast and nipple soreness
- Treatment of candidiasis involves treating both mother and infant simultaneously
- The infant should be treated with oral nystatin
- Treatment of the mother includes topical Nystatin, Miconazole or Ketoconazole cream applied on the nipple after each feeding

- For persistent candidiasis, oral fluconazole (diflucan) may be prescribed for the mother if the baby is at least 6 months of age
- In addition, pacifier, teats, teethers, breast pump parts, bras or reusable breast pads should be washed and boiled daily as spores are heat-resistant

Mastitis

- Mastitis is defined as a unilateral bacterial infection of the breast
- The diagnosis of mastitis is clinical
- Common organism is *Staphyloccus aureus*

Management of mastitis

1. Breast massage and clearing of plugged ducts if present
2. Application of cold pack on the affected area to reduce swelling
3. Increased fluids and bed rest
4. Prescribe antipyretics to reduce fever
5. Antibiotic therapy (Cloxacillin or Augmentin) for 7 to 10 days
6. Use trimethoprim-sulfamethoxazole (Bactrim), Erythromycin or Clindamycin if the mother is allergic to penicillin
7. Continue breastfeeding

Breast abscess

- Antibiotic treatment is necessary
- Fine needle aspiration or incision and drainage by a breast surgeon may be necessary
- The mother can continue breastfeeding on the unaffected breast
- The mother can hand-express or pump the milk from the affected breast to prevent engorgement and maintain milk supply

Increasing milk supply

- Ensure a good latch so that there is effective milk removal by the baby
- Breastfeed more frequently
- Using breast compression during feeding to help increase the intake of milk by the baby
- Expressing of milk after a feed to increase the milk supply

Pharmacological treatment to increase milk supply

1. *Metoclopramide*

- Metoclopramide increases prolactin level and thus improves milk supply
- Dosage: 10 mg tds orally for 7–14 days

- Effective for the initiation and maintenance of lactation
- Side-effects: Fatigue, irritability, depression and extrapyramidal side effects which may include tremor, bradykinesia (slow movements) and other dystonic reactions

Fenugreek (Herbal Supplement)

Fenugreek, also known as "venthaiyem" (in Tamil), "methi" (in Hindi) or "Halba" (in Malay), is the herb that is commonly used in cooking curry has been used traditionally to increase milk supply.

Fenugreek is considered safe for nursing mothers when used in moderation and is listed as GRAS (generally recognised as safe) by US FDA. However, excessive amount of fenugreek may cause loose stools in the mother.

Fenugreek tea can be taken four times a day by adding three teaspoons of fenugreek seeds into a glass of hot water to improve milk supply. Fenugreek capsules are available from health food outlets and pharmacies. It can be taken as two capsules four times a day or three capsules three times a day to improve milk supply.

Maintaining milk supply

- Regular breastfeeding usually will ensure adequate milk supply
- The milk supply increases with the baby's demand

- It is important for mothers to understand that substituting or delaying breastfeeding may reduce milk supply because of the reduction in stimulation of milk production which depends on infant's suckling and removal of milk from the breast
- Frequent regular feeding of 8–10 feeds a day is normal during the initial 4–8 weeks after birth
- Separation of mother and infant should be avoided whenever possible. However during separation, regular pumping of the breasts (every 3 hourly) should be sufficient to maintain milk supply. The expressed milk can be stored and given to the baby
- Expressed milk can be safely stored for up to 4 hours in room temperature, 48 hours in fridge (at 4 °C), 3–6 months in freezer (at –5 to –15 °C), 6–12 months in deep freezer (at –20 °C)
- Avoid excessive accumulation of milk in the breasts as this can affect milk supply.

Chapter 23

FREQUENTLY ASKED QUESTIONS ON PREGNANCY

1. Air Travel in Pregnancy

If pregnancy is uncomplicated, there is **no evidence that** flying is harmful in pregnancy.

- No changes in air pressure and humidity affect the foetus.
- Flying does not induce miscarriage, preterm labour or preterm prelabour rupture of membranes (PPROM)
- Flying does not increase the risk of miscarriage

There is increased risk of discomfort due to:

- Oedema
- Nasal congestion
- Pregnancy sickness

Risk of deep vein thrombosis (DVT) is increased in pregnancy

Recommendations to minimise the risks of DVT during air travel:

- Regular walks around the plane every 30 minutes.
- Hydration at frequent intervals
- Limiting caffeine/fizzy drinks/alcohol
- Use of elastic compression stockings (recommended if the duration of air travel is > 4 hours).
- Heparin in patients with additional risk factors for DVT

Flying is contraindicated in pregnancy if any of the following risk factors are present:

- Increased risk of preterm labour
- Severe anaemia
- Recent vaginal bleeding (placenta praevia major)
- Long bone fracture
- Recent major surgery
- Severe respiratory/cardiac problems
- Multiple gestation

2. Carrying heavy things in pregnancy

- It is common to hear that it is unsafe to lift heavy things in pregnancy. However, the risk of injury is usually directed at the mother and not the baby. The increase in the level of hormones during pregnancy causes the ligaments to soften, which leads to joints that may be less stable.
- The centre of gravity of pregnant mother shifts and this puts more stress on her back. These two factors make the mother more susceptible to injury when lifting heavy things.

3. Clothing in pregnancy

- As long as pregnant women are comfortable in their clothing and the clothing is not too restrictive or tight, it would not impede the development of the foetus.
- Exposing the belly has no known adverse effects on the foetus.

4. Dental health concerns in pregnancy

Periodontal disease (gum disease)

- Pregnancy increases the risk for developing gingivitis and periodontitis.

- Gingivitis is an inflammation of the gingiva (gums). The gingiva becomes erythematous, swollen and loses its normal shape. Bleeding also occurs easily, such as during toothbrushing.
- Periodontitis is a more severe form of gingivitis, involving destruction of the supporting bone structure surrounding the teeth, resulting in mobility and eventually, loss of the affected teeth.
- The increased susceptibility is due to the increase in oestrogen and progesterone during pregnancy. An increase in gingivitis frequently appears between the second and eighth months of pregnancy.
- Studies have shown a correlation between periodontal disease and preterm labour.
- Good dental hygiene is recommended in pregnancy.

Management

- Good oral hygiene: brush teeth after each meal, floss at least once a day, and use an anti-plaque mouth rinse.
- Visit the dentist regularly at least every 6 months for cleaning.

Caries (dental decay)

- Morning sickness and general malaise in the first trimester can result in poor oral health, increasing the susceptibility of the patient to caries.

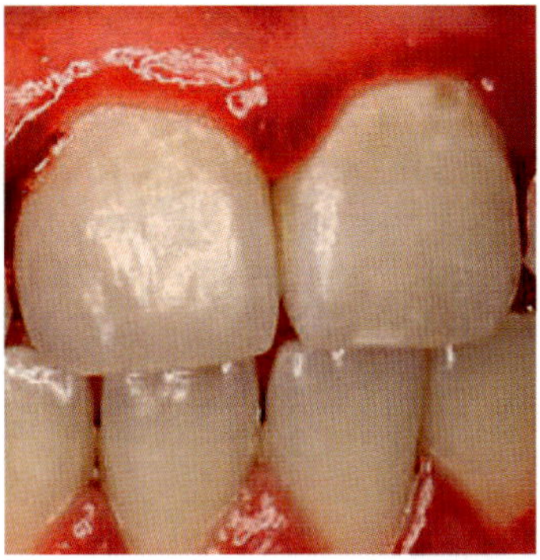

Figure showing gingivitis.

- Food cravings during pregnancy may result in higher or more frequent sugar intake, thus increasing the risk of developing caries.

Dental Procedures

- While regular check-ups and cleaning are highly recommended during pregnancy, major dental procedures (e.g. wisdom tooth removal, bleaching) that are not urgent should be postponed till after delivery of the baby.
- As the first trimester is the most critical period of the baby's development, dental treatment, if necessary, is best performed in the second trimester to minimise any potential risks.
- Treatment in the third trimester is not recommended due to the unfavourable supine position of the mother that may impede cardiac venous return.

Amalgam fillings (silver fillings)

- There has been a concern of mercury toxicity during the placement or removal of amalgam fillings in the pregnant woman, although there has been no evidence to prove this relationship.
- It is thus recommended that unnecessary procedures involving amalgam should be avoided.
- Alternative filling materials such as tooth-coloured restorations may be used.

Radiographs

- Dental X-rays are of very low dosage and pose little harm if any
- However, to be cautious, dental radiographs should only be taken during pregnancy if there is an emergency
- Examples of dental emergencies include infections that can cause toothache and may spread systemically, and dental trauma
- A lead apron over the abdomen should be worn to protect the foetus from radiation when dental radiographs are taken

Pregnancy Tumour

- Pregnancy tumour is also known as pyogenic granuloma or pregnancy epulis.
- This is a benign growth at the gingival margin that may enlarge substantially and bleed easily upon trauma.

- It is the result of an extreme inflammatory response to local irritation such as plaque and is most common in the second trimester.
- Large pregnancy tumour may be uncomfortable and makes speech and eating difficult.

Management of Pregnancy Tumour

- Pregnancy tumours usually resolve after delivery without intervention.
- If it causes discomfort or affects speech or eating, the pregnancy tumour may be excised surgically by a periodontist under local anaesthesia.
- Maintaining good oral hygiene and regularly receiving professional cleaning reduce the risk of pregnancy tumour.

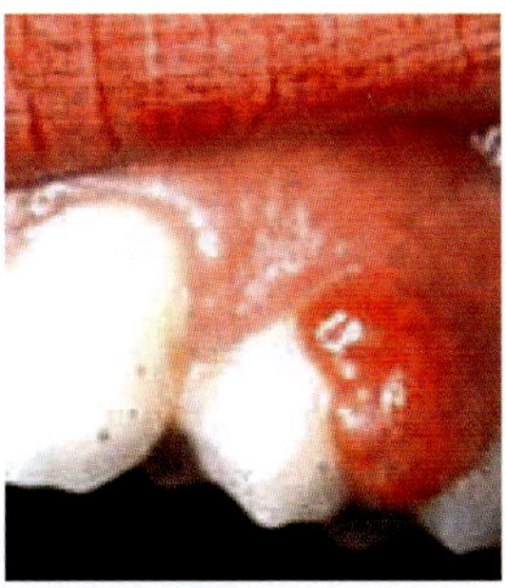

Figure showing a pregnancy tumour.

5. Does Epidural Cause Backache?

- Studies have failed to establish a link between long-term backache and epidural analgesia.

6. Exercise in Pregnancy

- Unless there are medical reasons to avoid it, pregnant women should exercise moderately for 20 minutes thrice a week.
- Exercise helps the pregnant woman to feel better and the calories spent help to prevent too much weight gain during pregnancy. They can consider brisk walking, dancing and swimming. Aerobics or yoga sessions designed specifically for pregnant women can also be explored.
- Activities should be conducted at a sub-threshold level before the woman becomes exhausted.
- Avoid activities that are at high risk for injury/contact sports, e.g. horseback riding, downhill skating, ice hockey, kickboxing, soccer or scuba diving.

7. Facial Treatments in Pregnancy

- Avoid those that contain relaxation oils as they may precipitate womb contraction.

8. Food, smoking and alcohol in pregnancy

Dos

i) *Folic acid supplementation*

Folic acid is a type of vitamin B that is needed for the formation of blood cells and the development of baby's nervous system. It has been shown to reduce the chance of a baby having neural tube defect. A simple way is to take a folate supplement (5 mg daily) for the first 12 weeks of pregnancy.

ii) Eat a variety of healthy food including food rich in iron, calcium and folate

Don'ts

i) *Smoking*

Smoking is associated with adverse effects on both the pregnant mother and her foetus. It can cause an increased risk of miscarriage, abruptio placentae, premature birth and low birth-weight baby. There is also a long-term relationship with decreased intellectual development of the infant and increased risk of sudden infant death syndrome (SIDS).

ii) *Alcohol consumption*

Alcohol consumption in pregnancy is linked to infants showing behavioural and learning difficulties. Excessive alcohol consumption is associated with foetal alcohol syndrome (FAS) where the infant may have varying effects, including multiple foetal malformations and decreased intellectual development.

iii) *Diet*

Do not focus on weight loss regime during pregnancy.

iv) *Caffeine*

Any drinks containing caffeine including coffee, tea and cola should be limited to one cup per day. Pregnant patients should also be informed about other sources of caffeine such as tea, colas, chocolate and over-the-counter drugs (e.g. headache and pain relief remedies, alertness drugs, some diuretics).

v) *Raw, uncooked or undercooked food*

Avoid raw or uncooked food to reduce the risk of food-borne infections such as listeriosis, toxoplasmosis, campylobacteria or salmonella infection. Do not eat:

a) Mould ripened cheese (e.g. brie, camembert or soft blue veined cheese, e.g. Danish blue, gorgonzola, Roquefort)
b) Raw or undercooked eggs and home made mayonnaise
c) Raw/unpasteurised milk
d) Raw/undercooked meat, refrigerated pate
e) Liver/liver products
f) Raw shell-fish/fish exposed to industrial pollutants and fish with mercury
g) Unwashed vegetables

9. Hair-Dyeing, Hair Rebonding and Perming in Pregnancy

- The concern about exposures to hair dye and hair straightening agents is that there may be absorption of chemicals into the bloodstream at the time of use. However, most chemicals are cleared from the bloodstream fairly quickly. Unfortunately, there have been only very few studies on the use of such products during pregnancy to quantify the risk of hair dye to a developing foetus.
- While no one can provide data about timing and safety, avoid dyeing or rebonding the hair once the woman has conceived.
- Perming hair during the second and third trimesters of pregnancy is a safe procedure and can make caring for hair less time consuming and easier. There are no studies that indicate that perming hair during pregnancy is detrimental to the foetus.

10. House Paint in Pregnancy

- Pregnant women may have an occupational exposure to paint, or they may be exposed to paint at home. The data from various studies are insufficient to show a cause-and-effect relationship between paint exposure and foetal harm. However, because oil based paints and paint thinners contain a number of aromatic organic solvents, exposure to these products should be limited or avoided, particularly during the first trimester of pregnancy.

- Brief exposure to water-based paints and similar compounds in a well-ventilated area should not pose a significant risk to the foetus.

11. Ideal Weight Gain in Pregnancy

- BMI <18.5 kg/m^2 (underweight)* — weight gain 12.5–18.0 kg
- BMI 18.5 to 24.9 kg/m^2 (normal weight)* — weight gain 11.5–16.0 kg
- BMI 25.0 to 29.9 kg/m^2 (overweight)* — weight gain 7.0–11.5 kg
- BMI ≥ 30.0 kg/m^2 (obese)* — weight gain 5–9.0 kg

**WHO International classification of BMI*

12. Insecticides in Pregnancy

- Most insecticides are readily absorbed, even with limited exposure. In general, pregnant women probably should not apply pesticides in the home or in the garden. They should avoid the use of fumigants.

13. Massage/Aromatherapy in Pregnancy

- Avoid excessive skin contact with essential oils especially in first trimester as it is absorbed through the skin into the bloodstream.

14. Mobile Phones in Pregnancy

- Insufficient data to comment on the safety of cellphone usage at the moment.

15. Sauna/Steam in Pregnancy

- Hyperthermia is contraindicated as there is an increased chance of miscarriage and birth defects like spinal cord and brain malformation.

16. Sex in Pregnancy

- Sex is safe during pregnancy as long as the woman adopts a position in which she is comfortable.
- Sex is best avoided if there are signs of threatened abortion or if there is presence of low lying placenta, premature contractions or preterm premature rupture of membranes.

17. Tattoos in Pregnancy

- The safety of the ink is unknown when injected into the skin. There exists the risk of local infection/allergy and small risk of transmission of blood borne infections like HIV, hepatitis B or C.

18. Use of Mosquito Repellants containing DEET in Pregnancy

- Less than 10% gets absorbed through the skin. Animal studies show no harm to the foetus.

19. Use of Over the Counter (OTC) Slimming Pills in Pregnancy

- Safety profile is not established, so should be avoided.

20. Working on Computers/Video Display Terminals/Photocopier/Printer in Pregnancy — Safe?

- Monitors have internal shielding that reduces non-ionising radiation to safe levels.
- Studies show no evidence that they cause miscarriage or harm the foetus.
- Avoid long hours in front of computers as it can predispose the woman to severe backache and/or deep vein thrombosis.

21. X-rays/Radiation Exposure in Pregnancy

- Avoid, unless benefits outweigh risks of radiation to the foetus.
- Radiation can cause developmental malformation, abnormal brain function, stunted growth, foetal malformations

and childhood cancers. Mothers who have had occasional exposure to X-ray may not be exposed to more than 0.5 rads. So, inadvertent exposure even in the first trimester may not necessarily be an indication to terminate the pregnancy. Exposure of up to 15 rads increases malformation risk and up to 50 rads can cause mental retardation.

- Critical period: 2 to 18 weeks of pregnancy (Centers for Disease Control & Prevention, 2011).
- CT scan (computer tomography)/Magnetic Resonance Imaging (MRI) — the amount of radiation is minimal. So, risk to the foetus is low.
- Passing through airport security as well as a metal detector is not known to pose any risk to the foetus.

Risk posed to foetus with imaging modalities

Imaging Modality	Foetal Radiation Exposure	
	mGy	Rads
Chest X-ray	< 0.01	< 0.001
CT scan abdomen	30	3
CT scan chest	0.16	0.016
Venography	< 0.50	< 0.05
Perfusion lung scan	0.06–0.18	0.006–0.018
Ventilation lung scan	0.01–0.35	0.001–0.035

1 Gy = 100 rads
1 mGy = 0.1 rads

22. Breastfeeding after Breast Augmentation Surgery

- If breasts have been surgically enlarged with silicone or saline implants, nipples may be more or less sensitive
- Breastfeeding success depends on the kind of the surgery but most approaches are compatible with breastfeeding
- If the surgery was for underdeveloped (hypoplastic) breasts, there may be trouble producing enough milk and may require use of pump after each nursing session to stimulate production.

Part 2

INVESTIGATIONS IN OBSTETRICS

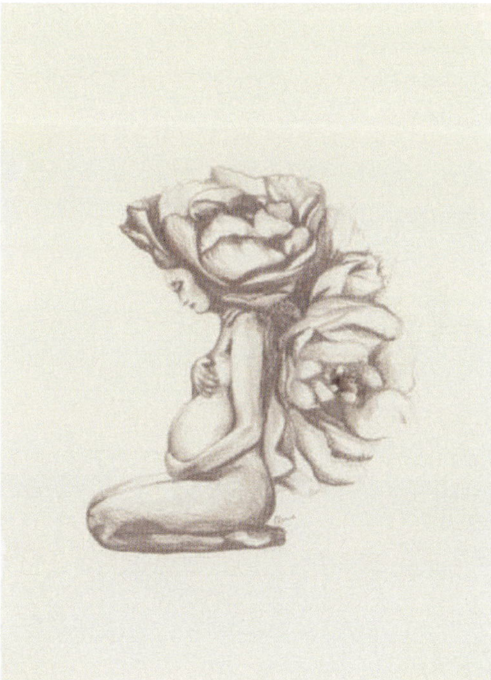

"Women" — 2013

Pencil on watercolour paper.

"Man can never know the loneliness a woman knows. Man lies in the woman's womb only to gather strength, he nourishes himself from this fusion, and then he rises and goes into the world, into his work, into battle into art. He is not lonely. He is busy. The memory of the swim in amniotic fluid gives him energy, completion. Woman may be busy too, but she feels empty. Sensuality for her is not only a wave of plessure in which she is bathed, and a charge of electric joy at contact with another. When man lies in her womb, she is fulfilled, each act of love a taking of man within her, an act of birth and rebirth, of child rearing and man bearing. Man lies in her womb and is reborn each time anew with a desire to act, to *be*. But for woman, the climax is not in the birth, but in the moment man rests inside of her." — Anais Nin

Chapter 24

ROUTINE ANTENATAL BLOOD INVESTIGATIONS AND INFECTIVE SCREENING

Routine Antenatal Blood Investigations

Also, refer to Chapter 31 on "Laboratory Values in Normal Pregnancy for Normal Range."

Test	Purpose	Interpretation and Management Guidelines
Full blood count		
Haemoglobin (Hb)	Check for anaemia	• Prescribe oral hematinics if <11 g/dL. • Refer to OBGYN for assessment and transfusion if Hb < 8 g/dL.
Mean corpuscular volume (MCV)	Thalassaemia screen	• If both patient & partner MCV ≤ 80 fL, refer to OBGYN • Refer to Chapter 25 on "Approach to Prenatal Screening for Thalassaemia"

(*Continued*)

(*Continued*)

Test	Purpose	Interpretation and Management Guidelines
Total white (TW) cell count	Infection	• In pregnancy, TW can be normal up to 17 x10^9/L.
Platelets	Thrombocytopaenia	• Refer to OBGYN if platelet < 150 x 10^9 /L • Watch for spontaneous bleeding if < 50 x 10^9 /L
	Pre-eclampsia	• Alert for HELLP syndrome. (Haemolysis, Elevated Liver enzymes, Low Platelets). • Refer to investigations for pre-eclampsia
ABO blood group and Rhesus (Rh) status	Screening for Rh negative patients and presence of abnormal blood antibodies	• If Rh negative and partner is Rh positive, **refer to OBGYN** • For prophylaxis, anti-D immunoglobulin, at 28 and 34 weeks gestation • Needs postnatal immunoglobulin if baby is RhD positive • Refer to Chapter 20 on "Medications in Pregnancy (Indications of Anti-D Immunoglobulin Administration in Pregnancy")

Routine Antenatal Infective Screening

<table>
<tr><th>Test</th><th colspan="2">Purpose</th><th>Normal</th><th colspan="2">Interpretation and Management Guidelines (KKH)</th></tr>
<tr><td rowspan="2">HepBsAg</td><td colspan="2" rowspan="2">Screen</td><td>Negative</td><td colspan="2">Recommend hepatitis B vaccination postnatally</td></tr>
<tr><td>Positive</td><td colspan="2">• For mother — consult hepatologist for follow up
• Recommend testing and vaccination for partner and family members
• For neonate-HBV immunoglobulin + first dose of HBV vaccine within 12 hours of birth
• Once immunisation is initiated, mother can breastfeed</td></tr>
<tr><td rowspan="4">Prevention</td><td colspan="3"></td><td>HBV vaccine</td><td>HBVIg</td></tr>
<tr><td>HbsAg +</td><td>HBeAg +</td><td>AntiHBe –</td><td>+</td><td>+</td></tr>
<tr><td>HBsAg +</td><td>HBeAg –</td><td>AntiHBe –</td><td>+</td><td>+</td></tr>
<tr><td>HBsAg +</td><td>HBeAg –</td><td>AntiHBe +</td><td>+</td><td>–</td></tr>
</table>

(Continued)

(*Continued*)

Test	Purpose	Normal	Interpretation and Management Guidelines (KKH)
HIV (human immuno-deficiency virus)	Screen	Negative	
		Positive	• Practise universal precautions • Notify (Infectious Diseases Act) • Referral to OBGYN and Communicable Disease Centre • Antiretrovirals (HAART-Highly Active Antiretroviral Therapy) • Avoid breastfeeding

(*Continued*)

(Continued)

Test	Purpose	Normal	Interpretation and Management Guidelines (KKH)
Syphilis	Screen CMIA (a chemil-uminescent immunoassay) on Abbott Architect analyser)	If CMIA is reactive, samples are tested for VDRL and TPPA (*Treponema Pallidum* Particle Agglutination test — this is a test for *Treponema Pallidum* antibodies as well)	<u>Active infection</u> • VDRL — reactive (high titres) • TPPA — reactive Treat with benzathine penicillin *<u>Past Infection</u>* • VDRL — often negative or at low titres • TPPA — reactive *If both VDRL and TPPA are negative or non reactive:* Two possibilities — 1) false positive CMIA 2) very early syphilis (before VDRL and TPPA seroconversion). • Recommend re-testing in 2 weeks, i.e. request for TPPA. • If both remain negative, then syphilis infection is excluded

(Continued)

Interpretation and Follow-up of Reverse Screening Results

Patient history	Test and result			Interpretation	Follow up
	EIA/CMIA/MFI	RPR	TPPA		
Unknown history of syphilis	Non-Reactive	N/A	N/A	No serologic evidence of syphilis	None, unless clinically indicated (e.g., early syphilis)
Unknown history of syphilis	Reactive	Reactive	N/A	Untreated or recently treated syphilis	Treat as per CDC guidelines
Unknown history of syphilis	Reactive	Non-reactive	Non-reactive	Probable false-positive screening test	No follow-up testing, unless clinically indicated
Unknown history of syphilis	Reactive	Non-reactive	Reactive	Possible syphilis (e.g., early or latent) or previously treated syphilis	Historical and clinical evaluation required
Known history of syphilis	Reactive	Non-reactive	Reactive or N/A	Past, successfully treated syphilis	None

CMIA, chemiluminescence immunoassay; EIA, enzyme immunoassay; MFI, multiplex flow immunoassay; N/A, not applicable; RPR, rapid plasma reagin; TPPA *Treponema pallidum* particle agglutination.
http://www.cdc.gov/std/treetment/2010

(Continued)

Test	Purpose	Normal	Interpretation and Management Guidelines (KKH)
Urine analysis (UFEME/ urine culture)	Screen for asymptomatic bacteriuria		If positive urine culture — treat with antibiotics Treatment reduces risk of : 1. preterm birth 2. low birth-weight baby 3. pyelonephritis in mother
Rubella	Screen for rubella antibodies	If IgG positive	• Suggests previous vaccination/ immunity
		If IgG negative	• Susceptible to rubella • Advise vaccination in postnatal period

Chapter 25

APPROACH TO PRENATAL SCREENING FOR THALASSAEMIA

Haemoglobinopathies are inherited disorders of haemoglobin involving haem or globin and may be divided into thalassaemia and the structural haemoglobinopathies.

Thalassaemia is a spectrum of inheritable haemoglobinopathies which result from a lack of normal adult haemoglobin (Hb) chains. It may range from mild to life-threatening form. It is transmitted in an **autosomal recessive** pattern.

Structural haemoglobinopathies include *sickle cell anaemia (HbSS)*, its variant *HbSC disease*, as well as *HbE disease.*

HbE is attributed to both a lack of normal haemoglobin as well as structurally abnormal haemoglobin chains.

The incidence of thalassaemia in Singapore is 4%.
3 common thalassaemia traits of greatest clinical concern locally are alpha-thalassaemia (α-thalassaemia), beta-thalassaemia (β-thalassaemia) and haemoglobin E traits (HbE traits).

The incidence of alpha-thalassaemia, beta-thalassaemia, and HbE trait are 3%; 1% and 0.5%, respectively.

Antenatal screening programme is essential for early detection of life-threatening haemoglobinopathies to the unborn foetus, to allow for appropriate genetic counselling to prospective parents and offering informed management choices.

Alpha-Thalassaemia

— Caused by mutations in alpha globin gene along short arm of chromosome 16

— **96% are caused by gene deletions, while 2.8% are caused by point mutations** (which include Hb Constant Spring mutation, Hb Quong Sze mutation)

— Clinical severity of alpha-thalassaemia depends on the number of functional alpha globin genes unaffected by gene deletion or mutation

Nomenclature	Genotype	Phenotype
Silent Constant Spring carrier	1 gene mutated (αα/αCSα)	– Normal phenotype
Homozygous Constant Spring	2 genes mutated (αCSα/αCSα)	– Similar to alpha thalassaemia trait
HbH-Constant Spring	2 genes deleted + Constant Spring point mutation (αCSα/--)	– Much more severe than HbH disease – Severe anaemia, severe splenomegaly, jaundice – Higher rates of transfusion and splenectomy

Nomenclature	Genotype	Phenotype
Alpha-2 thalassaemia [α+] **Silent alpha-thalassaemia carrier**	1 gene deleted (αα/α-)	— Normal phenotype — MCV normal
Alpha-1 thalassaemia [α°] **Alpha-thalassaemia trait**	2 genes deleted (αα/--) Commoner in Asian population or (α-/α-) Commoner in Black population	— Asymptomatic — Clinically similar to Beta-thalassaemia trait — Mild microcytic anaemia — Few HbH inclusion bodies — Normal Hb electrophoresis
HbH disease	3 genes deleted (α-/--)	— Moderately severe anaemia (Hb 7–10g/dL) — Chronic haemolysis with moderate pallor, jaundice, splenomegaly
*** HbH CS disease** *HbH Constant Spring disease* *Refer to Section on "Constant Spring"**	2 genes deleted + Constant Spring point mutation (αCSα/--)	— Much more severe than HbH disease — Severe anaemia, severe splenomegaly, jaundice — Higher rates of transfusion and splenectomy
Hb Bart's hydrops	4 genes deleted (--/--)	— Almost solely amongst Chinese — Lethal to foetus due to hydropic state usually resulting in intrauterine death or stillbirths — Severe maternal morbidity which includes pre-eclampsia, antepartum haemorrhage, postpartum haemorrhage

*Constant Spring

Constant Spring

— A clinically significant type of **point mutation** in **alpha-thalassaemia** which converts the stop codon to glutamine, resulting in a longer alpha-globin chain
— Results in unstable mRNA which is degraded prior to protein synthesis, as well as production of unstable alpha-globin chains, resulting in a lack of functional alpha-globin chains

Beta-thalassaemia

Caused by mutations in beta-globin gene along chromosome 11

— 96% caused by point mutations, 2% attributed to deletion mutations
— Results in reduced (B+) or complete absence (B°) of beta-globin chain synthesis
— Most beta-thalassemic syndromes locally are caused by a complete absence of beta-globin chain synthesis — (B°)
— Inadequate beta-globin chain production results in decreased amounts of normal adult haemoglobin (HbA) with subsequent increased production of HbA2 and HbF
— This leads to an imbalance in globin chain, forming unstable gamma-tetramer chains which interact with erythrocyte membranes and shorten their lifespan
— A low MCV of <80 fL has a high sensitivity but low specificity (A cut off of MCV <80 fL captures 99.7% of all

beta-thalassaemias; however, only 11.4% of microcytic anaemia with MCV <80 fL have beta-thalassaemia)

— Hb electrophoresis of beta-thalassaemia will show elevated HbA2 levels (3.4%–10%) and HbF levels
— A low MCV (microcytosis) could also reflect iron-deficiency anaemia but it is postulated that thalassaemia has a higher degree of microcytosis as compared to iron deficiency anaemia
— Patients with low MCV levels without beta-thalassaemia should still be assessed for alpha-thalassaemia and HbE traits

HbE Trait

— Commonest in the Malay population, accounts for 96% of HbE trait
— Caused by lysine replacing glutamate on codon 26
— Attributed by both a lack of normal haemoglobin chain production as well as structural defects in normal adult haemoglobin chains
— 20% of patients with HbE trait may not exhibit microcytosis below the discrimination level

* HbE/beta-thalassaemia disease

— 25% chance of inheriting HbE/beta-thalassaemia disease in a couple with one having HbE trait and the other a beta-thalassaemia carrier

Nomenclature	Genotype	Phenotype
Beta-thalassaemia trait	(B°/B) or (B+/B)	— Asymptomatic — Mild anaemia — Microcytosis, target cells
Beta-thalassaemia intermedia	(B+/B°) or(B+/B+)	— Moderately severe anaemia (Hb 7–9 g/dl) — Normal growth rates — Bone marrow hyperplasia — Splenomegaly with blood sequestration requiring splenectomy — Transfusion independent except during infection or pregnancy
Beta-thalassaemia major	(B°/B°)	— Present clinically at 3–6 months of age as HbA requires adequate beta-globin genes — Severe anaemia(Hb 3–4 g/dl) requiring monthly transfusions and iron chelation therapy — Iron overload may lead to cardiomyopathies and endocrinopathies

— wide spectrum of clinical syndromes which may range from mild anaemia to severe transfusion-dependent states

— up to 50% may require regular frequent blood transfusions

— up to 40% may require splenectomy

* HbE Disease

— Heterozygous HbE trait will resemble a person with beta-thalassaemia trait

— Homozygous HbE trait will have a clinical syndrome of mild anaemia

Alpha-thalassaemia/Beta-thalassaemia Coinheritance

— A diagnosis of beta-thalassaemia trait does not preclude co-existing alpha-thalassaemia

— A parent with silent alpha-thalassaemia carrier (αα/α-) or (αα/--) and a parent with beta-thalassaemia trait (B+/B) or (B°/B) have a 25% chance heterozygous alpha-thalassaemia/beta-thalassaemia coinheritance

— However, due to mechanisms resulting in a more balanced alpha-globin and beta-globin chain synthesis, patients with this coinheritence are compatible with a healthy lifestyle

Sickle Cell Disease

— ***Autosomal Recessive*** inheritance pattern

— Commonest in Africa, the Caribbean, Middle East, India, America

— Mutation in codon 6 of beta-globin gene (glutamic acid > valine)

— Mutated form of haemoglobin polymerises in deoxygenated conditions and results in sickling of erythrocytes; these sickled erythrocytes undergo haemolysis due to membrane rigidity and fragility resulting in widespread vaso-occlusion

— Comprises a spectrum which includes:

(i) Sickle cell anaemia (HbSS, homozygous HbS)

- 90% HbS, 2–10% HbF, minimal HbA2, no HbA
- Usually detected at birth
- Manifests clinically at age 6 months due to initial high concentrations of HbF (foetal Hb)
- 4 major clinical conditions:
  - (i) Haemolytic anaemia
  - (ii) Vaso-occlusion
  - (iii) Infection
  - (iv) End organ damage
    - — kidney, spleen, heart, lung, central nervous system, bone, eye, peripheral vascular system

(ii) Sickle cell trait (HbAS)

- 40% HbS, 60% HbA
- Usually asymptomatic

(iii) Variants (of which HbSC is most significant)

- HbSC
  - — Greatest clinical significance with moderate-severe clinical features
  - — Better outcome than sickle cell disease (HbSS) due to longer survival of HbSC compared to HbSS
- HbS-B°
  - — Clinically similar to sickle cell anaemia (HbSS) and HbSC disease
- HbS-B+
  - — Mild-moderate severity
- HbS-HbE
  - — Rare

Table of Thalassaemic Inheritance

Parent 1	Parent 2	Risk of Transmission	Action
Normal (αα/αα)	Alpha-2 thalassaemia (αα/α-)	• 50% normal • 50% alpha-2 thalassaemia	• Reassure
Alpha-2 Thalassaemia (αα/α-)	Alpha-2 thalassaemia (αα/α-)	• 25% normal • 25% alpha-1 thalassaemia • 50% alpha-2 thalassaemia	• Reassure
Normal	Alpha-1 thalassaemia o Homozygous (α-/α-) or o Heterozygous (αα/--)	• If homozygous (α-/α-) All alpha-2 thalassaemia • If heterozygous (αα/--) 50% normal, 50% alpha-1 thalassaemia	• Reassure
Alpha-1 thalassaemia heterozygous (αα/--)	Alpha-1 thalassaemia heterozygous (αα/--)	• 25% Bart's hydrops • 50% alpha-1 thalassaemia • 25% normal	• Refer for genetic counselling • Offer prenatal invasive testing
Alpha-1 thalassaemia homozygous (α-/α-)	Alpha-1 thalassaemia homozygous (α-/α-)	• All alpha-1 thalassaemia	• Reassure
Alpha-1 thalassaemia homozygous (α-/α-)	Alpha-1 thalassaemia heterozygous (αα/--)	• 50% HbH disease • 50% alpha-2 thalassaemia	• Refer for genetic counselling • Offer prenatal invasive testing

(Continued)

Table of Thalassaemic Inheritance (Continued)

Parent 1	Parent 2	Risk of Transmission	Action
Normal (αα/αα)	Silent Constant Spring carrier (αα/αCSα)	• 50% normal • 50% silent Constant Spring carrier	• Reassure
Silent Constant Spring carrier (αα/αCSα)	Silent Constant Spring carrier (αα/αCSα)	• 25% homozygous Constant Spring disease • 50% silent Constant Spring carrier • 25% normal	• Refer for genetic counselling • Offer prenatal invasive testing
Alpha-1 thalassaemia heterozygous (αα/--)	Silent Constant Spring carrier (αα/αCSα)	• 25% HbH Constant Spring disease • 25% alpha-1 thalassaemia • 25% Constant Spring carrier • 25% normal	• Refer for genetic counselling • Offer prenatal invasive testing
Normal	Beta thalassaemia trait (B°/B) or (B+/B)	• 50% Beta thalassaemia trait • 50% Normal	• Reassure
Beta thalassaemia trait (B°/B) or (B+/B)	Beta thalassaemia trait (B°/B) or (B+/B)	• 25% Beta thalassaemia major • 50% Beta thalassaemia carrier • 25% normal	• Refer for genetic counselling • Offer prenatal invasive testing

(Continued)

Table of Thalassaemic Inheritance (Continued)

Parent 1	Parent 2	Risk of Transmission	Action
Beta thalassaemia trait (B°/B) or (B+/B)	HbE carrier	• 25% HbE-beta thalassaemia disease • 25% beta thalassaemia carrier • 25% HbE trait • 25% normal	• Refer for genetic counselling • Offer prenatal invasive testing
Normal	HbE trait	• 50% HbE trait • 50% normal	• Reassure • Same if mother is the one with HbE trait and father is normal
HbE trait	HbE trait	• 25% homozygous HbE • 50% HbE trait • 25% normal	• Reassure
Alpha-2 thalassaemia (αα/α-)	Beta thalassaemia trait (B°/B) or (B+/B)	• 25% coinheritance alpha — beta thalassaemia • 25% beta thalassaemia trait • 25% alpha-2 thalassaemia • 25% normal	• Reassure
Alpha-1 thalassaemia (αα/--)	Beta thalassaemia trait (B°/B) or (B+/B)	• 25% coinheritance alpha — beta thalassaemia • 25% beta thalassaemia trait • 25% alpha-1 thalassaemia • 25% normal	• Reassure

(*Continued*)

Table of Thalassaemic Inheritance (Continued)

Parent 1	Parent 2	Risk of Transmission	Action
alpha-2 thalassaemia (αα/α-)	Coinheritance alpha–beta thalassaemia	• 25% HbH disease • 25% coinheritance alpha–beta thalassaemia • 25% alpha-1 thalassaemia • 12.5% beta thalassaemia • 12.5% normal	• Refer for genetic counselling • Offer prenatal invasive testing
Alpha-1 thalassaemia (αα/--)	Coinheritance alpha–beta thalassaemia	• 25% Bart's hydrops • 25% coinheritance alpha–beta thalassaemia • 25% alpha-1 thalassaemia • 12.5% beta thalassaemia • 12.5% normal	• Refer for genetic counselling • Offer prenatal invasive testing
Beta thalassaemia trait (B°/B) or (B+/B)	Coinheritance alpha–beta thalassaemia	• 25% beta thalassaemia major or intermedia	• Refer for genetic counselling • Offer prenatal invasive testing
Coinheritance alpha–beta thalassaemia	Coinheritance alpha–beta thalassaemia	• 50% Bart's hydrops, beta thalassaemia major or intermedia	• Refer for genetic counselling • Offer prenatal invasive testing
HbE trait	Coinheritance alpha–beta thalassaemia	• 25% HbE-beta thalassaemia disease	• Refer for genetic counselling • Offer prenatal invasive testing

(*Continued*)

Prenatal Invasive Testing

— Chorionic villous sampling (CVS) or amniocentesis

— If both parents have alpha-thalassemia trait, CVS is the preferred mode of prenatal invasive testing.

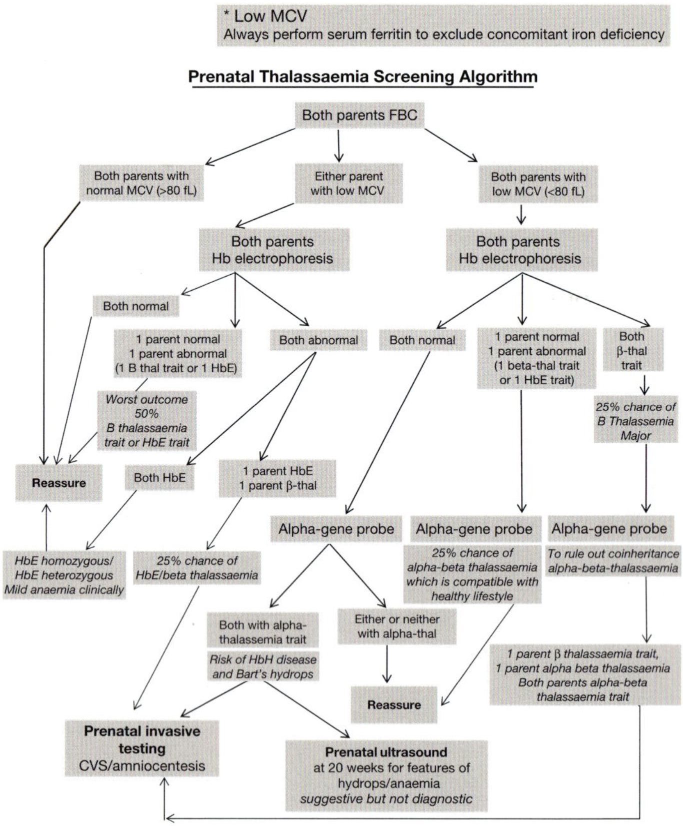

Ultrasound features suggestive of Hb Bart's hydrops foetalis

— Cardio-thoracic ratio >0.5, placental thickening >2SD, dilated umbilical vein, subcutaneous oedema, ascites, hepatosplenomegaly, oligohydramnios, cord oedema seen in 1/3 of affected pregnancies week 17–18 and are strongly suggestive of Hb Bart's hydrops foetalis

— Foetal anaemia can be predicted based on foetal middle cerebral artery (MCA)

— Peak systolic volume (PSV) >1.5 MoM

— Ultrasound scan cannot be utilised to detect beta-thalassaemia major as it only manifests clinically between 3–6 months of life

Chapter 26

MISCELLANEOUS ANTENATAL BLOOD INVESTIGATIONS

Refer to Chapter 31 on "Laboratory Values in Normal Pregnancy for Normal Range."

Miscellaneous Antenatal Blood Tests

Test	Purpose	Normal Range	Interpretation and Management Guidelines
Oral glucose tolerance test (OGTT) (75 g)	Exclude gestational diabetes (GDM)		*If risk factors present*, to perform OGTT at 24–28 weeks gestation. *Previous GDM* — screen at 16 to 18 weeks and repeat at 24—28 weeks, if the first OGTT is normal. Risk factors for diabetes include: • ≥35 years old • Race • Family history of diabetes • Previous history of GDM • Previous stillbirth • Previous/current macrosomia • Obesity • ≥2 episodes of glycosuria

(*Continued*)

(*Continued*)

Test	Purpose	Normal Range	Interpretation and Management Guidelines
Fasting glucose level		<5.5 mmol/L	If raised, **refer to OBGYN** for diabetic control
2 hour glucose level		<7.8 mmol/L	If raised, **refer to OBGYN** for diabetic control
Blood Sugar Profile		4.4–5.5 mmol/L	Pre-prandial
		5.5–7.0 mmol/L	2 hr post-prandial
Thyroid function test			
Free T4 (FT4)		9–26 pmol/L	*Hyperthyroidism* Propylthiouracil (PTU) • Limit use only to the first trimester* *Hypothyroidism*: Use thyroxine Refer to Chapter 15 on Medical Disorders and Potential Risk Factors in Pregnancy
Thyroid stimulating hormone (TSH)		0.3–5.5 miu/L	• Can be low in pregnancy, as long as free T4 is normal

*After the first trimester, switch to Methimazole (MMI) as there have been rare cases of liver damage in people taking PTU.

Pre-Eclampsia Blood/Urine Investigations

Test	Purpose	Interpretation and Management Guidelines
Pre-eclampsia blood tests	Assess evidence of end-organ damage	
Creatinine	Assess renal function	• Raised in renal impairment • In pregnancy, renal impairment if >80 μmol/L
Uric acid	Suggests pre-eclampsia	• Raised in pre-eclampsia • Rough estimate of upper limit = duration of gestation (in weeks) x 10
AST (Aspartate transaminase) ALT (Alanine transaminase)	Assess liver dysfunction	• Watch for HELLP syndrome (haemolysis, elevated liver enzymes and low platelets)
Bilirubin (Direct)		• Raised in jaundice, HELLP
Bilirubin (Total)		• Raised in jaundice, HELLP
Platelets	Assess coagulopathy	• If <150 x 10^9 /L, suggests consumptive coagulopathy • To exclude HELLP + other causes of thrombocytopaenia
Prothrombin time (PT)/activated partial thromboplastin time (APPT)/INR	Assess coagulopathy	• Prolonged in disseminated intravascular coagulopathy (DIVC)
24-hour urine total protein (UTP)	Helps to make management decisions based on severity of proteinuria	• Raised in pre-eclampsia (>300 mg/day) • Indicator of severity of pre-eclampsia • Predicts outcome in pre-eclampsia

Screening for Proteinuria in Pregnancy (Correlate with 24-hour urine total protein — UTP)	
Routine dipstick protein test	
Result	**Proteinuria mg/dL**
• Negative	
• Trace	Between 15—30 mg/dL
• +1	Between 30—100 mg/dL
• +2	Between 100—300 mg/dL
• +3	Between 300—1000 mg/dL
• +4	>1000 mg/dL
False positive test	Macroscopic/gross blood in urine
	Alkaline urine
	Semen
	Vaginal secretions

Urine Protein: Creatinine Ratio

Used as an alternative to 24 hr UTP.

The protein: creatinine ratio of ≥0.3 is an indicator of protein excretion of ≥300 mg/24 hr.

Sensitivity – 98.2%, specificity – 98.8%.

Chapter 27

SCREENING FOR CHROMOSOMAL DEFECTS

Introduction:

- Screening tests are **NOT** diagnostic tests
- Most women with a positive screening test have a normal baby
- The risk for abnormalities is just increased over the background risk
- Nevertheless, all women should be offered aneuploidy screening before 20 weeks of gestation and they should have the option of invasive testing, regardless of maternal age.

Various Screening Tests for Down Syndrome

Test	Type of Screening	Abnormal Result	Timing in Pregnancy	Down Syndrome Detection Rate
Nuchal translucency (NT)	Ultrasound scan of the width of the translucent gap at the back of the foetal neck	Thickened NT (NT > 95th percentile for crown rump length-CRL)	First trimester CRL (45–84 mm)	80% with false positive of 5%
Combined test	• *Ultrasound scan* for NT • *Blood test* βhcg PAPP-A • Maternal age	↑βhcg + ↓PAPPA = ↑Risk of Down syndrome	First trimester (11–13 + 6 weeks)	90% with false positive of 5%
Triple test	• Blood test at 15–20 weeks βhcg αFP uE3 • Maternal age	(↑αFP = ↑risk of neural tube defect) (↑βhcg + ↓αFP = ↑risk of Down syndrome)	Second trimester	70% with false positive of 5%
Quadruple test	• Blood test at 15–20 weeks βhcg αFP uE3 inhibin-A • Maternal age	↑βhcg + ↓αFP + ↑inhibin + ↓uE3 = ↑risk of Down syndrome	Second trimester	80% with false positive of 5%

(Continued)

(*Continued*)

Test	Type of Screening	Abnormal Result	Timing in Pregnancy	Down Syndrome Detection Rate
Integrated test	• *Ultrasound scan* for NT (first trimester) • *Blood test (first trimester)* PAPP-A • *Blood test at 15–20 weeks* βhcg αFP uE3 inhibin-A • Maternal age	Thickened NT and ↓PAPP-A + ↑βhcg + ↓αFP + ↑inhibin + ↓uE3 = ↑risk of Down syndrome	First trimester + second trimester	95% with false positive of 5%
Serum Integrated test	• *Blood test (first trimester)* PAPP-A • *Blood test at 15–20 weeks* βhcg αFP uE3 inhibin-A • Maternal age	↓PAPP-A + ↑βhcg + ↓αFP ↑inhibin + ↓uE3 = ↑risk of Down syndrome	First trimester + Second trimester	90% with false positive of 5%

Key:

NT	Nuchal translucency
CRL	Crown rump length
βhcg	Beta human chorionic gonadotrophin
PAPP-A	Pregnancy associated plasma protein-A
uE3	Unconjugated oestriol

The risk of Trisomy 21 based exclusively on maternal age

Maternal Age	Risk of Trisomy 21
18–20	1: 1500
30	1: 1000
35	1: 300
40	1: 100
44	1: 40

Various markers for aneuploidy screening

Various Markers	Interpretation
NT (subcutaneous space between the skin and cervical spine)	Thickened NT — to exclude trisomy 21/13/18 and other foetal anomalies, especially cardiac anomalies.
PAPP-A	↓–to exclude chromosomal abnormalities and adverse foetal outcome
βhcg	↑–to exclude Trisomy 21 ↓–to exclude Trisomy 13, 18
αFP	↑–to exclude foetal malformation (spina bifida/anencephaly) ↓–to exclude Trisomy 21/18
uE3	↓–to exclude Trisomy 21/18
Inhibin A	↑–to exclude Trisomy 21/13

First Trimester Screening Available in KK Hospital

Package	Type of Screening	Abnormal Result	Detection Rate	Abnormalities Screened
FTS	• Ultrasound scan between 11 and 13 weeks + 6 days (CRL 45–84 mm) • Blood test from 9 weeks (PAPP-A; βhcg) • Maternal age	Absent nasal bone Thickened NT ↑βhcg+ ↓PAPP-A = ↑Risk of Down syndrome	90%	• Trisomy 21/13/18

Cut-off for high risk is 1:300. If the woman is at high risk, **refer to OBGYN** for counselling on chorionic villous sampling, amniocentesis, or NIPT depending on the gestation.

Refer to Chapter 28 on "Prenatal Invasive Diagnostic Tests"

Screen negative (low risk)	• Patient's risk of having a baby with Down syndrome is less than cut off level (1:300) • No further testing is recommended
Screen positive (high risk)	• Patient's risk of having a baby with Down syndrome is above a cut-off level (1:300) • Denotes actual risk for patient • Offer foetal karyotype (chorionic villous sampling/ amniocentesis) for definitive diagnosis

Advantages of First Trimester Screening

- Early diagnosis allows the couple maximum time for decision making.
- Allows early termination of pregnancy if screened positive.

Pregnancy-Associated Plasma Protein A (PAPP-A)

Low levels of PAPP-A are more likely to be associated with chromosomal abnormalities and adverse foetal outcome (PAPP-A < 0.4 – 0.5 MoM)

a. Chromosomal abnormalities (e.g. Down syndrome)
b. Pre-eclampsia
c. Miscarriage
d. Intrauterine foetal death (IUD)
e. Intrauterine growth restriction (IUGR)
f. Preterm labour (PTL)
g. Neonatal death
h. Cerebral palsy

Management of Low PAPP-A

a. Growth scan between 34–37 weeks to see if interval growth is appropriate
b. Consider induction of labour at term if intrauterine growth restriction (IUGR) in foetus

Nuchal Translucency

Causes of Thickened Nuchal Translucency

1. Aneuploidy
   Down syndrome (trisomy 21)
   Turner syndrome (monosomy X)
   Trisomy 13 (Patau syndrome)
   Trisomy 18 (Edward syndrome)
2. Cardiac disorders
   Congenital heart disease (common — septal defect)
3. Structural defects
   Diaphragmatic hernia, renal anomalies, body stalk disruption , abdominal wall defects
4. Genetic syndromes (eg.congenital adrenal insufficiency (21-hydroxylase insufficiency, Noonan syndrome, Smith-Lemli-Opitz syndrome (SLOS), spinal muscular atrophy and Beckwith-Wiedemann syndrome)
5. Monochorionic twin with increased risk of twin-twin transfusion syndrome
6. Normal variant

Management for Thickened Nuchal Translucency

a. Foetal karyotyping (chorionic villous sampling and amniocentesis)
b. Foetal echocardiography (15–16 weeks) to rule out congenital heart defects.

Optimal time for cardiac evaluation is 18–22 weeks of gestation

c. Detailed foetal anatomic ultrasound scan (anomaly scan)
d. Serial foetal assessment for foetal well-being (growth scans)

Absent Nasal Bone (NB) : Trisomy 21 (rare in trisomy 18, 13)

Optimum time to measure nasal bone — CRL of 65 to 74 mm (i.e. after 12–13 weeks' gestation)

Maternal Serum Screening (MSS)

- Screen between 15–20 weeks of gestation
- Detection rate is about 70% with a false positive of 5%
- Upper limit for head circumference for MSS — 220 mm

Disadvantages

- Late diagnosis does not allow the couple the maximum time for decision making
- Mid-trimester termination of pregnancy has more complications including psychological problems

Maternal serum analytes and adverse obstetric outcome

		SM	PTL	IUGR	IUD (> 24 weeks)	GHTN	Abruptio
PAPP-A	↓	+	+	+	+	+ (PE)*	-
	↑	-	-	-	-	-	-
βhcg	↓	+	-	-	-	-	-
	↑	-	+	-	+	+ (PIH)	-
αFP	↓	-	-	-	-	-	-
	↑	+	+	+	+	-	+
uE3	↓	+	-	+	+	-	-
	↑	-	-	-	-	-	-
Inhibin–A	↓	-	-	-	-	-	-
	↑	-	+	+	+	+ (PIH)	-

* PE = Pre-eclampsia

Key:

GHTN — Gestational hypertension
IUGR — Intrauterine growth restriction;
IUD — Intrauterine death
PE — Pre-eclampsia
PIH — Pregnancy induced hypertension
PTB — Preterm birth
SM — Spontaneous miscarriage

Noninvasive Prenatal Testing (NIPT) for Foetal Aneuploidy

Patients at increased risk of aneuploidy can be offered testing with cell free foetal DNA. This technology can be expected to identify approximately 98% of cases of Down syndrome with a false-positive rate of less than 0.5%.

Indications for Considering the Use of Cell Free Foetal DNA

- Maternal age 35 years or older at delivery
- Foetal ultrasonographic findings indicating an increased risk of aneuploidy
- History of a prior pregnancy with a Trisomy
- Positive test result for aneuploidy, including first trimester, sequential, or integrated screen, or a quadruple screen.
- Parental balanced Robertsonian translocation with increased risk of foetal Trisomy 13 or Trisomy 21.

- Cell free foetal DNA testing should not be part of routine prenatal laboratory assessment, but should be an informed patient choice after pretest counselling.
- Cell free foetal DNA testing should not be offered to low-risk women or women with multiple gestations because it has not been sufficiently evaluated in these groups.

- Pretest counselling should include a review that although the cell free foetal DNA test is not a diagnostic test, it has high sensitivity and specificity. The test will only screen for the common trisomies and, at the present time, gives no other genetic information about the pregnancy.
- A family history should be obtained before the use of this test to determine if the patient should be offered other forms of screening or prenatal diagnosis for familial genetic disease.
- If a foetal structural anomaly is identified on ultrasound examination, invasive prenatal diagnosis should be offered.
- A negative cell free foetal DNA test result does not ensure an unaffected pregnancy.
- A patient with a positive test result should be referred for genetic counselling and offered invasive prenatal diagnosis for confirmation of test results.

  Cell free foetal DNA does not replace the accuracy and diagnostic precision of prenatal diagnosis with CVS or amniocentesis, which remain an option for women.

Harmony Prenatal Test (Directed DNA Test)

- Can assess the risk of foetal trisomies (T21, 18, 13)
- Can optimally analyse foetal sex and sex chromosome (X and Y) conditions
- Detection rate >99% for Down syndrome, 98% for T18 and 80% for T13 with a false positive rate of 0.1%.

Chapter 28

PRENATAL INVASIVE DIAGNOSTIC TESTS

	Chorionic Villous Sampling (CVS)	Amniocentesis (Amnio)	Cordocentesis (Foetal Blood Sampling)
1. Indications	• When first trimester screening test result is abnormal — or NIPT "high risk" • Chromosomal abnormality in a previous pregnancy • When both parents are thalassaemia carriers (refer to Chapter 25 on "Approach to Prenatal Screening of Thalassaemia" or both are carriers of a known genetic disease • If either parent has an unusual chromosome arrangement that can be inherited	• When first trimester screening test result indicates — or NIPT "high risk" status with regard to major chromosomal abnormalitiy • Baby/foetus born with chromosomal abnormality in a previous pregnancy (review anatomical aberration) • Screening scan or ultrasound markers that are suggestive of possible chromosomal abnormality	• Rarely done • Done when diagnostic information cannot be obtained through amniocentesis/CVS or the results of these tests are inconclusive

(*Continued*)

(*Continued*)

	Chorionic Villous Sampling (CVS)	Amniocentesis (Amnio)	Cordocentesis (Foetal Blood Sampling)
2. Uses	• Can diagnose nearly all chromosomal abnormalities • Can be used to detect other mendelian (single gene) conditions like cystic fibrosis, haemophilia, muscular dystrophies, Tay Sachs disease, haemoglobinopathies, e.g. thalassaemia, sickle cell anaemia.	• Can diagnose nearly all chromosomal abnormalities • Can provide information on neural tube defects (e.g. spina bifida or anencephaly) with elevation of αFP • Evaluation of degree of haemolytic anaemia • Assessment of foetal lung maturity (rarely done) • Amnioreduction in polyhydramnios	• Can detect – chromosomal abnormality (e.g. Down syndrome). – Blood disorders (i.e. foetal haemolytic disease) – Foetal infections, e.g. Toxoplasmosis, CMV or Rubella. – Foetal platelet count – Foetal anaemia – Isoimmunisation
3. Timing of Test	• 1st trimester (11–14 weeks)	• 2nd trimester (16–22 weeks)	• 2nd trimester (18–24 weeks)

(*Continued*)

(Continued)

	Chorionic Villous Sampling (CVS)	Amniocentesis (Amnio)	Cordocentesis (Foetal Blood Sampling)
4. Ultrasound Guided Procedure/ Sample	• Outpatient procedure • Choronic villi/placental cells that are derived from the same fertilised egg as the foetus • Local anaesthesia given • Transabdominal approach	• Outpatient procedure • 20 mL of amniotic fluid — contains cells that are shed primarily from foetal skin, bladder, gastrointestinal tract and amnion • Transabdominal approach	• Outpatient procedure • Foetal blood from umbilical vessels (usually from umbilical cord insertion site at placenta) • Transabdominal approach
5. Miscarriage risk	• 0.5%	• 0.3%	• 1–2%

(Continued)

(*Continued*)

	Chorionic Villous Sampling (CVS)	Amniocentesis (Amnio)	Cordocentesis (Foetal Blood Sampling)
6. Risks/ Complications	• Risk of miscarriage • Uterine infection (rare) (<0.1%) • Bleeding per vaginum. • Limb deficiencies or limb defects (if CVS done before 10 weeks' gestation). • Transplacental haemorrhage • Culture failure rate 0.5% • Mosaicism 1%	• Risk of miscarriage • Injury to foetus (rare because procedure is ultrasound guided) • Uterine infection (rare) — choriamnionitis (0.1%) • Leakage of amniotic fluid • Bleeding per vaginum	• As amniocentesis. *Other risks include* • Blood loss from puncture site. • Foetal bradycardia secondary to cord haematoma • Preterm premature rupture of membranes • Preterm delivery • Foetal loss 2–5%
7. Timing of Results	• Culture — 2 weeks • PCR: 48–72 hours	• FISH on uncultured amniocytes: 48–72 hours • PCR: 48–72 hours (trisomy 13, 18, 21, X, Y) • Culture amniocytes — 2 weeks	• 48–72 hours
8. Accuracy of Results	• 99.9%	• 99.9%	• 99.9%

(*Continued*)

(*Continued*)

	Chorionic Villous Sampling (CVS)	Amniocentesis (Amnio)	Cordocentesis (Foetal Blood Sampling)
9. Benefits of Test	• Earlier diagnosis. • Psychological benefit of earlier diagnosis. • Lower risk if termination of pregnancy is done when the result is abnormal • Ambiguous CVS result may indicate confined placental mosaicism which has been associated with adverse foetal outcome. Therefore, more informative than amniocentesis	• More commonly done • Can detect neural tube defects. (NTD can also be diagnosed with ultrasound scans). • Lower risk of maternal cell contamination or culture related mosaicism, therefore lower possibility of need for second prenatal diagnostic procedure	
10. Limitations of Test	• Slight increased risk of maternal cell contamination than amniocentesis • May need amniocentesis at a later date (if result indicates possible maternal contamination)	• Can only be done after 16 weeks. • Increased anxiety and stress waiting for diagnosis to be made • Second trimester termination is less desirable if amnio result is abnormal	

(*Continued*)

(*Continued*)

	Chorionic Villous Sampling (CVS)	Amniocentesis (Amnio)	Cordocentesis (Foetal Blood Sampling)
11. Signs & Symptoms to monitor after procedure	• Bleeding per vaginum • Increase vaginal discharge or leakage of amniotic fluid per vaginum • Fever • Nausea/vomiting • Pain in shoulder	• Same as CVS. • Leakage of amniotic fluid — rupture of membranes.	• Fever • Chills • Leaking of amniotic fluid • Bleeding per vaginum • Abdominal pain • Cessation of fetal movement
12. Precautions after procedure	• Avoid sexual intercourse/exercises • For 3 days — avoid lifting of heavy objects	• Avoid sexual intercourse/exercises • For 3 days — avoid lifting of heavy objects	• Same as amniocentesis

(*Continued*)

Additional Information

- For rhesus negative mothers, need intramuscular anti-D immunoglobulin after procedure to prevent Rh incompatibility if husband/partner is Rh positive. (Refer to Chapter 20 on "Medications in Pregnancy and Lactation".)
- A follow-up scan in one to two weeks post-procedure is recommended to rule out procedure-related complications.

Chapter 29

ULTRASONOGRAPHY AND FOETAL DOPPLER IN OBSTETRICS

1. Dating Scan

First trimester ultrasound screening is optimal for (1) pregnancy dating; (2) pregnancy location; (3) viability; (4) determining single or multiple pregnancies; (5) determining chorionicity in multiple pregnancies; (6) diagnosis of molar pregnancy; and (7) detection of anomalies like anencephaly, body stalk anomaly.

2. Screening Scan (Refer to Chapter 30 on "Approach to Screening Scan Foetal Abnormalities"

An ultrasound scan performed between 18 and 22 weeks is optimal for a survey of the foetal anatomy and placental location.

Routine second trimester ultrasound examination will reveal placental location and relationship to the internal cervical os. *Placenta praevia* complicates 0.3% to 0.5% of pregnancies. The majority (>90%) of low lying placenta diagnosed at 20 weeks resolve by term. Thus, a follow-up ultrasound in the third trimester, usually between 32 and 35 weeks, is warranted, as this information may influence delivery planning.

3. Growth Scan

This scan measures foetal head circumference (HC), foetal abdominal circumference (AC), femur length (FL), or biparietal diameter (BPD). It also measures amniotic fluid volume (AFI) and the estimated foetal weight (EFW).
Specific indications of growth scans include:

a. Growth-scan requests related to current pregnancy include:

- Concerns related to growth measurements
  - Static growth: no increase in sequential measurements
  - Slow growth: curve not following slope of any curve on the chart
  - Excessive growth: curve steeper than any curve on the chart
- Clinical suspicion of oligohydramnios or polyhydramnios
- Known or suspected foetal anomaly
- Late booker (20 + weeks gestation)

- Substance abuse
- Maternal smoking

b. Growth-scan requests related to obstetric history include:

- Previous birthweight(s) <5% customised centile
- Previous unexplained stillbirth

c. Growth-scan requests related to maternal medical history include:

- Pre-existing diabetes
- Chronic maternal disease

4. Foetal Doppler Studies in Obstetrics

Intrauterine growth restriction (IUGR) complicates 5–10% of all pregnancies and up to 30% of multiple pregnancies. In 60% of these pregnancies, the primary cause is placental insufficiency. Improvement in the identification of the foetus at risk of intrauterine death may lead to more successful management strategies.

What to Evaluate?

<u>Maternal Vessels</u>:

Uterine arteries

***Foetal Vessels*:**

Umbilical arteries

Middle cerebral arteries (MCA)

Ductus venosus

Umbilical vein

Common Indications for Doppler Flow Velocimetry Studies Include:

- Abnormalities of growth (both intrauterine growth restriction (IUGR) and excessive foetal growth (foetal macrosomia)
- Foetal anomalies (e.g. cystic hygromas, cardiac, thoracic, diaphragmatic, neural tube, renal and abdominal wall)
- Foetal hydrops
- Oligohydramnios (decreased amniotic fluid) and polyhydramnios (increased amniotic fluid)
- Poor obstetric history (e.g. pre-eclampsia, IUGR, previous stillbirth)
- Known maternal risk factors: hypertension, pre-eclampsia, diabetes, autoimmune disorders (overt and subclinical), thrombophilias (acquired and genetic)
- Abnormal maternal serum screening (e.g. elevated αFP and/or increased risk for foetal chromosomal abnormality)
- Multiple gestation

- Maternal trauma (foeto-maternal haemorrhage)
- Suspected placental abruption
- Known maternal isoimmunisation
- Exposure to parvovirus B19

Umbilical Artery Doppler should be available for assessment of the foeto-placental circulation in pregnant women with suspected severe placental insufficiency

Umbilical Artery Doppler to be performed if:

a. EFW $\leq$5% centile, or growth velocity has significantly reduced
b. Oligohydramnios, i.e. AFI <5 cm, single pocket <2 cm

Depending on other clinical factors, reduced, absent, or reversed umbilical artery end-diastolic flow is an indication for close foetal surveillance or delivery.

Umbilical artery doppler should not be used as a screening tool in healthy pregnancies, as it has not been shown to be of value in this group.

Middle Cerebral Artery (MCA) — Peak Systolic Velocity (PSV) Measurements

The gold standard for *foetal anaemia* assessment is foetal blood sampling. Unfortunately, this is the most invasive method and hence carries the highest risk. MCA PSV measurements may be carried out from 16–18 weeks' gestation up to 35 weeks. The MCA PSV is measured in the MCA closest to the maternal skin, with the foetal head in the transverse position. Other uses of MCA PSV are currently being investigated. These include applications in intrauterine growth restriction (IUGR), parvovirus, twin-to-twin transfusion, foeto-maternal haemorrhage, alpha thalassaemia and Kell allo-immunisation.

IUGR due to placental insufficiency is associated with chronic hypoxia, triggering a blood flow centralisation process in order to maintain blood flow to key organs such as the brain, chest and adrenal glands. Traditionally, this centralisation process has been identified as a reduction in the pulsatility index in the middle cerebral artery (MCA PI).

Ductus Venosus

The average shunting of blood through the ductus venosus normally decreases from 30% at 18–20 weeks to 18% at 31–34 weeks' gestation. The normal ductus venosus waveform pattern has a peak systolic, a peak diastolic and peak atrial velocity. The ductus venosus is the only venous vessel with forward flow during all phases of the cardiac cycle. With foetal deterioration, there is reversed flow during the atrial contraction of the ductus venosus and a markedly increased pulsatility index . This indicates a failure of compensatory mechanisms and the onset of right heart failure. Foetuses with reverse flow in the A-wave of the ductus venosus are not necessarily acidemic, and may survive for days to weeks *in utero*.

Chapter 30

APPROACH TO SCREENING SCAN FOETAL ABNORMALITIES

1. Head, neck and spine abnormalities
2. Abnormalities in the chest
3. Abnormalities in the abdomen
4. Abnormalities in the pelvis
5. Other ultrasound scan abnormalities

1. Head, Neck & Spine Abnormalities

Ultrasound Finding	Risk of Chromosomal Disorders	Action
Absent or short nasal bone (<4 mm) at 20 weeks	Likelihood ratio Down syndrome — 40-fold increase	• Offer karyotype
Absent vermis	Rarely diagnosed before 24 weeks	• Associated with loss of motor control, mental retardation
Acrania (absent cranium)	Lethal	• Offer termination • Preconceptual folic acid • Exclude DM
Anencephaly (absent partial brain & cranium)	Lethal	• Offer termination • Preconceptual folic acid • Exclude DM
Choroid plexus cyst (isolated)	• Risk only increased if presence of other abnormalities/ soft markers • Occurs in 1%. Usually resolves by 22–26 weeks	• Generally good prognosis if isolated finding
Cleft lip and/or palate	Increased risk of chromosomal disorders especially if presence of other structural abnormalities or bilateral cleft lip/ palate	• Offer karyotype • Prognosis good if isolated finding • Parental counselling with plastic surgeons — may require corrective surgery

(*Continued*)

(*Continued*)

Ultrasound Finding	Risk of Chromosomal Disorders	Action
Cystic hygroma (congenital malformation of lymphatic system)	Increased risk particularly Turner syndrome	• Offer karyotype • May be associated with hydrops, offer termination • Maternal and foetal investigations as per non-immune hydrops • Serial scans
Encephalocoele (failure of complete cranium closure with herniation)	Prognosis related to amount of herniated tissues and location	• Offer termination • Will require postnatal surgery if continuing pregnancy • May require *in utero* intervention e.g. if developed hydrocephalus • May be associated with Meckel-Gruber syndrome (autosomal recessive) • Preconceptional folic acid
Holoprosencepehaly (absence of forebrain development)	• Spectrum of disease — most are severe, leading to intrauterine death • May be associated with trisomy 13	• Offer termination • Offer karyotype
Intracranial calcification	Commonly associated with intrauterine infection	• TORCH investigation

(*Continued*)

(*Continued*)

Ultrasound Finding	Risk of Chromosomal Disorders	Action
Microcephaly (small foetal head)	Chromosomal risk not increased unless associated with other abnormalities	• Check for foetal alcohol syndrome, DM • Check infections e.g. varicella zoster, TORCH infection
Nuchal fold thickening in 2nd trimester (>6 mm after 15 weeks)	Likelihood ratio Down syndrome — 10-fold increase May be associated with Turner syndrome, Noonan syndrome, skeletal dysplasia, heart defect	• Offer karyotype • Screen for signs of hydrops • Serial scans at 28,32,36 weeks
Spina bifida (incomplete closure of spinal cord or its coverings)	No increased risk	• Prognosis/disability depends on level and length of defect, presence of neural tissue in meningeal sac • >90% long term survival • Parental counselling with neurosurgeon • Serial scans for polyhydramnios • Recurrence 1–5% • Preconceptual folic acid 5 mg
Ventriculomegaly (dilated lateral ventricles >10mm)	• 3–8% risk of aneuploidy • Likelihood ratio (LR) of Down syndrome — 9-fold	• Check cytomegalovirus (CMV) & Toxoplasmosis (Toxo) • Offer karyotype • Follow-up scans at 28 and 34 weeks • 10% risk of neurodevelopmental delay

2. Abnormalities in the Chest

Ultrasound Finding	Risk of Chromosomal Disorders	Action
Aberrant right subclavian artery (ARSA)	• Likelihood ratio Down syndrome — 20-fold increase • Increased risk of DiGeorge syndrome	• Offer karyotype & DiGeorge • May be associated with tracheal obstruction, swallowing difficulty
Congenital cystic adenomatoid malformation of lung (CCAM) New nomenclature is Congenital pulmonary airway malformation (CPAM)	No increased risk if isolated	• Prognosis depends on progression of lesions and presence of hydrops • Generally good prognosis if stable lesions • Serial scans • Small risk of requiring postnatal surgery • Postnatal CT scan of chest is recommended CXR is not reliable. *Differential diagnosis* • Bronchopulmonary sequestration (BPS) • Congenital diaphragmatic hernia (CDH).

(*Continued*)

(Continued)

Ultrasound Finding	Risk of Chromosomal Disorders	Action
Congenital diaphragmatic hernia (CDH)	• 10–20% increased risk of chromosomal disorders especially trisomy 18 • 50% have other structural abnormalities	• Offer karyotype • Variable prognosis — mortality may be up to 65% • Mortality increases if intrathoracic herniation of liver occurs • Joint counselling with neonatologists, paediatric surgeons • Planned delivery in tertiary centre
Congenital heart disease	• High risk of chromosomal disorders especially if AVSD • Increased risk of DiGeorge syndrome if conotruncal heart defects	• Offer karyotype ± DiGeorge • Joint counselling with neonatologists, cardiologists, paediatric surgeons • Foetal echocardiography • Serial scans • Planned delivery with neonatal team
Echogenic foci in ventricle of heart (hyperechogenicity attached to chordae tendinae)	No increased risk if isolated	• Most resolve spontaneously • If prominent and large, consider rhabdomyoma/ tuberous sclerosis
Pleural/pericardial effusion	Rare	• Maternal and foetal investigations as per non-immune hydrops including karyotype • Serial scans to monitor progression

3. Abnormalities in the Abdomen

Ultrasound finding	Risk of Chromosomal Disorders	Action
Absent stomach bubble	*Associated with oesophageal atresia 20% risk of chromosomal disorders if oesophageal atresia, VACTERL association	• Good prognosis if karyotype normal • Joint counselling with neonatal team • Pass nasogastric (NG) tube and chest X-ray (CXR) after delivery, avoid feeding
Calcification in liver	No increased risk if isolated	• Check for intrauterine infections — TORCH screen, Parvovirus • Generally good prognosis if isolated & stable
Choledochal cyst (cystic dilatation of bile ducts)	No increased risk	• Good prognosis • Risks of cholangitis and malignancy (2%)
Double stomach bubble	*Associated with duodenal atresia • 40% risk of chromosomal disorders (Down Syndrome) • 50% associated with other structural malformations	• Offer karyotype • Exclude other structural abnormalities • Joint counselling with neonatal team • Pass NG tube and CXR after delivery, avoid feeding

(*Continued*)

(*Continued*)

Ultrasound finding	Risk of Chromosomal Disorders	Action
Echogenic bowel (Grade 2 and above)	• Likelihood ratio of Down syndrome — 3–6-fold increase • Also associated with cystic fibrosis, foetal GIT bleeding, Cytomegalovirus (CMV) • Higher risk of foetal IUD, IUGR	• Offer karyotype if risk increased or presence of other structural abnormalities • DNA analysis for cystic fibrosis if positive family history • CMV screening • Serial scans — monitor growth, signs of foetal meconium peritonitis, foetal GIT bleeding
Gastroschisis (paraumbilical defect, free-floating bowel in amniotic cavity)	• Risk of chromosomal disorder low • <10% associated with other structural defects	• Karyotype not indicated if isolated finding • Exclude other structural abnormalities • Exclude substance abuse • Serial scans for growth, liquor, bowel appearance • Joint counselling with neonatologists, surgeons • Good prognosis > 80% survival • Increased risk of unexplained intrauterine death (IUD) near term • Surgical repair more urgent than omphalocele • Low recurrence risk

(*Continued*)

(Continued)

Ultrasound finding	Risk of Chromosomal Disorders	Action
Omphalocoele (persistence of herniation of gut — covered by peritoneum & amnion)	• 15–20% risk of chromosomal disorder • 60–80% associated with other structural defects	• Exclude other structural abnormalities • Offer karyotype • If normal karyotype → good prognosis, >75% survival • Require corrective surgery — joint counselling with neonatal surgeons • Serial scans — monitor growth restriction, polyhydramnios • Low recurrence risk
Single umbilical artery (SUA)	• No increased risk of chromosomal disorders. • Risk of intrauterine growth restriction (RR 2.1 fold)	• 0.2–2% of births • Exclude other malformations (10% association) • Good prognosis

4. Abnormalities in the Pelvis

Ultrasound Finding	Risk of Chromosomal Disorders	Action
Infantile polycystic kidneys (anhydramnios)	Autosomal recessive	• Poor prognosis • Offer termination

(Continued)

(*Continued*)

Ultrasound Finding	Risk of Chromosomal Disorders	Action
Multicystic dysplastic kidney disease	No increased risk	• Fatal if both kidneys affected • Survival depends on function of non-affected kidney • Serial scans at 28, 32, 36 weeks, weekly AFI thereafter
Pelvicalyceal dilatation (renal pelvis >5 mm) (if verified in 3rd trimester)	Low risk if isolated	• Karyotype not indicated if isolated finding • Serial scans — monitor progression, liquor volume • Only dilatations more than 10 mm after 28 weeks require postnatal exploration • Joint counselling with neonatologists
Renal agenesis	No increased risk	• Fatal if bilateral renal agenesis — offer termination

5. Other Ultrasound Scan Abnormalities

Ultrasound finding	Risk of Chromosomal Disorders	Action
Bilateral uterine artery notch on screening scan	Increased incidence of pregnancy-induced hypertension, pre-eclampsia and intrauterine growth restriction (IUGR)	• Monitor BP and growth of foetus • Can consider aspirin in high risk patients, e.g. advanced maternal age, past history of pre-eclampsia, bad obstetric history, high BMI, etc.

(*Continued*)

(*Continued*)

Ultrasound finding	Risk of Chromosomal Disorders	Action
Hydrops foetalis (accumulation of fluid in 2 or more serous cavities)	5% due to chromosomal abnormalities	• Maternal and foetal investigations for hydrops • Prognosis depends on underlying cause • Multidisciplinary care — neonatologists, cardiologists, surgeons • Treat underlying cause • Serial scans — monitor progression • May require *in utero* transfusions (if foetal anaemia suspected) • Planned delivery with neonatal team
Maternal pool in placenta	No increased risk	• Largely normal with good prognosis • Consider chorioangiomas/ tumours with possibility of haemorrhage/abruption • Growth scan — monitor growth and signs of hydrops
Oligohydramnios (reduced amniotic fluid volume) AFI < 5 cm or Single vertical pocket: <1 cm = severe 1 – 2 cm = mild	Increased risk if associated with other structural abnormalities or severe IUGR	• Exclude structural abnormalities/IUGR (look for foetal bladder/ kidney/stomach) • Offer karyotype if indicated • Exclude PPROM (leaking liquor) (counsel risks of pulmonary hypoplasia, limb contractures/absence of digits if PPROM <22 weeks)

(*Continued*)

(*Continued*)

Ultrasound finding	Risk of Chromosomal Disorders	Action
		• Infection screen • Prognosis depends on cause • Manage in tertiary centre
Polyhydramnios (pool depth > 8 cm or amniotic fluid volume (AFI) > 25 cm	Increased risk of T13, 18, 21	• Offer karyotype • Exclude structural abnormalities, e.g. tracheoesophageal fistula • Screen for diabetes • TORCH screen, Parvovirus • Thalassaemia screen • Manage in tertiary centre
Skeletal abnormalities/ Dysplasia	Low risk unless presence of other structural abnormalities	• Overall detection rate by ultrasound >90% • Lethality depends on rib cage involvement and pulmonary hypoplasia
Uterine shelf (free edge of uterine tissue within uterine cavity)	No increased risk Could mimic uterine septum	• Generally does not cause problems. Good prognosis • Consider chorioamniotic/ membrane separation • Monitor foetal growth • Increased risk of retained placenta

Chapter 31

LABORATORY VALUES IN NORMAL PREGNANCY

Normal physiological adaptations during pregnancy can alter biochemical results and should be taken into consideration before interpretation of results. In addition, the list below is comprehensive but not exhaustive.

Haematology

	Non-Pregnant Adult	First Trimester	Second Trimester	Third Trimester	Comments on the Effect of Pregnancy
Full Blood Count					
Haemoglobin (g/dL)	12.0–15.8	11.6–13.9	9.7–14.8	9.5–15.0	May ↓
Haematocrit (%)	35.4–44.4	31.0–41.0	30.0–39.0	28.0–40.0	↓
Mean cell volume (MCV) (fL)	80–100		80–100		↔
White blood cell count (x 10^9/L) - Neutrophils (x 10^9/L)*	3.5–9.1 1.4–4.6	5.7–13.6 3.6–10.1	5.6–14.8 3.8–12.3	5.9–16.9 3.9–13.1	WBC ↑ due to rise in neutrophils *Neutrophil levels increase by 35% 24 hours following administration of betamethasone. This is associated with a 25% decrease in lymphocyte count. The effect is transient and resolves back to baseline within 3 days
Platelets (x 10^9/L)	165–415	174–391	155–409	146–429	↓ or ↔

(Continued)

(*Continued*)

	Non-Pregnant Adult	First Trimester	Second Trimester	Third Trimester	Comments on the Effect of Pregnancy
Iron studies					
Iron, Serum (pmol/L)	7–25	13–26	8–32	5–35	Relatively ↔
Ferritin (pmol/L)	22–337	14–292	5–216	0–373	Generally ↓
Transferrin (μmol/L)	2.5–5	3.1–4.2	2.7–5.4	3.5–6.5	↔
Transferrin Saturation (%)	22–46	Not reported	10–44	5–37	↓
Folate, Serum (nmol/L)	12–41	6–34	1.8–54	3–47	↓ or ↔
Vitamin B12 (pmol/L)	206–713	87–323	96–484	73–388	↓
Coagulation Studies					
Partial thromboplastin time, activated (aPTT) (sec)	26.3–39.4	24.3–38.9	24.2–38.1	24.7–35.0	↓
Prothrombin time (PT) (sec)	12.7–15.4	9.7–13.5	9.5–13.4	9.6–12.9	↓
INR	0.9–1.04	0.89–1.05	0.85–0.97	0.80–0.94	↓

Inflammatory Markers

	Non-Pregnant Adult	First Trimester	Second Trimester	Third Trimester	Comments on the Effect of Pregnancy
C-Reactive Protein (CRP) (mg/L)	0.2–3.0	Not reported	0.4–20.3	0.4–8.1	May ↑ physiologically in the second trimester

Biochemistry

	Non-Pregnant Adult	First Trimester	Second Trimester	Third Trimester	Comments on the Effect of Pregnancy
Renal Function					
Urea (mmol/L)	2.5–7.5	2.8–4.2	2.5–4.1	2.4–3.8	↓
Creatinine (µmol/L)	65–101	52–68	44–64	55–73	↓
Potassium (mmol/L)	3.5–5.0	3.6–5.0	3.3–5.0	3.3–5.1	↔
Sodium (mmol/L)	136–145	133–148	129–148	130–148	↔
Chloride (mmol/L)	102–109	101–105	97–109		↔
Bicarbonate (mmol/L)	22–30	20–24			↓
Uric acid, serum (mmol/mL)	180–350	140–230	140–290	210–380	↓ In first and second trimester
24-hour urine total protein (g/24 hour)	<0.15	<0.3			
24-hour creatinine clearance (mL/min)	70–140	140–162	130–169	119–139	↑

(Continued)

(Continued)

	Non-Pregnant Adult	First Trimester	Second Trimester	Third Trimester	Comments on the Effect of Pregnancy
Liver Function					
Bilirubin (μmol/L)	0–17	4–16	3–13	3–14	↓
Bile acids (μmol/L)	0.3–4.8	0–4.9	0–9.1	0–11.3	Values will rise significantly after a meal so it is best to measure fasting level
Aspartate transaminase (AST) (IU/L)	12–38	3–23	3–33	4–32	↓
Alanine transaminase (ALT) (IU/L)	7–41	3–30	2–33	2–25	↓
Gamma-glutamyl transpeptidase (GGT) (IU/L)	9–58	2–23	4–22	3–26	↓

(Continued)

(*Continued*)

	Non-Pregnant Adult	First Trimester	Second Trimester	Third Trimester	Comments on the Effect of Pregnancy
Alkaline phosphatase (IU/L)	33–96	17–88	25–126	38–229	↑ (due to alkaline phosphatase from placental origin)
Albumin (g/L)	41–53	31–51	26–45	23–42	↓
Total protein (g/L)	67–86	62–76	57–69	56–67	↓
Others					
Amylase (IU/L)	20–96	24–83	16–73	15–81	↔

Note:

∗Blood tests to investigate for *severe pre-eclampsia* include serum creatinine, AST, ALT, uric acid, full blood count and coagulation studies.

∗*Acute fatty liver of pregnancy* (*AFLP*) is associated with elevated AST, ALT and bilirubin with associated decreased blood glucose level. Jaundice is rarely seen in other forms of pregnancy-related hepatic injury. There may also be prolongation of PT with low fibrinogen and low antithrombin levels which may be mistaken as disseminated intravascular coagulopathy — however, the coagulopathy of AFLP is due to decreased production of clotting factors by the liver rather than excessive consumption of clotting factors.

∗Unexplained abnormalities of ALT, AST, GGT and/or bile salts is considered sufficient to diagnose *obstetric cholestasis*. The increase in alkaline phosphatase in pregnancy is usually placental in origin and so does not normally reflect liver disease. However, other causes of abnormal liver function tests must first be excluded by thorough history and examination prior to making the diagnosis of obstetric cholestasis.

Endocrine Values

	Non-Pregnant Adult	First Trimester	Second Trimester	Third Trimester	Comments on the Effect of Pregnancy
Fasting blood glucose (mmol/L)	4.2–5.5	4.2–4.4	4.2–4.4	4–4.3	• Corticosteroids induce an increase in fasting maternal blood glucose to >5mmol/L for 4 days after the first course. • A standard 2-dose course of betamethasone may result in an abnormal glucose challenge test within 7 days of administration. • Administration of intravenous beta-agonist for tocolysis may cause a rise in serum blood glucose.
HbA_1c(%)	4–6	4–6	4–6	4–7	↔ or ↓ • HbA_1c is not a reliable indicator of glycaemic control in the second and third trimesters of pregnancy because of physiological changes that occur in all pregnant women which can lead to reduced HbA_1c in women without diabetes

(Continued)

(Continued)

	Non-Pregnant Adult	First Trimester	Second Trimester	Third Trimester	Comments on the Effect of Pregnancy
Thyroxine , free (fT4) (pmol/L)	9–26	10–16	9–15.5	8–14.5	↔ • In pregnancy, the values influenced by the serum thyroid binding hormone level (i.e. total thyroxine, total triiodothyronine, and resin triiodothyronine uptake) change significantly • hcg shows some cross-reactivity to TSH receptor and can stimulate production of thyroid hormones Therefore, in the first trimester, there is a possibility of gestational hyperthyroidism from increased hcg levels

(Continued)

(Continued)

	Non-Pregnant Adult	First Trimester	Second Trimester	Third Trimester	Comments on the Effect of Pregnancy
Triiodothyronine, free (fT3) (pmol/L)	2.6–5.7	3–7	3–5.5	2.5–5.5	↔
Thyroid stimulating hormone (TSH) (mU/L)	0.3–4.2	0–5.5	0.5–3.5	0.5–4	↔
Prolactin, serum (μg/L)	0–20	36–213	110–330	137–372	↑ with increasing gestation age

Lipids

	Non-Pregnant Adult	First Trimester	Second Trimester	Third Trimester	Comments on the Effect of Pregnancy
Cholesterol, total (mmol/L)	<5.2	3.7–5.4	4.6–7.7	5.7–9.0	↑ with increasing gestational age, mainly due to rise in LDL-cholesterol
– HDL-cholesterol (mmol/L)	1.04–1.55	1.04–2.02	1.35–2.25	1.24–2.25	↔
– LDL-cholesterol (mmol/L)	<2.6	1.6–4.0	2.0–4.8	2.6–5.8	↑
– VLDL-cholesterol (mmol/L)	0.16–1.0	0.26–0.46	0.34–0.60	0.54–0.93	↔
Triglycerides (mmol/L)	<1.7	0.45–1.8	0.85–4.3	1.5–5.1	↑ with increasing gestational age

Tumour Markers

	Non-Pregnant Adult	First Trimester	Second Trimester	Third Trimester	Comments on the Effect of pregnancy
CA 125 (U/mL)	<35	0–51.5	0–30.8	0–56.3	May ↑
Alpha-foetoprotein (αFP) (μg/L)	<15	19–119	96–302	160–550	↑ • ↑ αFP may be due to: 1. Pregnancy — physiologically up to 2.5 MoM — Multiple gestation 2. Foetal/placental abnormality — Placental abruption — Neural tube defect — Abdominal wall defect 3. Tumour — Germ cell tumours — Hepatocellular cancer • ↓αFP <0.5 MoM is associated with: — Down syndrome (T21) — Edward syndrome (T18)

Chapter 32

AN OVERVIEW OF SERUM HUMAN CHORIONIC GONADOTROPHIN (HCG)

- hcg is produced by trophoblastic cells
- Several isoforms of hcg exist in the circulation
  - 2 main forms are regular hcg and hyperglycosylated hcg (hcg-h)

Sources

Pregnancy

— Syncytiotrophoblasts produce regular hcg which promotes progesterone production by corpus luteum until placental progesterone production becomes established after 12 weeks of gestation

— Extravillous cytotrophoblasts produce hcg-h which promotes invasion of extravillous cytotrophoblast into the uterine wall to form anchoring villi and into the spiral arteries to create high flow, low resistance vessels

Gestational Trophoblastic Disease (GTD)

— Levels of serum hcg > 200 000 IU/L strongly suggest GTD
— hcg-h promotes trophoblast growth and invasion
— Invasion may be controlled as in implantation of a normal pregnancy and in complete/partial molar pregnancies or uncontrolled as in malignant choriocarcinoma

Pituitary Gland

— Normal pituitary gland produces a small amount of hcg (1–32 IU/L)
— May occur prior to ovulation and cause false positive result

Non-Trophoblastic Malignancy

— Breast, germ-cell, bladder, renal, prostate, lung, gastrointestinal, head and neck, haematological, and neuroendocrine origins

hcg Level in Pregnancy

- hcg level usually increases by at least 66% in 48 hours in a normal pregnancy

Gestation via last menstrual period	Levels of HCG (IU/L)
3	5–50
4	5–426
5	18–7340
6	1080–56 500
7–8	**7650–229 000**
9–12	**25 700–288 000**
13–16	13 000–254 000
17–24	4060–165 400
25–40	3640–117 000

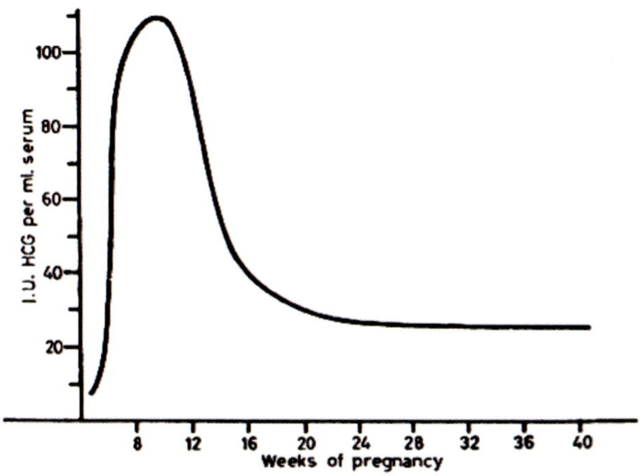

hcg level in pregnancy.

- hcg level peaks during 10–12 weeks gestation
- Decline of hcg to undetectable level after pregnancy
  - Depends on gestation (and hcg level) at the time of termination
  - Ranges from 7–60 days
  - Decline is rapid for the first several days (half life 9–31 hours), then more slowly (half-life 55–64 hours)

hcg Level in Relation to Spontaneous Miscarriage

- Level of hcg rises suboptimally (does not increase by at least 66% over 48 hours) or falls
- Level returns to negative by 2–4 weeks after surgical evacuation
- Persistent elevation of hcg should always raise the suspicion of choriocarcinoma or placental site trophoblastic tumour if retained products of conception have been ruled out
- Serum hcg level is not routinely measured after a spontaneous miscarriage unless patient has had a history of GTD or persistent vaginal bleeding

hcg Level in Relation to Gestational Trophoblastic Disease (GTD)

- Level >200 000 IU/L usually suggests GTD
- Level takes 99 days to normalise after a complete GTD and 59 days to normalise after a partial GTD

- Persistent GTD
  - 15–20% after complete GTD; 3–5% after partial GTD
  - Suspect if
    - (i) serum hcg reaches a plateau (decline of <10% for 4 values over 3 weeks)
    - (ii) serum hcg rises (increase > 10% of 3 values over 2 weeks)
    - (iii) persistence of detectable serum hcg for >6 months after molar evacuation
- 90% of persistent GTD are invasive mole, and <10% are choriocarcinomas

hcg Level in Relation to Ectopic Pregancy

- *Discriminatory zone* — An intrauterine gestational sac (IUGS) should be visible via *transvaginal ultrasound scan* at βhcg level of **1500 IU/L.** Conversely, absence of an intrauterine gestation at βhcg >1500 is termed pregnancy of unknown location (PUL), and a diagnosis of ectopic pregnancy has to be ruled out
- Most ectopic pregnancies have suboptimal hcg rise, BUT a normal rise in βhcg does not exclude an ectopic pregnancy ~ 20% of ectopic pregnancies can have a normal hcg rise
- Trending of βhcg level after Methotrexate (MTX) treatment

  - βhcg Days 5 and 12 after MTX administration and then weekly till negative to rule out persistent disease

- Trending of HCG level after surgical treatment
  - Weekly measurement of hcg is recommended after salpingostomy (tube preserved) till levels undetectable to rule out persistent disease
  - hcg is not routinely trended after salpingectomy

- Persistent levels of hcg after treatment of ectopic pregnancy
  - Failure of MTX treatment (15–25%)
  - Rare incidences of heterotopic pregnancy (concomitant intrauterine gestation and ectopic gestation) 1:7000 more commonly associated with artificial reproductive techniques

Beta hcg Test

- Earliest time of a positive hcg test is about 8 days after conception. However, this is only possible in about 5% of women.
- Most women have a positive hcg test by 11–12 days after conception, i.e. day 25–26 of last menstrual period

Urine hcg Test

- Qualitative test (positive or negative)
- Positive at levels of 25 IU/L

Serum hcg Test

- Quantitative test
- Lowest detectable level is 1.2 IU/L
- *False negative result*
    - "Hook effect" where extreme high levels may cause the antibodies to be saturated and result in an artifactually low value of hcg
    - Local laboratories have an automatic detector to perform the test at 1:1000 dilution when hcg level is >15 000 IU/L
    - Recent exposure to mononucleosis, patients with Ig A deficiency syndrome may have heterophilic antibodies leading to false positive result
    - Patients with previous history of gestational trophoblastic disease may also have subsequent false positive result

Part 3

GYNAECOLOGY

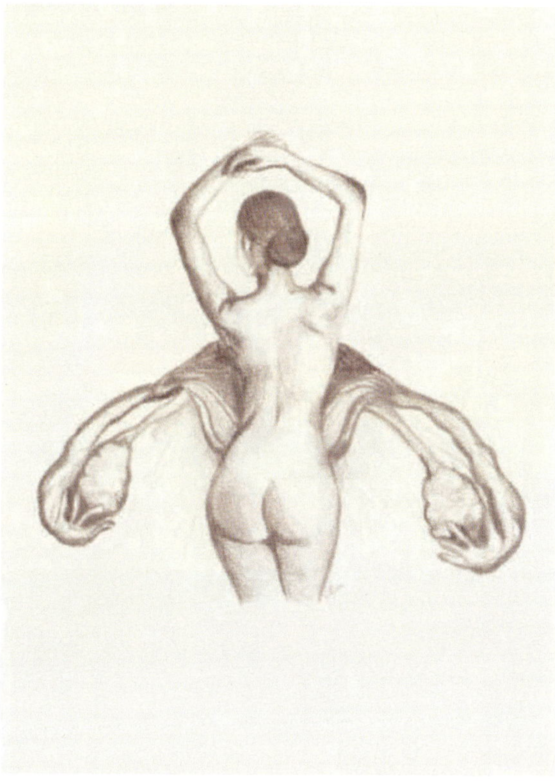

"Female" — 2013

Pencil on watercolour paper.

"She is the mermaid with her fish-tail dipped in the unconscious". — Anais Nin

Chapter 33

AMENORRHOEA

Primary Amenorrhoea

Definition

— Never experienced menstrual period by age 16

— Usually due to a genetic or anatomic condition

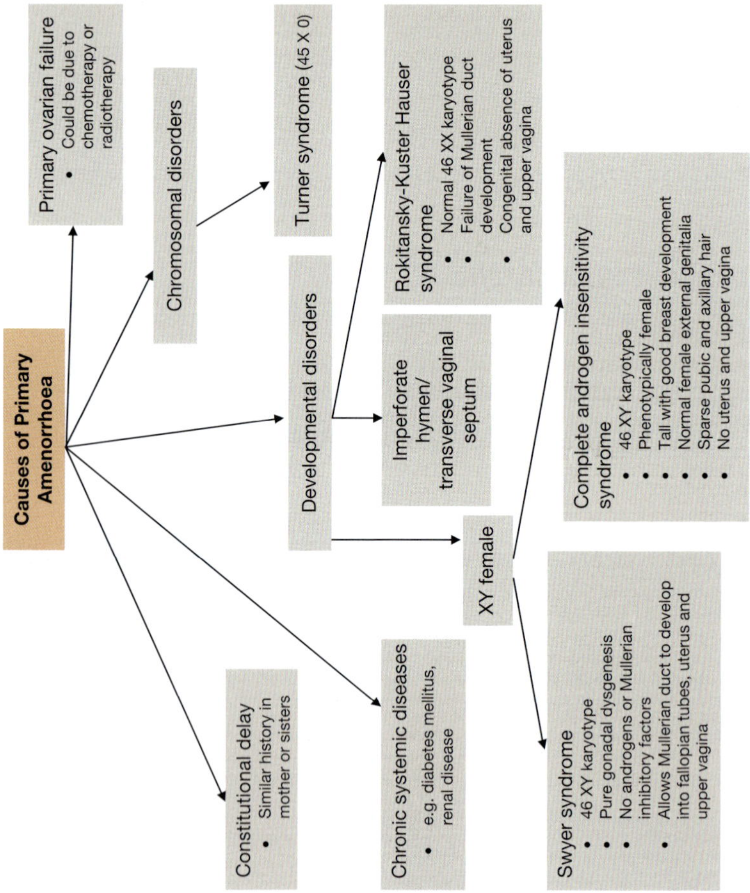
Causes of Primary Amenorrhoea
Primary ovarian failure
• Could be due to chemotherapy or radiotherapy
Chromosomal disorders
Turner syndrome (45 X 0)
Developmental disorders
Rokitansky-Kuster Hauser syndrome
• Normal 46 XX karyotype
• Failure of Mullerian duct development
• Congenital absence of uterus and upper vagina
Imperforate hymen/ transverse vaginal septum
XY female
Complete androgen insensitivity syndrome
• 46 XY karyotype
• Phenotypically female
• Tall with good breast development
• Normal female external genitalia
• Sparse pubic and axillary hair
• No uterus and upper vagina
Swyer syndrome
• 46 XY karyotype
• Pure gonadal dysgenesis
• No androgens or Mullerian inhibitory factors
• Allows Mullerian duct to develop into fallopian tubes, uterus and upper vagina
Chronic systemic diseases
• e.g. diabetes mellitus, renal disease
Constitutional delay
• Similar history in mother or sisters

Management of Primary Amenorrhoea

- **Refer to OBGYN** for investigations and management of primary amenorrhoea
- For constitutional delay, no treatment is needed except reassurance.
- For chromosomal disorders and primary ovarian failure, small dose of ethinyl oestradiol 1 µg daily can be started for 6 months, increasing to 2, 5, 10 and eventually 20 µg with increments at six monthly intervals. This is then followed by combined oral contraceptive pills.
- For vaginal and Mullerian agenesis, vaginal reconstruction is necessary. This can be achieved by vaginal dilators or surgical procedures like William's vulvo-vaginoplasty, McIndoe's procedure or skin graft.
- For XY female, counselling the parents is important to discuss psychological issues of gender of rearing and gender identity. Management includes gonadectomy as the dysgenetic testes have a high lifetime risk of malignancy (30%).

Secondary Amenorrhoea

Definition

Cessation of menses for >6 months in a woman who was previously menstruating.

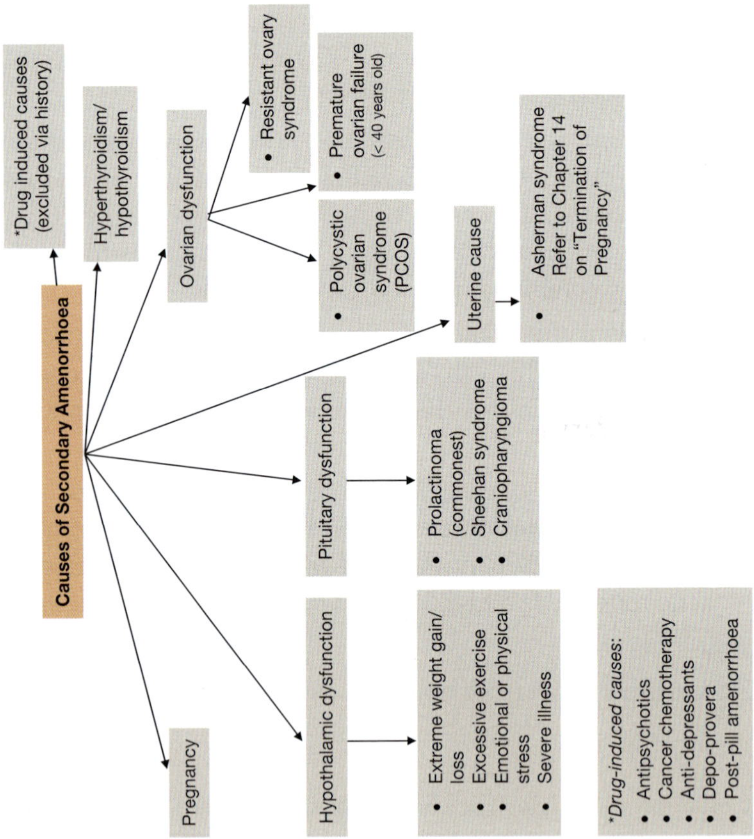
Causes of Secondary Amenorrhoea
Pregnancy
Hypothalamic dysfunction
• Extreme weight gain/ loss
• Excessive exercise
• Emotional or physical stress
• Severe illness
Pituitary dysfunction
• Prolactinoma (commonest)
• Sheehan syndrome
• Craniopharyngioma
Uterine cause
• Asherman syndrome Refer to Chapter 14 on "Termination of Pregnancy"
Ovarian dysfunction
• Polycystic ovarian syndrome (PCOS)
• Premature ovarian failure (< 40 years old)
• Resistant ovary syndrome
Hyperthyroidism/ hypothyroidism
*Drug induced causes (excluded via history)
*Drug-induced causes:
• Antipsychotics
• Cancer chemotherapy
• Anti-depressants
• Depo-provera
• Post-pill amenorrhoea

Investigations for Secondary Amenorrhoea:

1. Urine pregnancy test to exclude pregnancy.
2. Follicular stimulating hormone (FSH)/luteinising hormone (LH)
   - Suggests ovarian failure if FSH > 30 IU/L
   - Low levels suggest hypothalamic/pituitary dysfunction
   - Reversal of LH/FSH ratio > 3:1 suggests PCOS.
3. Serum prolactin level
   - Hyperprolactinaemia could cause secondary amenorrhoea.
4. Thyroid function test
   - Hyperthyroidism or hypothyroidism could cause secondary amenorrhoea.
5. Progestogen challenge test
   - Ensure not pregnant
   - Give oral norethisterone 5 mg bd for 5 days/Duphaston 10 mg om for 7 days
   - If there is withdrawal bleeding with progestogens, e.g. norethisterone, this indicates the presence of oestrogen. The patient would need cyclical progestogen for withdrawal bleeding to protect the endometrium from endometrial hyperplasia and carcinoma.
   - If there is no withdrawal bleeding with progestogen, then combined oral contraceptive pill would be needed for added oestrogen stimulation (oestrogen and progesterone challenge test).

- **Refer to OBGYN** for investigations and management of secondary amenorrhoea after excluding pregnancy
- Further treatment depends on the cause of the secondary amenorrhoea
- Prolonged amenorrhoea in young women causes decreased oestrogen levels resulting in bone loss (osteopenia/osteoporosis). Consider calcium supplementation to reduce boss loss.

Chapter 34

ABNORMAL UTERINE BLEEDING (AUB)

The normal menstrual cycle lasts between 21 and 35 days with menstrual flow lasting 2–7 days.

Definition of AUB

Any menstrual bleeding from the uterus that is either abnormal in volume (excessive duration or heavy flow), regularity, timing (delayed or frequent) or is non-menstrual (IMB, PCB or PMB).

Acute AUB	Excessive AUB bleeding that requires immediate intervention to prevent further blood loss
Chronic AUB	AUB has been present for the majority of the past 6 months

There was near unanimity for FIGO to recommend to discard the term "dysfunctional uterine bleeding" and to use AUB instead.

FIGO AUB Classification also recommends other terminologies which replace the earlier ones.

1. Heavy menstrual bleeding (HMB) previously — menorrhagia	HMB is defined as excessive menstrual blood loss leading to interference with the physical, emotional, social and material quality of life of a woman, and which can occur alone or in combination with other symptoms. Adverse outcome is greater in women with total menstrual blood loss (MBL) that exceeds 80 mL or menses duration exceeding 7 days
2. Intermenstrual bleeding (IMB)	Uterine bleeding that occurs between clearly defined cyclic and predictable menses
3. Postmenopausal bleeding (PMB)	Any uterine bleeding in a menopausal woman (other than the expected cyclic bleeding that occurs in women taking sequential postmenopausal hormone therapy). (Menopause is one year of amenorrhoea after the final menstrual period)
4. Postcoital bleeding (PCB)	Non-menstrual genital tract bleeding immediately (or shortly) after intercourse

Classification of AUB-FIGO

PALM:
polyp; adenomyosis; leiomyoma, malignancy or hyperplasia
Leiomyoma category (L) is subdivided:

- submucosal myoma (L_{SM})
- myomas that do not impact the endometrial cavity (L_O)

COEI:
coagulopathy; ovulatory dysfunction; endometrial; iatrogenic

N: not yet classified.

Polyp
Adenomyosis
Leiomyoma
Malignancy and hyperplasia

Sub**m**ucosal
Other

Coagulopathy
Ovulatory dysfunction
Endometrial
Iatrogenic
Not yet classified

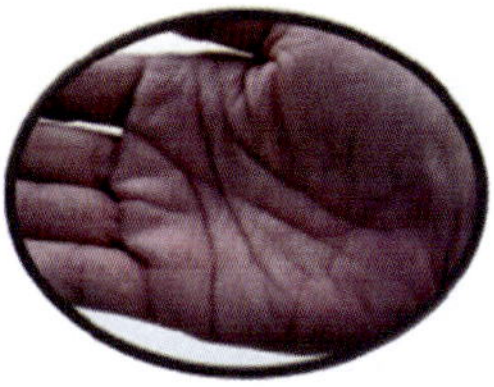

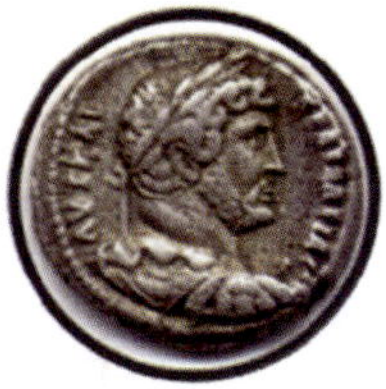

Approach to Management of AUB

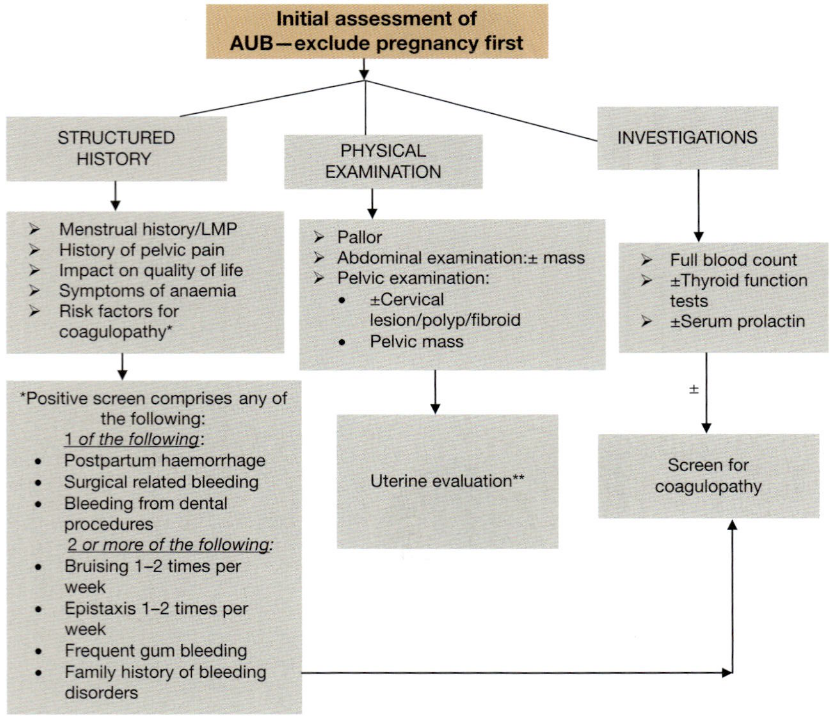

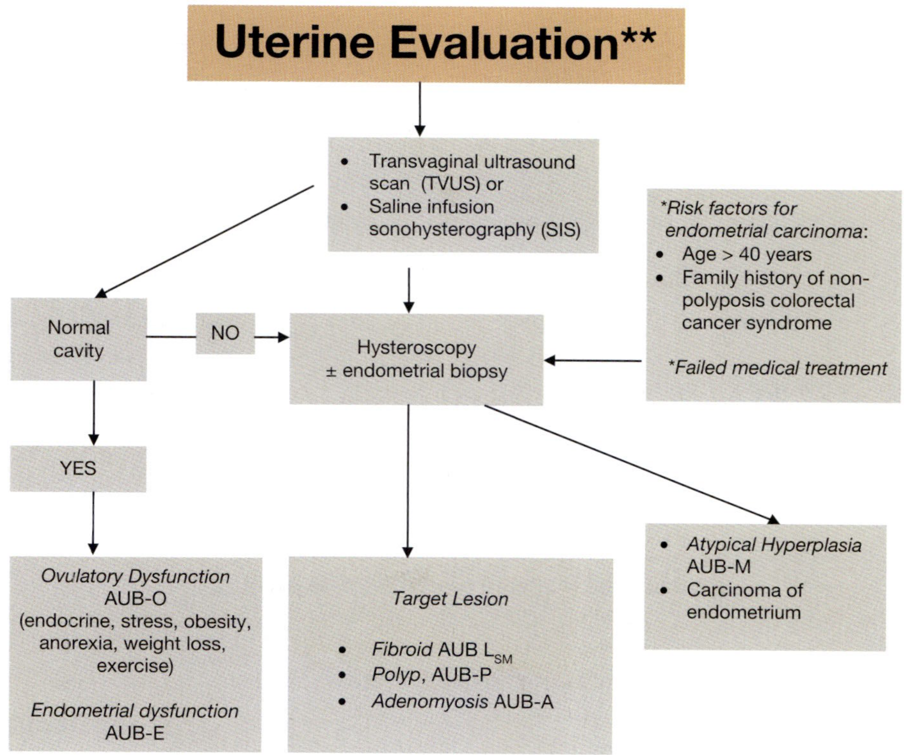
Uterine Evaluation**
Transvaginal ultrasound scan (TVUS) or
Saline infusion sonohysterography (SIS)
*Risk factors for endometrial carcinoma:
Age > 40 years
Family history of non-polyposis colorectal cancer syndrome
*Failed medical treatment
Normal cavity
NO
Hysteroscopy ± endometrial biopsy
YES
Ovulatory Dysfunction AUB-O (endocrine, stress, obesity, anorexia, weight loss, exercise)
Endometrial dysfunction AUB-E
Target Lesion
Fibroid AUB L SM
Polyp, AUB-P
Adenomyosis AUB-A
Atypical Hyperplasia AUB-M
Carcinoma of endometrium

Treatment for AUB

Treatment	Effect on Fibroid Size	Decrease in HMB	Effect on Fertility
1. First-step treatment (medical treatment)			
Tranexamic acid	Nil	30–50%	No effect
NSAIDs (e.g. mefenamic acid)	Nil	20–40%	No effect
Combined oral contraceptive (synthetic oestrogen)	—	40%	Contraceptive
Combined oral contraceptive Qlaira® (natural oestrogen)	—	90% after 6 cycles	Contraceptive
Oral progestogen (high-dose)	Nil	60%	No effect
Intrauterine progestogen (LNG-IUS)	Decrease 30%	70–100%	Contraceptive
GnRH analogues (3–6 months with/without add-back HRT)	Decrease 30%	60–100% (cause amenorrhoea in 80–90% of women)	Contraceptive
Progestogen-only implant (Implanon-NXT®) or Progestogen-only injectable (Depoprovera)®	—	30–100% (cause amenorrhoea in 15–20%)	Contraceptive

(Continued)

(*Continued*)

Treatment	Effect on Fibroid Size	Decrease in HMB	Effect on Fertility
2. Second-step treatment (minimally invasive uterus-conserving surgery)			
Hysteroscopic fibroid resection	Excision and removal of intracavitary fibroids	50–80%	Improved if submucous fibroid excised
Endometrial ablation	No effect	80%	No effect
Transcervical resection of endometrium	Will be able to excise and remove intracavitary fibroids	80%–100%	No effect
Laparoscopic myomectomy	Excise subserosal and non-deeply embedded intramural fibroids	No effect or may decrease up to 30%	May improve fertility
Uterine artery embolisation	Decrease 30%	60–80%	Not suitable if desires fertility
3. Third-step treatment/major surgery			
Abdominal myomectomy	Excise subserosal, intramural and intracavitary lesions	60–80%	May improve
Hysterectomy	Complete cure	Complete cure	Permanent, irreversible contraception

Goals of treatment for heavy menstrual bleeding (HMB)

- Alleviate acute bleeding. Give intramuscular progesterone 100 mg stat
- Prevent future episodes of non-cyclic bleeding. Aim to give a bleed which is predictable in timing and amount
- Decrease the risk of long-term complications, e.g. development of endometrial cancer

Medications Used for AUB

1) NSAIDs

e.g. Mefenamic acid 500 mg tds. Add antacids for gastric protection

2) Antifibrinolytic agents

e.g. *Tranexamic acid* 500 mg–1g tds
Side Effect — can cause venous thrombosis

3) Combined oestrogen and progestogen preparation

- Combined oral contraceptive pill (COCP)
- Qlaira® (oestradiol valerate/dienogest)
- Progyluton®

Qlaira®

- First oral therapy approved for heavy menstrual bleeding (HMB) with contraceptive effect
- Novel dosing regimen of 26 + 2 (i.e. 26 days of active pills and 2 days of placebo pills, which provides good cycle control)
- Reduces menstrual blood loss by 90% after 6 cycles of treatment
- Rapid and significant reduction of menstrual blood loss by 70% after two cycles
- Low discontinuation rate of 3% with favourable safety profile

Progyluton®

- Cyclical sequential combined hormonal replacement therapy with 2 mg oestradiol valerate for first 11 days and 2 mg oestradiol valerate with 0.5 mg norgestrel for next 10 days
- Regulates menstrual cycle and does not affect endogenous hormone production
- Does not interfere with ovulation
- Can be used by pre- and peri- menopausal patients

4) Cyclic progestogen (at least 10–14 days per cycle or up to 21 days)

- Norethisterone 5–10 mg bd
- Provera 5–10 mg bd
- Dydrogesterone (Duphaston® 10 mg bd)

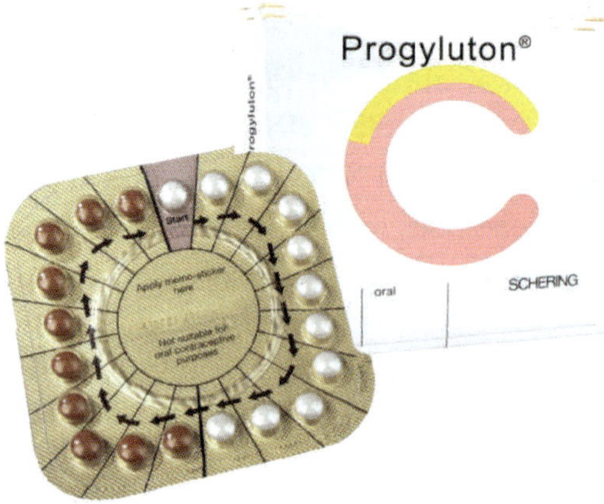

5) Mirena®/Levonorgestrel (LNG)-releasing intrauterine system

- Releases 20 mg of LNG daily which affects the endometrium locally
- Lasts 5 years
- Low local hormonal effect in the endometrium which provides shorter and lighter menses and reduces dysmenorrhoea
- 50% amenorrhoea after 1 year, 75–95% decrease in objectively measured MBL (mean blood loss)
- 20% intermittent per-vaginal spotting in first 6 months
- Lower risk of pelvic inflammatory disease and ectopic pregnancy as compared with copper-IUCD

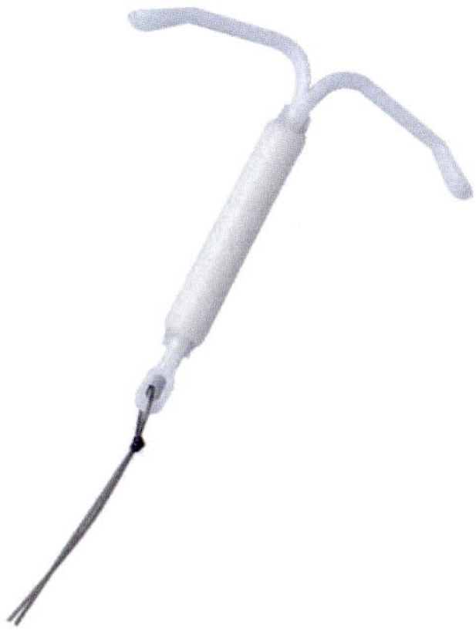

Mirena intrauterine system.

Compliance

	Mirena	No treatment
At 1 year	68% continued with Mirena	32% had hysterectomy
At 5 years	58% continued with Mirena	42% had hysterectomy
Cost-benefit analysis	Mirena was 40% cheaper than hysterectomy	

6) Gonadotrophin releasing hormone analogue (GnRHa)

- Continuous treatment with GnRHa causes down-regulation of pituitary gland and subsequent decrease in gonadotrophins and ovarian steroids
- Causes amenorrhoea (90%)

- *Side-effects* are related to hypooestrogenism and post-menopausal in type (hot flushes, insomnia, mood swings)
- Not recommended for more than 6 months of continuous usage due to the risk of osteoporosis unless used with hormonal add-back therapy
- Subcutaneous Zoladex (goserelin) 3.6 mg monthly, subcutaneous Lucrin (leuprorelin) 3.75 mg monthly/11.25 mg 3-monthly, intramuscular Decapeptyl (triptorelin) 3.75 mg monthly

7) Depot Provera®

- Intramuscular Depot Provera 150 mg 3 monthly
- Induce endometrial atrophy and amenorrhoea
- Irregular bleeding in first 3 months
- *Side-effects*: abdominal bloating, breast tenderness, weight gain, depression, water retention

8) Danazol

- Induce amenorrhoea in the majority if taken in moderate/high doses (>400 mg daily)
- If taken at low dose (200–400 mg daily), it will induce amenorrhoea in some while others may experience light but often unpredictable bleeding.

- *Masculinising side-effects*: hirsutism, acne, voice change (irreversible)

Surgical Management of AUB

- As a last resort for patients with failed medical treatment

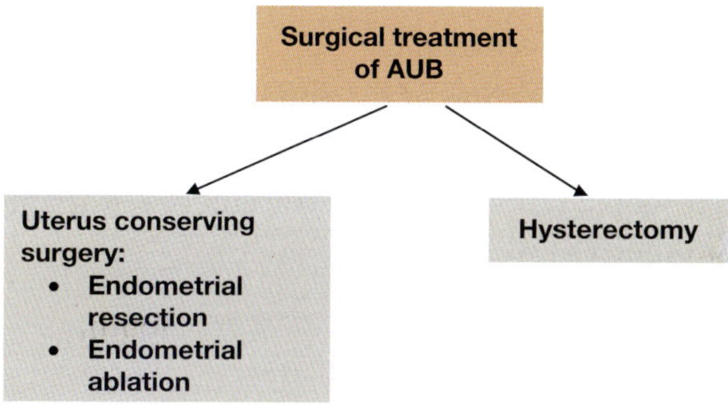

a. Endometrial resection and endometrial ablation

Prerequisite

- HMB is severe enough to affect quality of life
- the woman has completed her family
- uterine cavity length <10 cm
- with benign histology

Indications

- Failed medical treatment (including Mirena LNG-IUS) for menorrhagia
- Wish to conserve uterus

Techniques of endometrial ablation

1) *First-generation techniques*:

- Transcervical resection of the endometrium [TCRE]
- Ablation (rollerball) of the endometrium under direct hysteroscopic vision using electrocautery (either monopolar or bipolar).

Disadvantages

- Experienced operator required
- Complications dependent on both operator experience (e.g. uterine perforation) and method itself (e.g. dilutional hyponatraemia or fluid overload if using glycine uterine distension).

2) *Second–generation techniques*:

- Thermal balloon endometrial ablation (Thermachoice®)
- Impedance bipolar radiofrequency ablation (NovaSure®)
- Hydrothermablation (HydroThermAblator®)
- Endometrial cryotherapy (Her Option®)

Advantages

- Performed as day-surgery procedure
- Some can be under local anaesthesia (with or without sedation)

b. Hysterectomy

Indications

- Other treatment options have failed or are inappropriate
- Women have completed their families
- Desire for amenorrhoea

Chapter 35

ADOLESCENT ABNORMAL UTERINE BLEEDING (AUB)

Incidence and Facts

1. Mean age of menarche is about 12 years of age in Singapore
2. 50% of girls have irregular periods in first year after menarche
3. 50% of cycles are anovulatory
4. 20% of girls have irregular periods up to 5 years of menarche

Presenting Complaints

1. Unexpected and often heavy vaginal bleeding
2. Irregular periods every 3 to 6 months

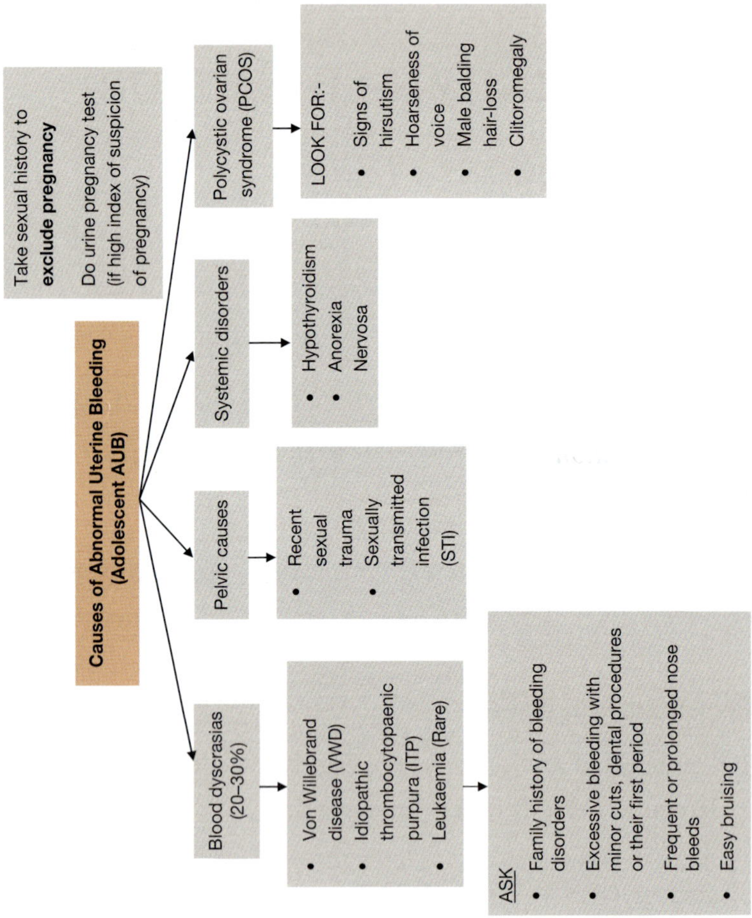
Take sexual history to exclude pregnancy
Do urine pregnancy test (if high index of suspicion of pregnancy)
Causes of Abnormal Uterine Bleeding (Adolescent AUB)
Blood dyscrasias (20–30%)
• Von Willebrand disease (VWD)
• Idiopathic thrombocytopaenic purpura (ITP)
• Leukaemia (Rare)
ASK
• Family history of bleeding disorders
• Excessive bleeding with minor cuts, dental procedures or their first period
• Frequent or prolonged nose bleeds
• Easy bruising
Pelvic causes
• Recent sexual trauma
• Sexually transmitted infection (STI)
Systemic disorders
• Hypothyroidism
• Anorexia Nervosa
Polycystic ovarian syndrome (PCOS)
LOOK FOR:-
• Signs of hirsutism
• Hoarseness of voice
• Male balding hair-loss
• Clitoromegaly

Investigations of Adolescent AUB:

1. *Full blood count* — useful to reveal anaemia and thrombocytopaenia
2. *Prothrombin time (PT), activated partial thromboplastin time (aPTT), and bleeding time* — if blood dyscrasias and clotting disorders suspected
3. *Urine pregnancy test* — must be performed even in patients who deny sexual activity if there is a high index of suspicion
4. *Cervical swabs* — to exclude chlamydia and gonorrhoea infection, especially if sexual activity is confirmed
5. *Thyroid-stimulating hormone (TSH) and free thyroxine concentration (fT4)* — to screen for thyroid disease
6. *Dehydroepiandrosterone sulfate (DHEAS), free testosterone* — to evaluate for PCOS
7. *VWF Ag (Von Willebrand factor antigen), VWF RCo (Von Willebrand factor ristocetin cofactor) and factor VIII* — if Von Willebrand disease is suspected
8. *Pelvic ultrasound scan* — to exclude pelvic pathology like fibroids and polycystic ovaries
9. *Hysteroscopy and uterine curettage* — *rarely* indicated in the adolescent with AUB. This procedure is usually reserved for women with significant and prolonged haemorrhage unresponsive to medical therapy.

Management of Adolescent AUB:

1. *Oral hematinics* if haemoglobin <11g/dL
2. *Oral tranexamic acid* (250 mg tds) to treat heavy bleeding days
3. *Add oral NSAIDs* (e.g. *mefenamic acid, 250 mg tds*) if bleeding persists
4. Consider *hormonal treatment* such as *oral contraceptive pills or cyclical progestins* [e.g. Dydrogesterone (Duphaston®) 10 mg on for 21 days].

Chapter 36

PREMENSTRUAL SYNDROME (PMS)

Definition of Different Types of Premenstrual Syndrome

Type	Definition
Premenstrual syndrome (PMS)	Cyclical symptoms leading up to menstruation and completely relieved by the end of menstruation
• **Mild**	No interference with personal/social and professional life
• **Moderate**	Suboptimal performance in personal/social/ professional life
• **Severe**	Withdrawal from personal/social/professional life
Premenstrual dysphoric disorders (PMDD)	Severe form of PMS in which symptoms of anger, irritability and internal tension are prominent

Epidemiology

- Affects 50%–75% of women with regular menstrual cycles
- Significant PMS affects up to 50% of women
- PMDD affects 5% of this group

Risk Factors

- Strong **genetic** component: preliminary evidence that PMDD is associated with genetic variation in the oestrogen receptor *alpha gene, ESR1*
- **Environmental** factors: cigarette smoking, history of traumatic events or anxiety disorder

Clinical Features of PMS

- **Symptoms** always start after ovulation, worsens as menstruation approaches, and resolves within the first few days of bleeding without recurrence until at least day 12 of cycle.
- **Physical:** breast swelling and discomfort, abdominal bloating, oedema, weight gain, headaches, extreme fatigue, deterioration in asthma, migraine or epilepsy
- **Emotional and behavioural:** aggression, anger, irritability, tearfulness, low mood, anxiety, altered eating habits, disturbed sleep, relationship difficulties, occupational problems

Diagnosis of PMS

- Prospective recording of symptoms, at least over two cycles; using a symptom diary as retrospective recall of symptoms is unreliable
- **Symptom free interval** from day 4 to 12 of the idealised 28 day menstrual cycle
- If symptoms persist **throughout** menstrual cycle, then an alternative diagnosis is likely e.g. mood or anxiety disorder

Assessment of PMS

- **History:**
  - focus on regularity of menstrual cycles
  - prospective symptoms inventories, e.g. **Calender of premenstrual experiences (COPE)**.
- **Physical examination**
- **Bloods:** not necessary for diagnosis of PMS or PMDD

CALENDAR OF PREMENSTRUAL EXPERIENCES

Name ______________________ Month/Year __________ Age ________ Unit # ________

Begin your calendar on the *first* day of your menstrual cycle. Enter the calendar date below the cycle day. Day 1 is your *first* day of bleeding. Shade the box above the cycle day if you have bleeding (■). Put an X for spotting (×).

If more than one symptom is listed in a category, ie, nausea, diarrhea, constipation, you do not need to experience all of these. Rate the most disturbing of the symptoms on the 1-3 scale.

Weight: Weigh yourself before breakfast. Record weight in pounds in the box below date.

Symptoms: Indicate the severity of your symptoms by using the scale below. Rate each symptom at about the same time each evening.

0 = **None** (symptom not present) 2 = **Moderate** (interferes with normal activities)

1 = **Mild** (noticeable but not troublesome) 3 = **Severe** (intolerable, unable to perform normal activites)

Other Symptoms: If there are other symptoms you experience, list and indicate severity.

Medications: List any medications taken. Put an X on the corresponding day(s).

Bleeding	■	■	■	×	×	×	×	×	×	×	×		×								
Cycle Day	1	2	3	4	5	6	7	8	9	10	11	12	13	14	15	16	17	18	19	20	21
Date	11/23	11/24	11/25	11/26	11/27	11/28	11/29	11/30	12/1	12/2	12/3	12/4	12/5	12/6	12/7	12/8	12/9	12/10	12/11	12/12	12/13
Weight	123	124	122	123	123	123	123	122	123	120	122	123	124	122	124	124	122	122	122	122	121
SYMPTOMS																					
Acne	1	1	1	1	1	1	1	1	0	1	1	0	1	1	0	0	0	1	1	1	1
Bloatedness	1	0	0	0	0	0	0	0	0	0	0	0	1	0	1	0	0	0	0	0	0
Breast tenderness	1	1	0	0	0	0	0	0	0	0	0	0	0	1	1	1	1	1	1	1	0
Cramping, abdominal	1	1	1	0	0	0	0	0	0	0	0	0	0	0	0	0	0	0	0	0	0
Fatigue	2	2	1	1	0	0	0	0	0	1	0	0	0	0	1	0	0	1	1	1	0
Headache	1	1	0	0	1	0	0	1	3	0	1	0	0	0	0	0	0	0	0	0	0
Swelling (hands, ankles, breast)	1	1	0	0	0	0	0	0	0	0	0	0	0	0	1	1	1	1	1	1	1
Angry outbursts, arguments, violent tendencies	0	0	0	0	0	0	0	0	0	0	0	0	1	0	0	0	0	0	0	0	0
Anxiety, tension, nervousness	2	0	0	0	0	0	0	0	0	0	0	0	1	1	1	1	1	1	1	1	1
Clumsiness	1	0	0	0	0	0	0	0	0	0	0	0	1	0	0	0	0	0	0	0	0
Confusion, difficulty concentrating	1	0	0	0	0	0	0	0	0	0	0	0	1	0	0	0	0	0	0	0	0
Crying easily	1	0	0	0	0	0	0	0	0	0	0	0	1	0	0	0	0	0	0	0	0
Depression	1	0	0	0	0	0	0	0	0	0	0	0	1	0	0	0	0	1	0	0	1
Food cravings (sweets, salts)	1	0	0	0	0	0	0	0	0	0	0	0	1	0	0	0	1	1	1	1	1
Forgetfulness	0	0	0	0	0	0	0	0	0	0	0	0	0	0	0	0	0	0	0	0	0
Irritability	1	0	0	0	0	0	0	0	0	0	0	0	1	1	1	0	0	1	1	1	1
Increased appetite	1	0	0	0	0	0	0	0	0	0	0	0	1	0	0	0	1	1	1	1	1
Mood swings	2	0	0	0	0	0	0	0	0	0	0	0	1	0	0	0	0	0	0	0	0
Sexual desire/activity change	0	0	0	0	0	0	0	0	0	0	0	1	1	1	0	0	0	0	0	0	0
Wish to be alone	1	0	0	0	0	0	0	0	0	0	0	0	1	0	0	0	0	0	0	0	0
Other Symptoms																					
1. Nausea	1	1	0	0	0	0	0	0	3	0	1	0	0	0	0	0	1	1	0	0	0
2.																					
Medications																					
1. Acetaminophen		×			×					×	×										
2. Aspirin/Butalbinal									×												
3. Pseudoephedrine															×	×					

Treatment of PMS

FIRST LINE	Exercise, diet, stress reduction Cognitive behavioural therapy, vitamin B6 dose (100 mg om) Combined new generation pill e.g. Yaz® (cyclical or continuous) Continuous or luteal phase (day 15–28) low dose SSRI

↓

SECOND LINE	Oestradiol patches (100 mcg) with oral progestogens Day 17–28 Higher dose SSRI continuously or in luteal phase

↓

THIRD LINE	GnRH analogues with addback HRT (continuous combined oestrogen and progesterone or tibolone) (if used for more than 6 months)

↓

FOURTH LINE	Hysterectomy and bilateral oophorectomy with addback HRT (including testosterone)

- Consider referral to a psychiatrist if women have marked underlying psychopathology

Selective Serotonin Reuptake Inhibitors (SSRIs)

- Overall response rate: 60–75%
- Superior in relieving both common physical symptoms and mood symptoms
- *Possible side effects*: headache, anxiety, nausea — incidence about 15%
- SSRI treatment should be prescribed by psychiatrists and used with caution

- Gradual withdrawal is needed if given on a continuous basis
- Luteal phase therapy has the advantage of being less expensive and has fewer side effects, but higher dose of SSRI might be needed in some women to adequately treat physical symptoms
- Examples:
  - fluoxetine 20–60 mg/day
  - sertraline 50–150 mg/day
  - paroxetine 20–30 mg/day
  - citalopram 20–30 mg/day

GnRH Analogues

- "Medical oophorectomy"
- Side effects related to hypoestrogenism including hot flushes and loss of bone mineral density
- The efficacy of GnRH analogues is maintained when low-dose oestrogen and progesterone are added back. However, it is essential that oestrogen and progesterone are given in a continuous fashion and not as a cyclical regime, as the latter may reproduce PMS symptoms
- Long-term use of GnRH agonists is possible with oestrogen-progesterone addback with no loss of bone mineral density and continuous resolution of symptoms.

Chapter 37

DYSMENORRHOEA

Causes

1. Primary — no pelvic pathology, usually in perimenarche
2. Secondary
   a. Endometriosis
   b. Adenomyosis
   c. Fibroids
   d. Pelvic inflammatory disease
   e. Uterine abnormalites — non-communicating accessory uterine cavity with functioning endometrium
   f. Cervical stenosis
   g. Pelvic congestion syndrome

1. Typical Symptoms of Primary Dysmenorrhoea

a. Menstrual pain — crampy or dull
b. Localised to lower quadrants of abdomen
c. Associated with nausea/vomiting/fatigue/backache/dizziness/diarrhoea
d. Occurs at onset or a few days prior to onset of menses and persists for one to three days
e. Usually young

2. Typical Symptoms of Secondary Dysmenorrhoea

a. Onset after ovulatory cycles become established
b. Crampy — intermittently intense menstrual pain/continuous dull aching pain
c. Lower abdominal in location, usually midline
d. Associated with nausea, fatigue, diarrhoea, headache

3. Findings Suggestive of Pelvic Pathology Consistent with Secondary Dysmenorrhoea include:

a. Onset of non-midline pelvic pain
b. Abnormal uterine bleeding
c. Dyspareunia/dyschezia
d. Progression in severity

Management of Dysmenorrhoea

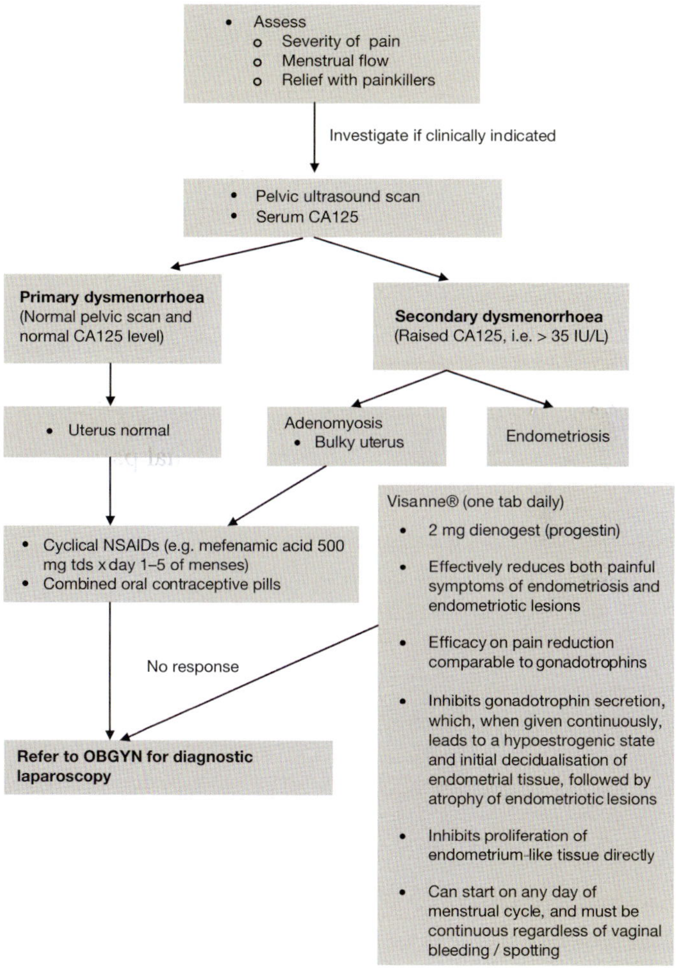

Chapter 38

CHRONIC PELVIC PAIN (CPP)

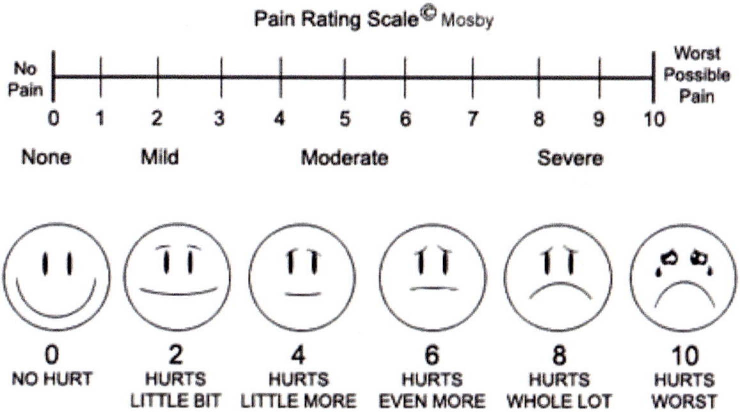

Pain Score Chart.

CAUSES OF CHRONIC PELVIC PAIN

Gynaecological Causes
- Endometriosis Adenomyosis (pain varies markedly over the menstrual cycle)
- Pelvic adhesions
- Pelvic inflammatory disease (PID)
- Advanced gynaecological malignancy

Urinary Causes
- Chronic urinary tract infection
- Interstitial cystitis

Gastrointestinal Causes
- Irritable bowel syndrome

Other Causes
- Musculoskeletal
- Pelvic organ prolapse
- Nerve entrapment in scar tissue, fascia, narrow foramen

Investigations for Chronic Pelvic Pain

- Pelvic ultrasound to exclude pelvic pathology like endometriotic cyst or adenomyosis
- Magnetic resonance imaging (MRI)
- Screen for infection (refer to Chapter 54 on "Pelvic Inflammatory Disease")
- Urine microscopy and culture to exclude chronic urinary tract infection
- Diagnostic laparoscopy to exclude pelvic endometriosis, adhesions, etc.

Management of Chronic Pelvic Pain

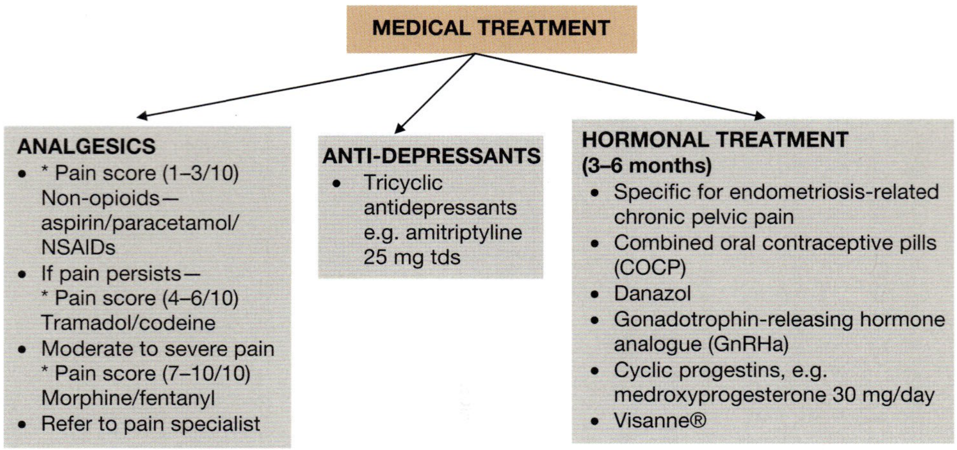

Refer to OBGYN if

- Evidence of pelvic pathology like endometriotic cyst or adenomyosis
- Failed first-line medical treatment
- Chronic pelvic pain related to menstrual cycle

Consider Laparoscopy

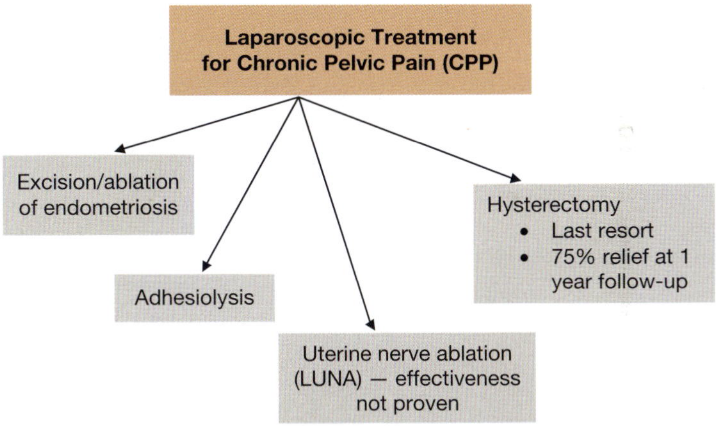

Other Treatments

- Transcutaneous nerve stimulation
- Acupuncture

Chapter 39

POLYCYSTIC OVARIAN SYNDROME (PCOS)

Definition based on the Rotterdam Criteria

- Polycystic ovaries (either 12 or more peripheral follicles or increased ovarian volume greater than 10 cm^3)
- Oligo- or anovulation
- Clinical and/or biochemical signs of hyperandrogenism
  - Clinical: hirsutism, acne or male balding pattern
  - Biochemical: high serum androgen concentration

Fulfillment of **two of the three** above criteria is diagnostic of PCOS

Epidemiology

- Occurs in 5–10% of women

High Risk Groups

- Women with anovulatory infertility
- Obesity or insulin resistance
- Type I or II diabetics
- First-degree relatives with PCOS

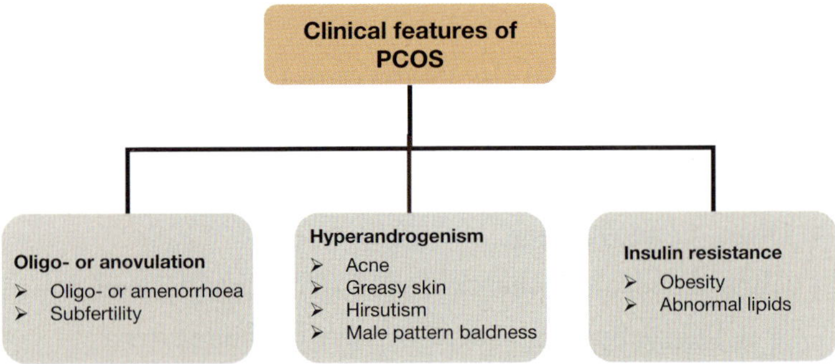

Assessment of PCOS

- **History**
  - Menstrual history: usually **oligomenorrhoea or secondary amenorrhoea**
  - Obstetric history: possible subfertility, recurrent miscarriages, gestational diabetes

- Past medical history: possible diabetes mellitus or hyperlipidaemia or cardiovascular disease
- Others: complaints of daytime fatigue, hypersomnolence, weight gain, hirsutism, acne, male pattern balding

• Physical Examination

- Body mass index (BMI): obesity is common
- Blood pressure
- Acne
- Hirsutism

• Investigations

Blood tests

- Female hormone profile (not necessary for diagnosis)
  - ↑ LH:FSH ratio> 3:1
  - testosterone ≥2.5 nmol/L
- Serum FSH, thyroid function tests and prolactin are usually normal
- If testosterone ≥5 nmol/L, and clinical evidence of hyperandrogenism is present, 17-hydroxyprogesterone should be sampled and androgen-secreting tumours should be excluded

- If clinical suspicion of Cushing syndrome, this should be further investigated
- Offer oral glucose tolerance test if obese (BMI ≥ 30), age ≥40 or strong family history of type II diabetes mellitus

Ultrasound scan of pelvis (required for diagnosis)

- Typical features of polycystic ovaries

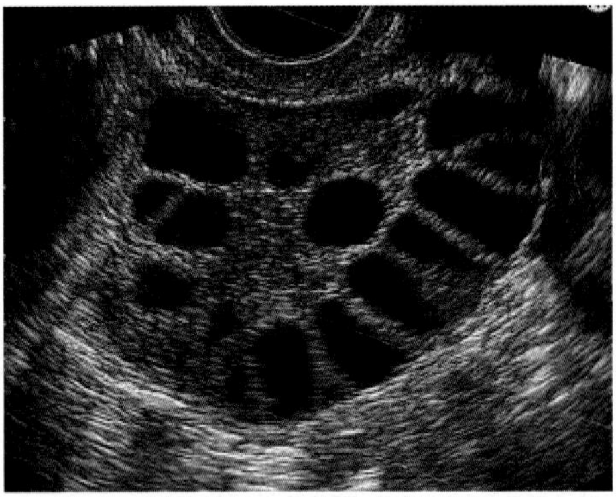

Appearance of polycystic ovaries containing more than 12 follicles arranged at the periphery of a dense stroma core.

Management of PCOS

- Treatment should be individualised based on

- o Severity of symptoms
- o Desire for fertility

Management of PCOS

Conservative

- ➢ **Lifestyle changes**
  - Diet
  - Exercise
- ➢ Loss of 5% of body weight has been reported to result in
  - Spontaneous resumption of ovulation
  - Improvement in fertility

Medical

- ➢ **Menstrual regulation**
  - Combined oral contraceptive pills (COCP)
  - Consider Diane-35® if concurrent treatment for hirsutism and acne is needed
- ➢ **Subfertility**
  - Ovarian stimulation with **clomifene citrate or laparoscopic ovarian drilling**
- ➢ **Insulin resistance**
  - **Metformin** has been suggested to reduce insulin resistance

Use of clomiphene citrate

- Action: Increases production of gonadotrophins by inhibiting negative feedback on hypothalamus
- Indication: subfertility
- Success: 40–60% conception rate after 6 months
- *Common side effects*: hot flushes, abdominal discomfort, dose dependent visual blurring
- Ovarian hyperstimulation syndrome occurs in 1% of these women

- Starting dose: 50 mg daily from day 2–6 of cycle. Adjust the dose according to response. Maximum dose is 150 mg per day.
- Limit to 6 ovulatory cycles due to increased risk of ovarian cancer from repeated ovarian stimulation
- *Indications*
  - Anovulatory infertility
    - Appears to be similar to laparoscopic ovarian drilling for inducing ovulation
- Does not increase risk of major malformations when used in first trimester of pregnancy

Use of Metformin

Indications

First line medical therapy after weight loss

- Anovulatory infertility
- Usually used with clomiphene citrate
- Useful if evidence of glucose intolerance
- Appears to be similar to laparoscopic ovarian drilling for inducing ovulation
- Common side effects: diarrhoea, nausea, vomiting, indigestion, flatulence, abdominal discomfort

- Does not increase risk of major malformations when used in first trimester of pregnancy
- Dose used: 500 mg bd or tds

Laparoscopic Ovarian Drilling

- Unknown mechanism of action
- Usually after failed clomiphene treatment
- Pregnancy rates: ~80%
- *Disadvantage*: surgical and anaesthetic risks, postoperative adhesion, theoretical risk of premature ovarian failure
- Similar efficacy with gonadotrophin treatment.

Long-term Complications of PCOS

- Type 2 diabetes mellitus
- Cardiovascular disease including hypertension and hyperlipidaemia
- Gestational diabetes
- Endometrial hyperplasia and possible carcinoma. (Refer to Chapter 46 on "Thickened Endometrium").

Commonly Used Medications for Treatment of PCOS

				Efficacy				
Drug	Example	Active ingredient	Mechanism	Hirsutism	Menstrual Irregularity	Insulin Lowering	Indications	Comments
Combined oral contraceptive pill (COCP)	Diane 35®	Ethinyl oestradiol 35 µg ÷ cyproterone acetate 2 mg	Suppress ovarian function	+	+		Menstrual irregularity, hirsutism	Contraindicated in patients with venous thrombosis, uncontrolled hypertension
	Yasmin®	Ethinyl oestradiol 30 µg ÷ drospirenone			+			
Progestin	Provera®	Medroxy-progesterone acetate	Suppress gonadotrophin		+		Menstrual irregularity	Less efficacious than COCP
	Duphaston®	Dydrogesterone						
Gonado-trophin releasing agonists	Depot Lucrin®	Leuprolide acetate depot	Suppress gonadotrophin	+	+		Alternative to COCP	Contraindicated in patients with osteoporosis without hormonal add-back therapy

(Continued)

(*Continued*)

				Efficacy				
Drug	Example	Active ingredient	Mechanism	Hirsutism	Menstrual Irregularity	Insulin Lowering	Indications	Comments
Antiandrogens	Spironolactone	Spironolactone	Competitive inhibitor of androgen receptor binding	+	+/–		Severe hirsutism	Use only with appropriate contraception because of adverse effects on foetus. Contraindicated in kidney or liver failure
	Cyproterone acetate	Cyproterone acetate	Competitive inhibitor of androgen receptor binding	+	+/–		Severe hirsutism	Use only with appropriate contraception because of adverse effects on foetus
	Finasteride	Finasteride	Competitive 5α reductase inhibitor	+	+/–		Severe hirsutism	Use only with appropriate contraception because of adverse effects on foetus
Biguanide	Glucopage® Glucopage XR®	Metformin	Reduces hepatic glucose production		+/–	+	Obesity and insulin resistance; type II DM	Efficacy poor without weight control
Selective oestrogen receptor modulator	Clomid®	Clomiphene citrate	Increase production of gonadotrophins by inhibiting negative feedback on hypothalamus				Subfertility	Be aware of ovarian hyperstimulation syndrome and multiple pregnancy. Maximum of 6 ovulatory cycles: risk of ovarian carcinoma from repeated ovarian stimulation

Chapter 40

APPROACH TO GYNAECOLOGICAL CANCERS

In Singapore, cancer ranks as the top cause of death. Gynaecological cancers such as cancer of uterus, ovary and cervix are ranked 4th, 5th and 9th respectively, among the 10 most frequent cancers in Singapore females from 2007 to 2011.

Special Considerations

a. *Fertility-sparing treatment in gynae-oncology*

As women delay childbearing, there is an increase in diagnosis of cancer in women still desiring fertility. Fertility-sparing treatment is hence becoming more important but it should not compromise on survival.

b. *Cancer in pregnancy*

Some women develop cancer while pregnant. The incidence is 1 in 1000 and the most common cancers are cervical cancer, breast cancer and melanoma. The patient should be cared for and counselled by a multidisciplinary team. Management decisions will be based on a few factors, including the gestational age at diagnosis, stage of disease, mother's autonomy regarding treatment options and future childbearing desire. The benefits of treatment to the mother should be weighed against the risks of treatment in pregnancy.

1. Carcinoma of the Cervix

Type of Cancer	Risk Factors	Protective Factors	Histological Subtypes	Screening
Cervix 9th most frequent cancer in Singapore females Lifetime risk 0.68% High-risk age group: 30–34 and 80–84 years old	– HPV infection – Multiple sexual partners – Early age of sexual debut – Smoking – Immune suppression – COCP use >5 years – DES exposure – Family history	– Cervical screening (Pap smear) – HPV vaccines-Cervarix®, Gardasil®	• *Squamous* (70–80%) • Others include adenocarcinomas (15%), small cell neuroendocrine, adenosquamous	Cervical smear screening

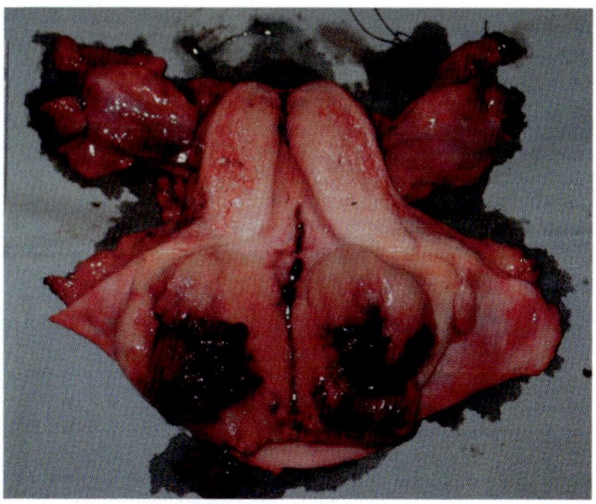

Carcinoma of the cervix.

Carcinoma of the Cervix (*Continued*)

Presenting Symptoms & Physical Examination	Investigations	Treatment	Fertility Preservation
Presenting symptoms: — Irregular vaginal bleeding — Post-coital bleeding — Dyspareunia — Vaginal discharge — If advanced: pain, loss of weight/appetite *Physical examination:* — May be normal in microinvasive disease — Cervical abnormalities include gross erosion, ulcer, or friable, irregular mass with contact bleeding	Colposcopy and cervical biopsy *Cancer staging:* EUA, cystoscopy, proctoscopy *Imaging:* — CXR — U/S pelvis — CT abdomen — MRI pelvis — PET-CT scan where indicated	Early stage disease ($1A_1$–$2A_2$): surgery Postoperative adjuvant radiotherapy if indicated Locally advanced disease (2B & 4A): chemoradiation, radical radiotherapy. Metastatic/ recurrent disease: chemoradiation, systemic chemotherapy, palliative surgery	Stage $1A_1$ — large cone biopsy with clear margins. Stage$1A_2$–$1B_1$– radical trachelectomy with pelvic lymph node sampling

PCOS — Polycystic ovarian syndrome; AGUS — Atypical glandular cells of undetermined significance; HPV — Human papilloma virus; COCP — Combined oral contraceptive pills; DES — Diethylstilbestrol; MRI — Magnetic resonance imaging; EUA — Examination under anaesthesia

2. Carcinoma of the Fallopian Tube

Type of Cancer	Risk Factors	Histological Subtypes	Screening
Fallopian tube High-risk age group: 5th – 6th decade	— Nulliparity — History of infertility	Epithelial, adenocarcinomas, sarcomas, secondaries	No proven screening tool at present

Carcinoma of the Fallopian Tube (*Continued*)

Presenting Symptoms & Physical Examination	Investigations	Treatment	Fertility Preservation
Presenting symptoms — Asymptomatic — Classical triad of abdominal pain, hydrops tubae profluens, pelvic mass — Finding in hysterectomy specimen — Abnormal vaginal bleeding — Urinary or bowel symptoms — Unexplained abnormal cervical cytology (e.g. AGUS smear) *Physical examination:* — Pelvic mass — Profuse watery vaginal discharge — Ascites	*Laboratory:* — CA125 *Imaging:* — CXR — U/S Pelvis — CT abdomen/ pelvis	Management principles similar to ovarian cancer Primary debulking surgery, adjuvant chemotherapy if indicated	Unilateral salpingo-oophorectomy in Stage 1A, grade 1

3. Carcinoma of the Ovary

Type of Cancer	Risk Factors	Protective Factors	Histological Subtypes	Screening
Ovary — 5th most frequent cancer in Singapore females Lifetime risk 1–2% High-risk age group: 60–70 years old	— Nulliparity — Infertility — Endometriosis — Previous history of breast, uterine or colorectal cancer — Strong family history (5–10% has inherited predisposition of breast and ovarian cancer (BRCA 1 and 2) and colon cancer (HNPCC 2)	— Pregnancy — Breastfeeding — Use of combined oral contraceptive pills (COCPs) — Salpingectomy/ Tubal ligation	*Epithelial ovarian cancers* (80%). • Most common subtype is serous (50%) followed by endometrioid, mucinous, clear cell, transitional, mixed and undifferentiated. *Sex cord-stromal tumours* (7%). • 70% are granulosa cell tumours, secretes oestrogen potentially leading to endometrial hyperplasia and carcinoma. • Other subtypes include: Sertoli-Leydig cell tumours and gynandroblastomas *Malignant germ cell tumours*. • Occurs mostly in young females. • Dysgerminoma is most common (others: yolk sac tumour, embryonal carcinoma, polyembryoma, non-gestational choriocarcinoma and immature teratoma).	No good screening test at present. Most commonly used are CA 125 and U/S pelvis Trials have not shown that screening for ovarian cancer is effective BRCA testing may be done in women at high risk Salpingo-oophorectomy in women who have a mutation in the BRCA1 and BRCA2 genes may reduce the risk of developing ovarian cancer, although there is still a risk of primary peritoneal carcinoma

Carcinoma of the Ovary (*Continued*)

Presenting Symptoms & Physical Examination	Investigations	Treatment	Fertility Preservation
Presenting symptoms: — Pelvic or abdominal pain — Abdominal distension — Early satiety — Changes in bowel habit — Urinary frequency *Physical examination*: — Often normal — In advanced disease: Cachexia — Abdominal or pelvic mass — Ascites.	*Laboratory*: Ovarian cancer profile (CA125, βhcg, CEA, AFP, LDH. Levels are difficult to interpret in pregnancy) *Imaging*: — U/S pelvis — CXR — CT scan abdomen/pelvis (and thorax if clinically indicated) *Histopathology*: Cytology of ascitic or pleural fluid	*Surgery* Staging laparotomy, peritoneal washings, THBSO, omentectomy and pelvic lymphadenectomy Appendicectomy if mucinous tumour *Chemotherapy* (first-line: platinum-based drug with taxane, second-line doxorubicin, topotecan, etc.) *Novel chemotherapeutic agents* may be considered if failed conventional treatment or recurrent disease. (targeted treatment such as bevacizumab)	8% of stage 1 epithelial ovarian cancers <35 years Disease confined to one ovary: unilateral salpingo-oophorectomy, omental biopsy, ipsilateral pelvic lymph node dissection May require adjuvant chemotherapy. (may try to conceive 6 months after completion)

BRCA 1,2 — Tumour suppression gene. A mutation in this gene is associated with a high risk of breast and other cancers; HNPCC — Hereditary non-polyposis colorectal cancer; COCP — Combined oral contraceptive pill; CA 125 — Carbohydrate antigen 125; βhcg — Beta human chorionic gonadotrophin; CEA — Carcinoembryonic antigen; AFP — Alpha-fetoprotein; LDH — Lactate dehydrogenase; U/S — Ultrasound; CXR — Chest X-ray; CT — Computed tomography; THBSO — Total hysterectomy bilateral salpingo-oophorectomy; GnRHa — Gonadotrophin releasing hormone analogues

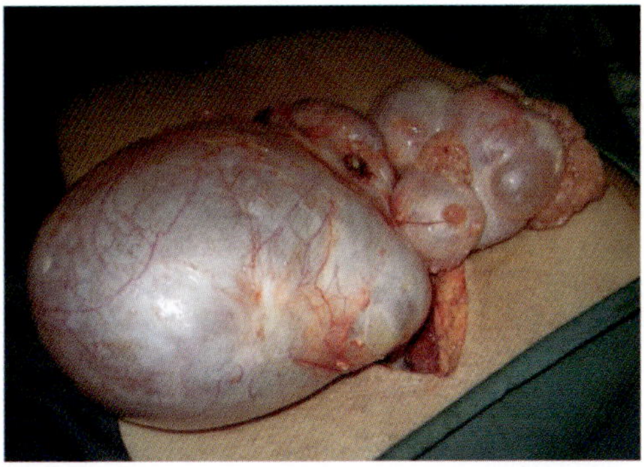

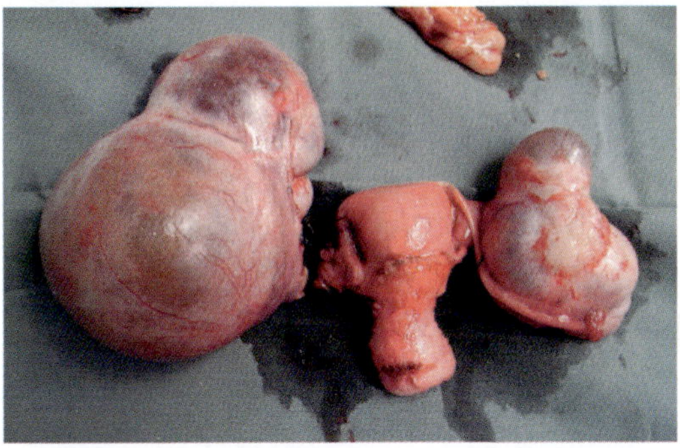

Carcinoma of the ovary.

4. Carcinoma of the Uterus (endometrium)

Type of Cancer	Risk Factors	Protective Factors	Histological Subtypes	Screening
Uterus 4th most frequent cancer in Singapore female Lifetime risk 2.5% High-risk age group: 50–69 years old	— Obesity — Nulliparity — PCOS — Unopposed oestrogen stimulation — Tamoxifen use — Family history of uterine, breast or colon cancer — 5% hereditary (HNPCC 40–60% lifetime risk)	Parity	*Endometrioid* cancer (80%) usually arises on background of endometrial hyperplasia. — Serous, clear cell, squamous and undifferentiated, Malignant Mixed Mullerian tumour (MMMT); endometrial stromal sarcoma (ESS) and leiomyosarcoma (LMS) are less common	No proven screening tool at present

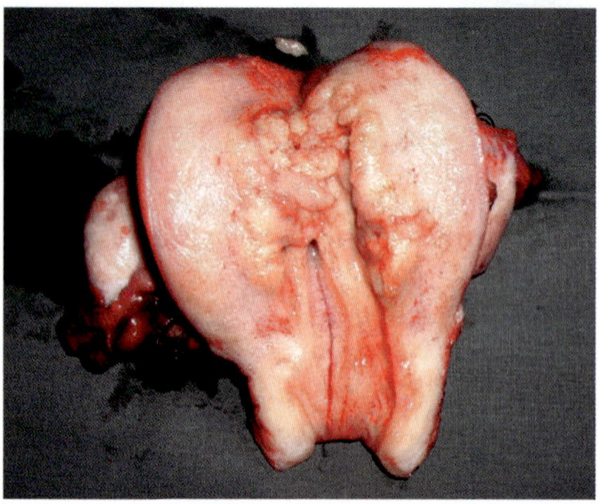

Carcinoma of the endometrium.

Carcinoma of the Uterus (endometrium) (*Continued*)

Presenting Symptoms & Physical Examination	Investigations	Treatment	Fertility Preservation
Presenting symptoms (>80% *present in early stage*): — Abnormal uterine bleeding — Postmenopausal bleeding — Persistent postmenopausal vaginal discharge — Abnormal cells on cervical cytology (e.g. AGUS smear) *Physical examination:* — May be normal — Abdominal or pelvic mass — If advanced: ascites, hepatomegaly	*Laboratory:* *Imaging:* — CXR — U/S pelvis — CT abdomen/ pelvis *Histology:* Endometrial biopsy (gold standard is hysteroscopy, dilatation and curettage Alternative: office endometrial sampling with Pipelle or Explora)	*Surgery* Staging laparotomy, THBSO, bilateral pelvic lymph node dissection, omentectomy. Extended staging including para-aortic lymph node dissection in selected cases *Adjuvant radiotherapy* Brachytherapy +/– external beam radiotherapy based on risk stratification *Chemotherapy* (platinum-based drugs, Anthracyclines, taxanes) for advanced disease or palliation; hormonal treatment if hormone receptor positive	High dose progestogens (e.g. Megace, medroxyproge-sterone acetate for apparent early stage grade 1 disease. Risk of recurrence 25–50% Complete hysterectomy after family completed

5. Carcinoma of the Vulva/Vagina

Type of Cancer	Risk Factors	Histological Subtypes	Screening
Vulva High-risk age group: post-menopausal (80% > 60 years old)	– HPV infection – Smoking – VIN – Paget's disease	*Squamous cell* (90%) Melanoma, adenocarcinoma, basal cell, sarcoma, verrucous	No proven screening tool at present
Vagina High-risk age group: Post-menopausal	– HPV association – CIN – VAIN – Multiple sexual partners – Early age of sexual debut – Smoking – DES exposure (offspring; clear cell carcinoma) – Previous history of cervical cancer	Squamous (81.5%) adenocarcinoma (10.5%); others (melanoma, sarcoma, small cell, lymphoma, undifferentiated), metastasic lesions from other sites (e.g. bladder, urethra)	No proven screening tool at present

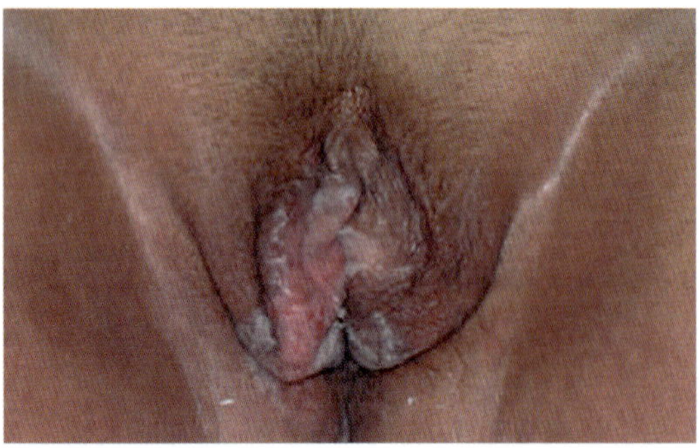

Carcinoma of the vulva.

Carcinoma of the Vulva/Vagina (*Continued*)

Presenting Symptoms & Physical Examination	Investigations	Treatment	Fertility Preservation
*Presenting symptoms of **vulva** carcinoma* – Vulvar lump or ulcer – Vulvar pruritus – Bleeding or discharge from vulva lesion – Dysuria – Lump in groin *Physical examination:* – Ulcer, fleshy/irregular mass or leucoplakia on labia majora – Enlarged groin nodes	Colposcopy, Keye's punch biopsy for histopathology, Pap smear *Imaging:* – CXR – CT abdomen/pelvis	Early and resectable for locally advanced tumour: surgery (i.e. Radical vulvectomy and groin node dissection). May require postoperative radiotherapy Unresectable tumour (resection would require a stoma): chemoradiation or primary radiotherapy followed by limited resection of tumour	
*Presenting symptoms of **vagina** carcinoma* – Vaginal bleeding or discharge – Pelvic pain – Urinary symptoms – Tenesmus *Physical examination:* – Exophytic lesions usually.	*Histopathology:* Colposcopic directed biopsy. *Imaging:* – CXR – CT Abdomen – MRI Pelvis Cystoscopy, Proctoscopy	Radiotherapy is treatment of choice. Role of surgery limited	Ovarian transposition if radiotherapy is required

VIN — Vulval intraepithelial neoplasia; CIN — Cervical intraepithelial neoplasia; VAIN — Vaginal intraepithelial neoplasia

Chapter 41

PAP SMEAR SCREENING AND MANAGEMENT OF ABNORMAL PAP SMEARS

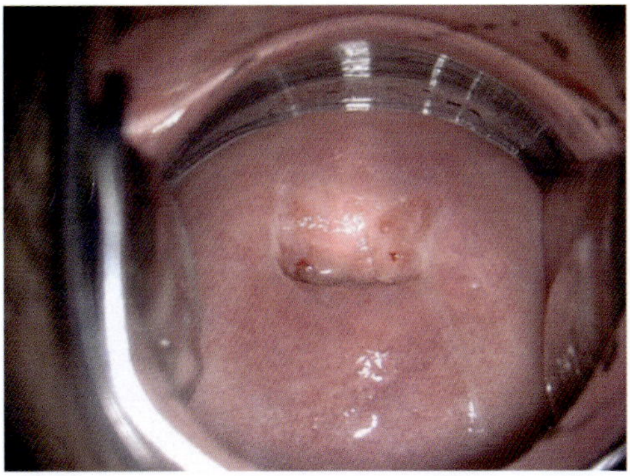

Figure 1. Nulliparous cervix.

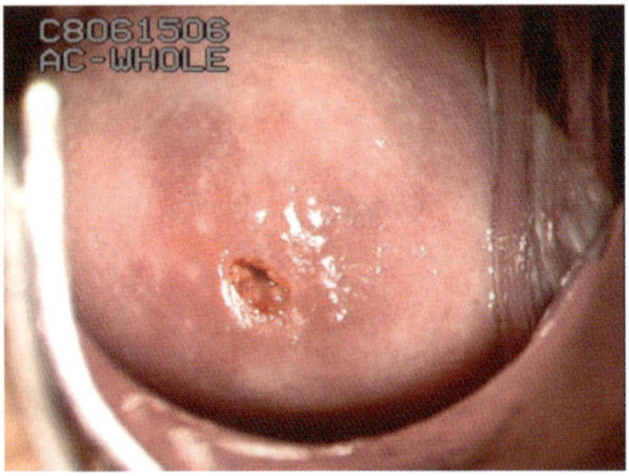

Figure 2. Parous cervix with slit shaped os.

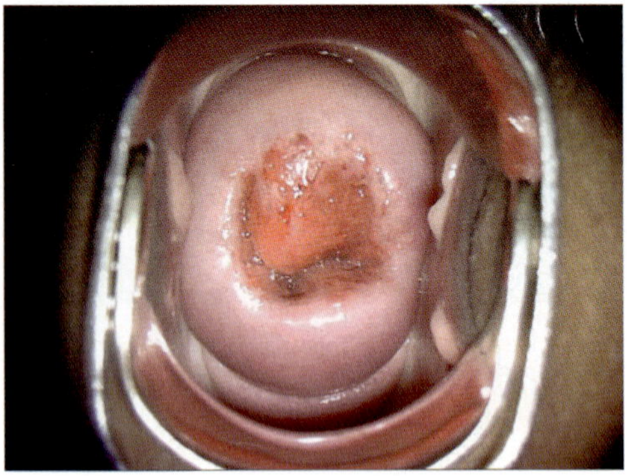

Figure 3. An ectropion.

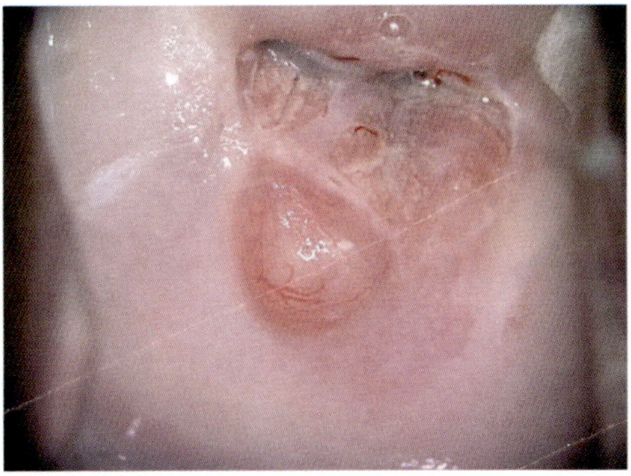

Figure 4. Nabothian follicle. Note the prominent blood vessels on the surface showing a normal regular branching pattern.

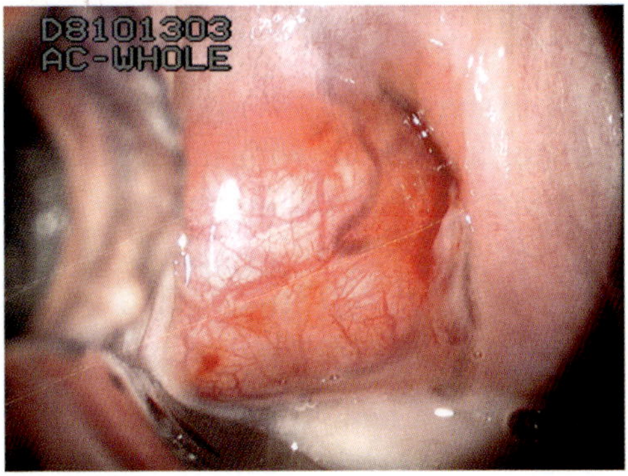

Figure 5. Cluster of nabothian follicles distorting the cervix.

Cervical Screening Singapore programme

1. Who to be screened — all women who have ever had sex are advised to have their first Pap smear by age 25.
2. Frequency of screening — once every 3 years if no risk factors.
3. Discharge from screening at 65 years of age if the smear taken at age 65 is negative and there was a previous negative smear within the last 3 years.
4. Women who have a history of CIN 2/CIN 3/adenocarcinoma *in situ* and who have been appropriately treated (or disease has spontaneously regressed) should be routinely screened for at least 20 years following diagnosis even if this extends screening past age 65 years.
5. *Women who have undergone hysterectomy*

   - If subtotal hysterectomy — women have same risk of cervical cancer as those with intact uterus and cervix. So continue routine screening protocol.
   - If indication was CIN 2/3 — stop screening if three consecutive annual smears subsequent to hysterectomy have been normal.
   - If indication was a benign condition of uterus and not cervical cancer precursors/cancer — stop screening.
   - If the histology is not known — do one baseline vault smear and if this is negative, there is no need for further screening.

6. *For concurrent testing with cytology and HPV tests*

   In women more than 30 years of age:

   Not more frequently than three years.

   Can screen every five years.

7. *For immunocompromised women* (e.g. *HIV*)

   Screen twice a year in the first year and annually thereafter.

8. *For women who never have had sexual intercourse* — do not require routine screening, but, if they develop some gynaecological symptoms, they should be referred to **OBGYN**.

High Risk Factors for Cervical Cancer

- Early onset of sexual interocourse
- Multiple sexual partners
- Human Papilloma Virus infection (HPV)
- Human Immunodeficiency Virus infection (HIV)
- History of sexually transmitted infections (STIs)
- Immunosuppression such as on long-term steroids

Bethesda 2001 Cervical Cytology Classification — Negative for Squamous Intraepithelial Lesion or Malignancy

Epithelial cell abnormalities: Squamous Cell

Atypical squamous cells of undetermined significance (ASCUS)

Atypical squamous cells, cannot exclude HSIL (ASC-H)
Low-grade Squamous intraepithelial lesion (LSIL)
 encompassing: HPV/mild dysplasia/CIN 1
High-grade squamous intraepithelial lesion (HSIL)
 encompassing: moderate and severe dysplasia, CIS/CIN 2 & CIN 3 — with features suspicious for invasion (if invasion is suspected)
Squamous cell carcinoma (SCC)

Epithelial Cell Abnormalities: Glandular Cell

Atypical glandular cells (AGC)
 — endocervical cells (NOS)
 — endometrial cells (NOS)
 — glandular cells (NOS or specify in comments)
Atypical glandular cells (AGC)
 — endocervical cells, favour neoplastic
 — glandular cells, favour neoplastic
Endocervical adenocarcinoma *in situ*
Adenocarcinoma
 — endocervical
 — extrauterine
 — endometrial
 — not otherwise specified (NOS)

Comparison of the WHO and Bethesda System Terminology

WHO Histopathologic Terms	Bethesda Cytology Terms
CIN 1/mild dysplasia	LSIL
CIN 2/moderate dysplasia	HSIL
CIN 3/severe dysplasia	HSIL
CIN 3/carcinoma *in situ*	HSIL

∗LSIL: low-grade squamous intraepithelial lesion.

∗HSIL: high-grade squamous intraepithelial lesion.

Sampling Devices for Pap Smear

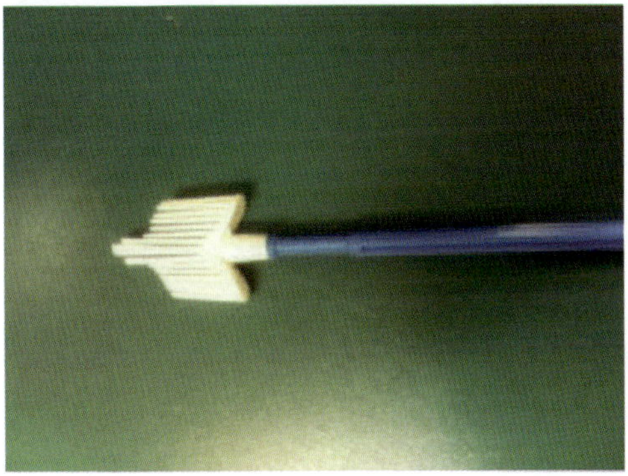

Figure 6. Cytobrush for PAP smear.

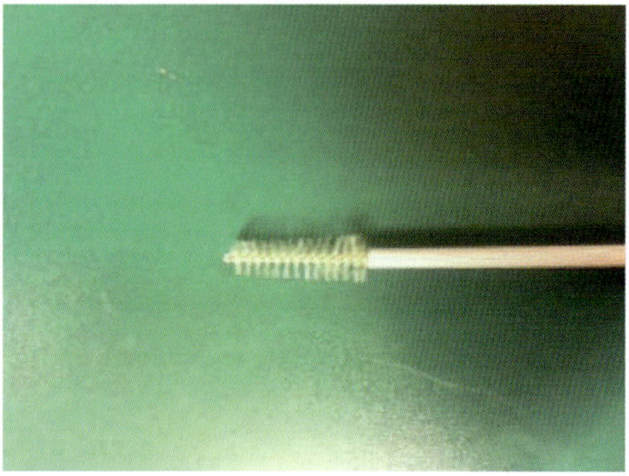

Figure 7. Endocervical brush for PAP smear.

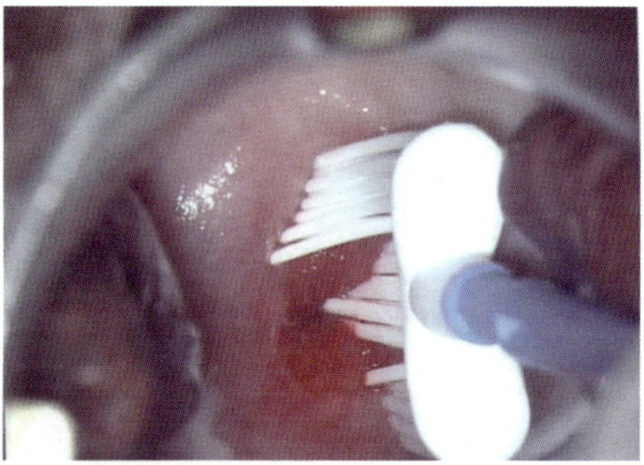

Figure 8. PAP smear with the cyto-brush. Care should be taken to sample both the ectocervix and the endocervix.

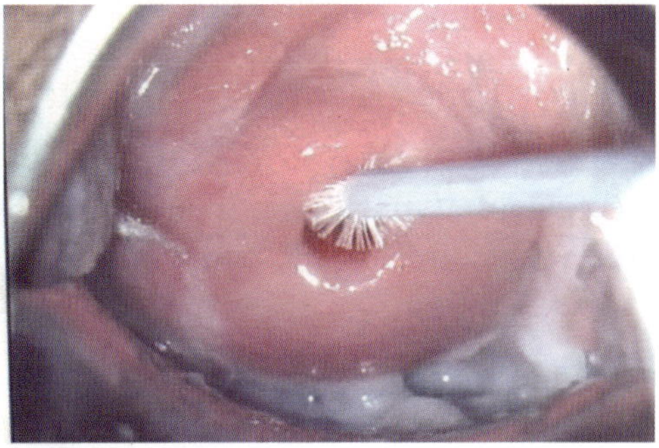

Figure 9. Pap smear with the endocervical brush. The endocervix may need additional sampling with the endocervical brush if the cytobrush cannot reach the endocervix.

How to Obtain Samples

Insert central bristles of the cytobrush into the endocervix with the outer bristles in contact with the ectocervix. Rotate the brush in the same direction for five turns.

Sample Preparation

(a) Conventional pap smear — smear the sample on a slide promptly and fix the slide.

(b) Liquid-based thin layer cytology — place the brush in the liquid fixative solution (used in KKH).

Advantages of Liquid-Based Cytology

1. Greater specimen adequacy (especially with bleeding or inflammation).
2. Better detection of atypical glandular cells, ASCUS, LSIL as compared with conventional pap smear.
3. Can do concurrent HPV testing.
4. Less fixation and drying artifact.

Factors Thought to Affect or Interfere with Pap Smear Sampling

1. Menses — does not affect sample cellularity but ideally not to be done during menses
2. Gels/lubricants/semen/spermicidal agents/intravaginal medications — less likely to affect liquid-based thin layer cytology (clean cervix with a large cotton swab to remove the obscuring blood/discharge/lubricants before taking sample)
3. Douching
4. Tampon use
5. Barrier contraception
6. Vaginal intercourse

(Items 4–6: No data available)

ASCUS = atypical squamous cells of undetermined significance
LSIL = low grade squamous intra-epithelial lesion

Specimen Adequacy/Unsatisfactory Pap smear

- *Adequate smears* have adequate number of well preserved squamous cells and endocervical cells.
- *Unsatisfactory specimens* include inadequate squamous cells obscurred by blood and inflammation — unreliable for the detection of cervical epithelial cell abnormalities.

Follow-Up Management of Pap Smears

1. Normal — repeat smear in three years — routine screening
2. Inflammatory — repeat smear in six months (colposcopy after three consecutive inflammatory smears)
3. Borderline nuclear changes — repeat in six months (colposcopy after three consecutive smears)
4. Endometrial cells (<40 years old) — check last menstrual period. Repeat in six months (if needed).
5. Atrophic smear — routine screening
6. Mild dyskaryosis — colposcopy (30% CIN II–III)
7. Moderate dyskaryosis — colposcopy (50%–75% CIN II–III)
8. Severe dyskaryosis — colposcopy (80%–90% CIN II–III)
9. Invasion suspected — urgent colposcopy
10. Abnormal glandular cells — urgent colposcopy

11. Presence of normal cytologically benign appearing endometrial glandular cells in women ≥40 years — endometrial biopsy is recommended if patient has symptoms or risk factors for endometrial cancer.

Follow Up Management of Pap Smears

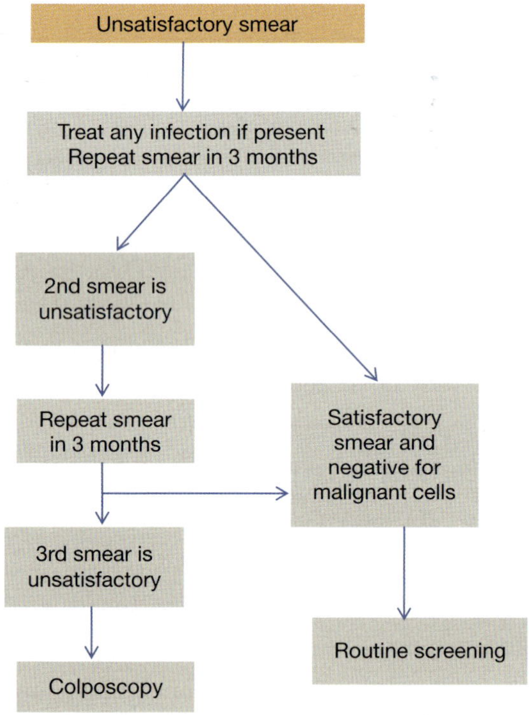

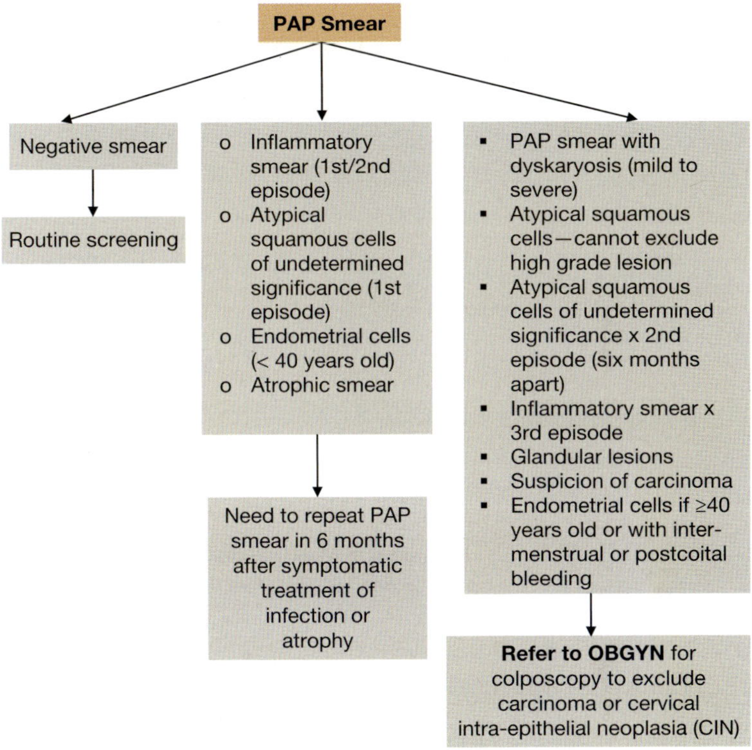
PAP Smear
Negative smear
Routine screening
o Inflammatory smear (1st/2nd episode)
o Atypical squamous cells of undetermined significance (1st episode)
o Endometrial cells (< 40 years old)
o Atrophic smear
Need to repeat PAP smear in 6 months after symptomatic treatment of infection or atrophy
▪ PAP smear with dyskaryosis (mild to severe)
▪ Atypical squamous cells—cannot exclude high grade lesion
▪ Atypical squamous cells of undetermined significance x 2nd episode (six months apart)
▪ Inflammatory smear x 3rd episode
▪ Glandular lesions
▪ Suspicion of carcinoma
▪ Endometrial cells if ≥40 years old or with inter-menstrual or postcoital bleeding
Refer to OBGYN for colposcopy to exclude carcinoma or cervical intra-epithelial neoplasia (CIN)

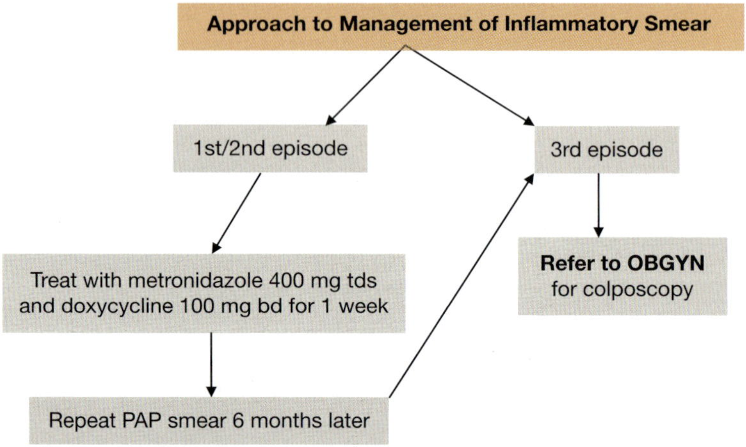
Approach to Management of Inflammatory Smear
1st/2nd episode
3rd episode
Treat with metronidazole 400 mg tds and doxycycline 100 mg bd for 1 week
Refer to OBGYN for colposcopy
Repeat PAP smear 6 months later

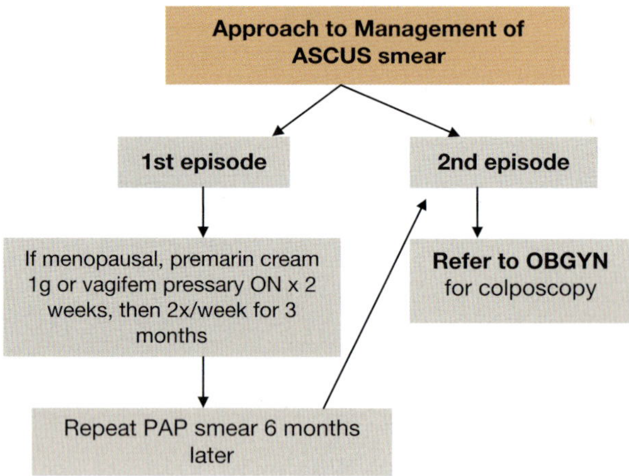
Approach to Management of ASCUS smear
1st episode
2nd episode
If menopausal, premarin cream 1g or vagifem pressary ON x 2 weeks, then 2x/week for 3 months
Refer to OBGYN for colposcopy
Repeat PAP smear 6 months later

Approach to Management of Endometrial Cells in PAP Smear

↓

Correlate with age, last menstrual period (LMP) and clinical findings

↓

- Age ≥40 years old
- History of intermenstrual or postcoital bleeding
- PAP smear taken >15 days of LMP

↓

Refer to OBGYN for endometrial assessment

Approach to Management of Atrophic Smear

↓ If symptomatic (postmenopausal bleed and cancer excluded)

Vagifem pessary every night x 2 weeks then 2 times per week for 3 months

↓

Repeat PAP smear 6 months later
If normal, return to normal screening interval

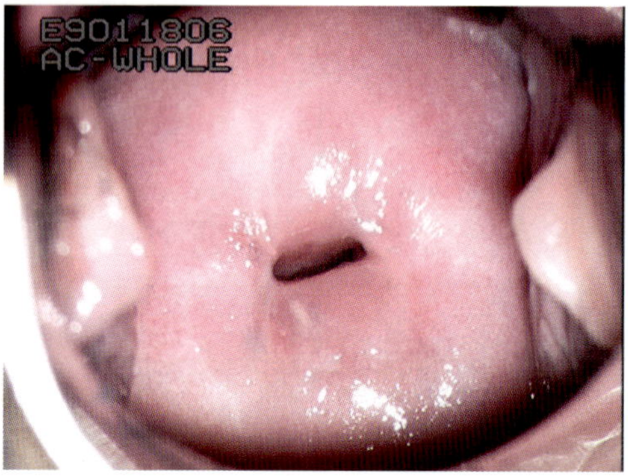

Figure 10. Atrophic cervix, showing the squamocolumnar junction retracted into the endocervix.

Referral Criteria for Colposcopy

- Any single smear showing mild/moderate/severe dyskaryosis
- Any smear suggestive of glandular abnormality
- Three consecutive inadequate smears
- Three consecutive inflammatory smears
- Three consecutive borderline smears
- Any smear suggestive of malignancy
- History of postcoital bleeding
- Abnormal looking cervix
- Keratinising cells

What is Colposcopy? How to explain to our patients?

It is a simple outpatient procedure.

A colposcope is an instrument that shines a beam of light on the cervix and magnifies the view. At the beginning of the examination, you lie on your back and place your feet in the stirrups as you would for a Pap smear. The doctor inserts a speculum into your vagina and opens it to visualise your cervix. Then the doctor applies a vinegar solution (acetic acid) to the cervix and vagina with a cotton ball. The vinegar will make abnormal tissues white so that the doctor can identify the abnormal areas that may need further evaluation.

If the doctor detects areas of abnormal tissue, he or she will perform a biopsy. A specialist doctor called a pathologist will then examine these samples.

Management of CIN 1

Counselling regarding the natural history of disease

- Low premalignant potential
- Virtually all women with LSIL have HPV infection
- 60% revert to normal
- 15% progress to CIN 3
- Lesions less likely to regress in immunocompromised
- Management — either observation or treatment
- Treatment — excision/ablation

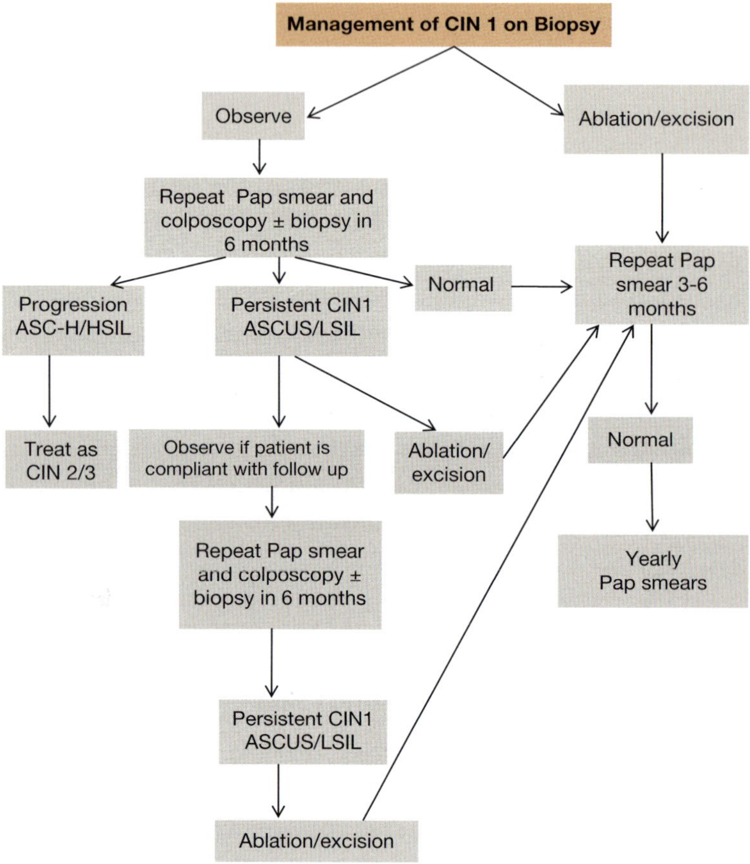
Management of CIN 1 on Biopsy
Observe
Ablation/excision
Repeat Pap smear and colposcopy ± biopsy in 6 months
Progression ASC-H/HSIL
Persistent CIN1 ASCUS/LSIL
Normal
Repeat Pap smear 3-6 months
Treat as CIN 2/3
Observe if patient is compliant with follow up
Ablation/ excision
Normal
Repeat Pap smear and colposcopy ± biopsy in 6 months
Yearly Pap smears
Persistent CIN1 ASCUS/LSIL
Ablation/excision

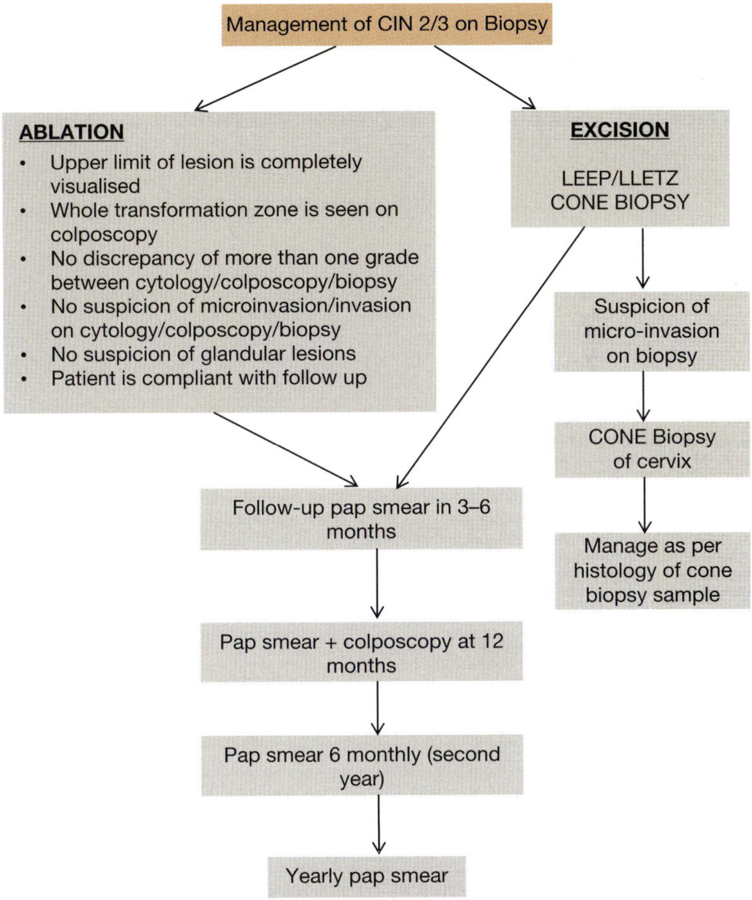
Management of CIN 2/3 on Biopsy
ABLATION
Upper limit of lesion is completely visualised
Whole transformation zone is seen on colposcopy
No discrepancy of more than one grade between cytology/colposcopy/biopsy
No suspicion of microinvasion/invasion on cytology/colposcopy/biopsy
No suspicion of glandular lesions
Patient is compliant with follow up
EXCISION
LEEP/LLETZ
CONE BIOPSY
Suspicion of micro-invasion on biopsy
CONE Biopsy of cervix
Manage as per histology of cone biopsy sample
Follow-up pap smear in 3–6 months
Pap smear + colposcopy at 12 months
Pap smear 6 monthly (second year)
Yearly pap smear

Summary of Treatment for Pre-Invasive Cervical Lesions

- Ablative treatment — cryotherapy, LASER
- Excision
- LEEP (loop electrosurgical excision procedure)
- Laser cone biopsy
- Knife cone biopsy

LEEP (Large Loop Excision of Transformation Zone)

- Transformation zone (TZ) excised to depth of 7–8 mm
- Provides tissue diagnosis
- Easy to perform, done as outpatient setting
- Well tolerated by patients, low morbidity, high patient acceptability
- Success rates 90–96%

Procedure

- Excise TZ with high current using thin electrode
- Size and shape of the loop should be tailored to the size and extent of TZ and extension to endocervical canal
- *Complications* include intraoperative and postoperative bleeding, infection
- Cervical stenosis (1–3%)
- Increases the risk of subsequent PROM, PTL LBW infants

Contraindications of LEEP

- Active cervical, vaginal and pelvic infection
- Suspected invasive cancer

Cone Biopsy

Indications

- Cytologic abnormality not consistent with histological diagnosis
- Unsatisfactory colposcopy
- Microinvasion on biopsy, to rule out invasive cancer
- Adenocarcinoma *in situ* (AIS)

Methods:

- Cold knife cone biopsy
- Laser cone biopsy

Complications of Cone Biopsy

- Bleeding, infection and trauma to the cervix

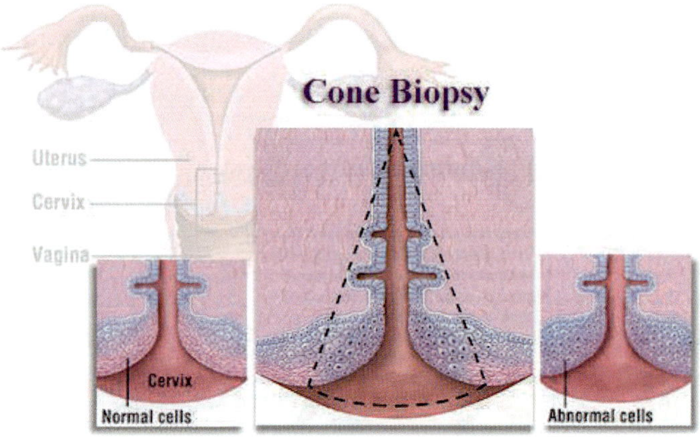

Figure 11. Cone biopsy of cervix.

Atypical Glandular Cells

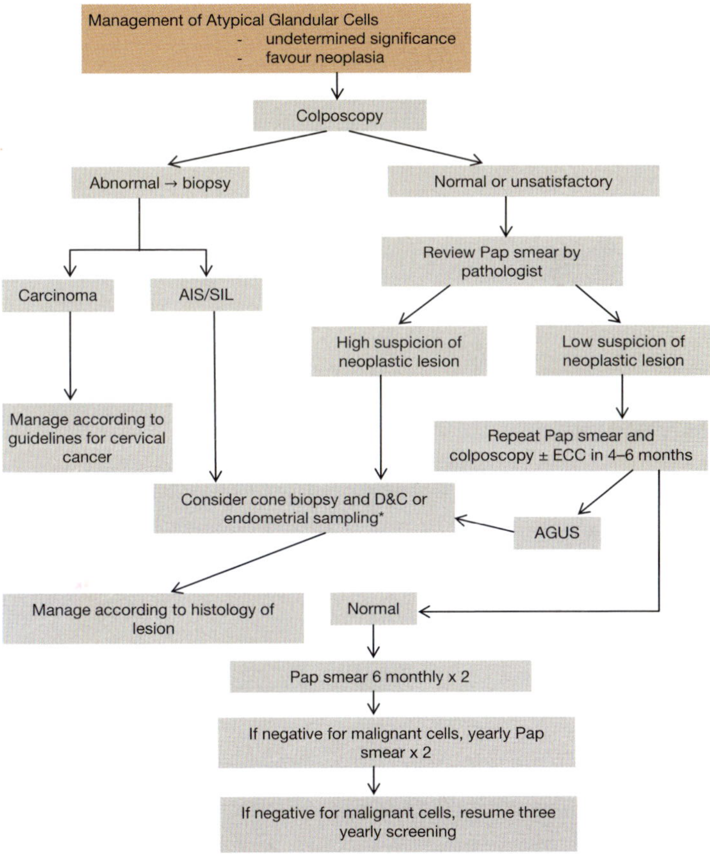

*If risk factors for Ca endometrium are present or the patient is symptomatic or ≥40 years → D&C (± hysteroscopy) is advised for endometrial tissue evaluation.
Note: If histology of cone biopsy and D&C normal → to investigate for disease in ovary, fallopian tubes and peritoneum.
AGUS – Atypical glandular cells of undetermined significance.
AIS – Adenocarcinoma *in situ*.
ECC – Endocervical curetting.
SIL – Squamous intra-epithelial lesion.

Adenocarcinoma *in situ* (AIS)

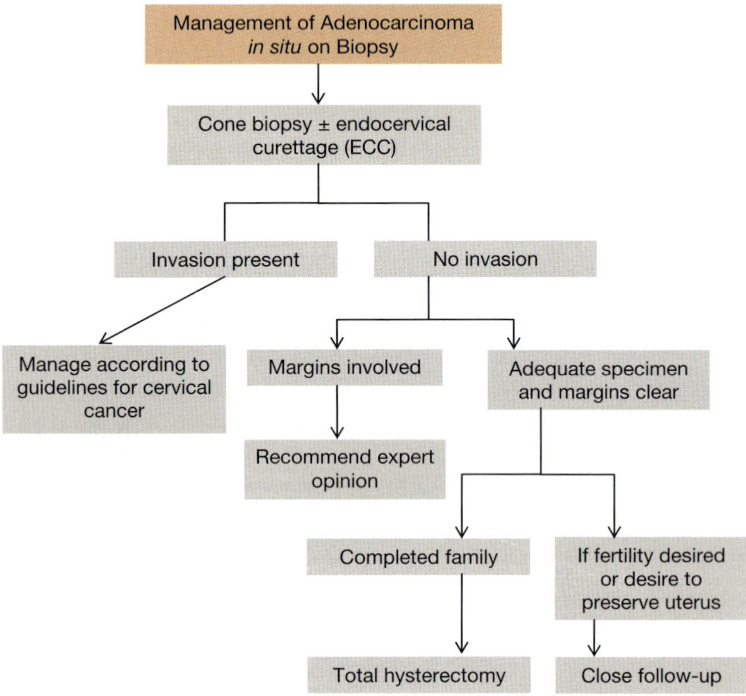

Note: For cone biopsy for adenocarcinoma *in situ*, a single large specimen with clear margins is necessary for adequate histopathological interpretation. A LEEP may not be adequate. A cold knife cone under anaesthesia is preferred.

Chapter 42

POSTCOITAL BLEEDING (PCB)

Causes of PCB

- Cervical cancer/cervical intra-epithelial neoplasia (CIN)
- Cervical ectropion/polyps
- Cervicitis (e.g. Chlamydia is most common; bacterial vaginosis)
- Atrophic vaginitis
- Genital prolapse — secondary to ulceration
- Benign vascular neoplasms (e.g. haemangioma/arterio-venous malformation)

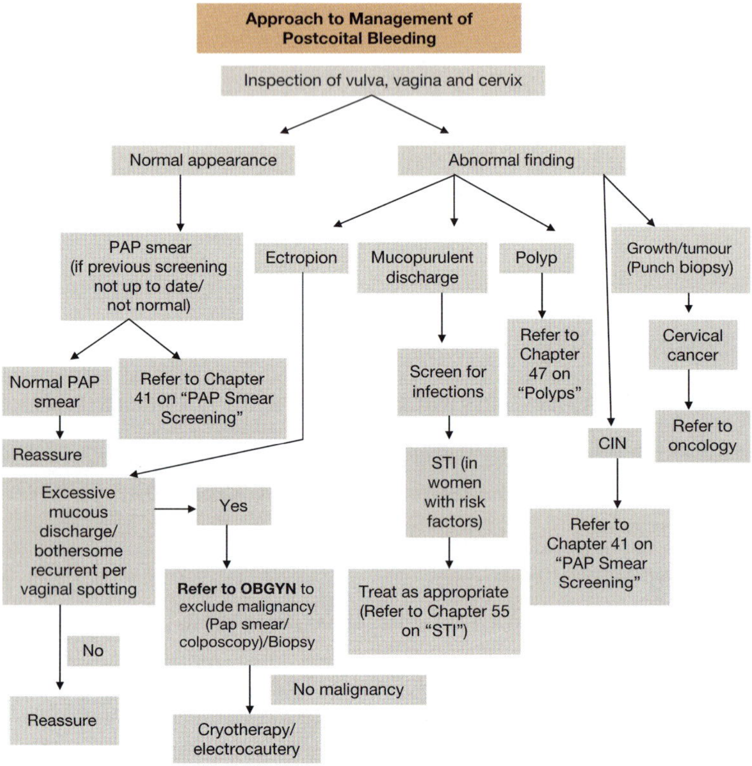

Note: If postcoital bleeding is persistent, refer for colposcopy and evaluation of endometrium.

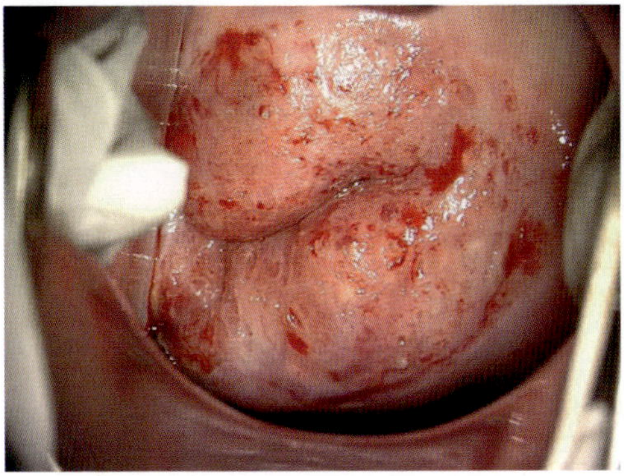

Figure 1. Atrophic cervicitis, showing petechial haemorrhages and contact bleeding.

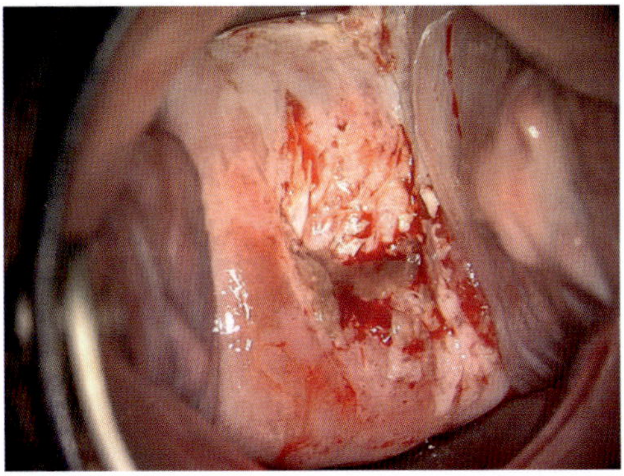

Figure 2. Early cancer of the cervix. Note the eroded surface and contact bleeding.

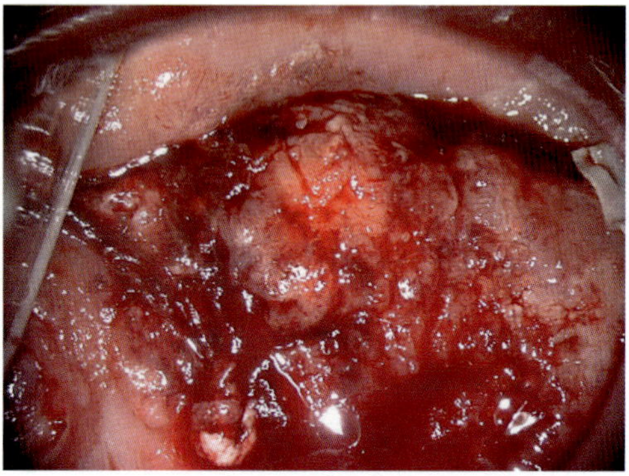

Figure 3. Advanced cancer of the cervix occupying the entire cervix and extending to the vagina.

Chapter 43

HUMAN PAPILLOMA (HPV) VACCINES AND HPV TESTING — SALIENT FACTS FOR CLINICAL PRACTICE

Facts about Cervical Cancer

- Cervical cancer is the 2nd commonest cancer among women in many Asian countries, after breast cancer.
- Highly preventable cancer.

Human Papilloma Virus and Cervical Cancers and Other Cancers

- HPV causes the majority of cervical cancer.
- HPV DNA is found in almost 100% of cervical cancers.
- More than 100 types of HPV can infect humans.
- 15 HPV types are considered high oncogenic risk HPV (hr-HPV).

- The hr-HPV types 16 and 18 account for 70% of cervical cancers.
- The other commoner hr-HPV causing cervical cancers are types 31, 33, 45, 52, and 58.
- HPVs have also been implicated in causing cancers of the vulva, vagina, anus, penis, and head and neck.

Human Papilloma Virus and Genital Warts

- HPV types 6 and 11 account for 90% of genital warts.
- Genital warts are benign and do not lead to cancer.
- However, genital warts are highly infective and can be persistent and debilitating (refer to Chapter 55 on "STI").

Clinical Manifestations

- HPV infection usually occurs in the late teens and early adulthood.
- CIN usually occurs between ages of 25–40 years.
- Cervical cancer usually presents after 40 years old.

Natural History of hr-HPV Infection and pathogenesis of Cervical Cancer

- HPV infection of the cervix occurs commonly but is usually transient in young women.

- In 80% of women infected with HPV, HPV infection regresses spontaneously.
- Persistent hr-HPV infection of the cervix predisposes it to develop pre-cancer and then cancer.

The Cervical Epithelium and Cervical Cancers

- The epithelium of the ectocervix (visible) is made of squamous epithelium.
- The epithelium of the endocervix (not visible) is made of glandular epithelium.
- The epithelium between the endocervix and ectocervix that is transformsed from glandular cells to squamous cells is called transformation zone (TZ).
- The transformation zone of the cervix is prone to carcinogenesis.

Cervical Intraepithelial Neoplasia (CIN) and Squamous Cell Carcinoma (SCC)

- Cervical intraepithelial neoplasia (CIN) — pre-cancers of the squamous epithelium.
- Three grades of CIN : CIN-I, CIN-II and CIN-III.
- The majority of CIN-I will regress spontaneously.
- High grade CIN (CIN-II and III) has a significant risk of developing SCC.

Adenocarcinoma *In situ* (AIS) and Adenocarcinoma — Why does it Need Special Attention?

- Adenocarcinoma develops from the glandular epithelium of the endocervix.
- Adenocarcinoma *in situ* (AIS) is pre-cancer of the endocervical glandular epithelium.
- HPV-16 is responsible for the majority of adenocarcinoma.
- HPV-18 and HPV-45 are responsible for adenocarcinomas in a greater proportion, as compared with that for squamous cell carcinomas.
- Screening for adenocarcinoma of the cervix is more difficult because:
  - The endocervix is not visible for clinical examination.
  - Unlike the squamous epithelium, the endocervical glandular epithelium does not exfoliate therefore making Pap smear screening less reliable.
- Hence, adenocarcinoma of the cervix tends to present at a later stage of the disease when the disease is bulky.

Overview of Treatment for Cervical Pre-Cancers

- Patients with low-grade CIN have options of close observation or treatment.
- Patients with high-grade CIN are usually treated.

- Patients with adenocarcinoma *in situ* (AIS or suspected AIS) must always be treated.
- CIN can be treated by the following methods, as appropriate:
    - Excision of cervix by
        - LEEP — loop electrosurgical excision procedure
        - Laser cone biopsy
        - Knife cone biopsy
    - Ablation of cervix
        - Laser vapourisation of the cervix
- AIS is normally treated by cold knife cone biopsy.
- Total hysterectomy is only performed if there is co-existing gynaecological disease, e.g. symptomatic uterine fibroids causing severe menorrhagia.

Pap Smear Screening

- For more than 50 years, Pap smear screening has been the sole screening method for cervical pre-cancers and cancers.
- Pap smears is a cytological test which detects pre-cancerous or cancerous cells from cervical specimen of a grossly normal cervix.

High-Risk(hr-) HPV Testing

- Cervical hr-HPV tests are now available and increasingly being used in clinical practice.

- It has greater sensitivity and better predictive value of cervical disease.
- If the woman is tested negative for hr-HPVs, she has a negligible risk of having a cervical pre-cancer or cancer.
- However, as not all hr-HPV positive women have cervical disease, the use of hr-HPV tests for routine screening purposes has a tendency for over-call and increased referrals for further cervical evaluation.

Self-Sampling for Cervical Screening

- Despite the Pap smear screening being available for many years, many women still do not go for routine or regular screening.
- These unscreened and under-screened women are at high risk of getting cervical cancers.
- An effective way to help the unscreened and under-screened women is self-sampling of the cervical specimen under clinical supervision. This provides convenience, privacy and minimal discomfort.
- In the Netherlands, a self-screening device called the Delphi Screener has been subjected to large clinical trials with favourable results.
- Recently, the Delphi Screener has been introduced to Singapore and will be made available to the Asia-Pacific countries.

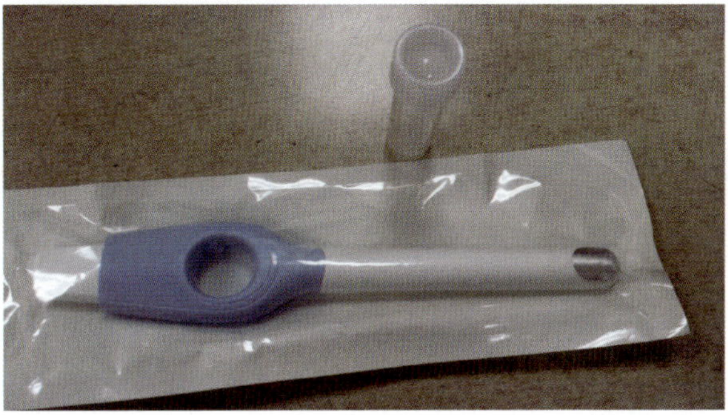

Delphi Screener — vaginal self-sampler.

HPV Vaccination

- There are two brands of HPV vaccines available, namely: Cervarix® and Gardasil®.
- Both Cervarix® and Gardasil®contain vaccines against cancer-causing HPVs-16 and 18.
- They are prophylactic and not therapeutic vaccines.
- The basic constitutional difference between the two brands of HPV vaccines is:
    - Cervarix® contains a proprietor adjuvant, ASO4, which induces greater immunogenic responses, resulting in higher antibody titres against HPV 16 and 18.
    - Gardasil® contains vaccines against HPV-6 and 11, which are responsible for 90% of genital warts.
- Both vaccines are given in 3 doses:
    - Cervarix® : 0, 1, 6 months
    - Gardasil® : 0, 2, 6 months

- Both vaccines have very good safety profiles.
- The commonest side-effects are: transient mild fever and pain at the injection site.

- **Common guidelines for vaccination of women**
  - The vaccines are best given before the onset of sexual activity.
  - Mid-adult women have been shown to exhibit strong immune serological responses and demonstrated vaccine efficacy against HPV-related infection or CIN.
  - Vaccinated women should continue with routine cervical cancer screening.
  - Sexually active women can still benefit from the vaccines against any of the vaccine-HPV types with which they are not currently infected.
  - Likewise, women with current or prior HPV infection or CIN can also benefit from the vaccines against any of the vaccine-HPV types with which they are not currently infected.
  - The HPV vaccine is made of viral-like protein. It does not contain any HPV virion or DNA.
  - Women who are immunocompromised, e.g. those who are on steroids or have HIV infection may be vaccinated, but their immune response to the vaccine may be poorer.

- Lactating women can be vaccinated.
- While the HPV vaccines are not recommended in women who are pregnant or planning to get pregnant, there has been no demonstrable increased adverse outcome of pregnancies of vaccinated women in the vaccines trials.
- Termination of pregnancy is not indicated for vaccinated women who become pregnant.
- These women should defer the remaining dose(s) of the vaccines until pregnancy is completed.
- There is no need to restart the entire vaccination schedule but there should not be a delay of more than 12 months between the 2nd and 3rd dose.

- **Vaccination of males**
  - Males can be vaccinated on request.
  - Vaccination of males may induce herd immunity.
  - Early data showed that Gardasil® vaccine can protect men against genital warts.

Chapter 44

VULVAR AND VAGINAL LESIONS

Vulvar Disorders

General principles of evaluation and management of vulvar disorders

- Patient education — provide information leaflets
- Address anxiety /psychosexual dysfunction/fear of malignancy/fear of sexually transmitted infection
- Exaggerated lithotomy position to expose perineum.
- Examine cutaneous and mucosal surfaces systematically
- Control secondary infection by oral antibiotics
- Oral antifungals when necessary
- Reduce irritation on vulva (do not prescribe multiple creams)
- Night sedation for pruritic vulvar conditions
- Replace oestrogens if atrophy
- Follow up for flares and side effects of medication
- Persistent Bartholin cysts even if asymptomatic in postmenopausal women warrant removal as the risk of malignancy is higher

- Pigmented lesions — perform excision biopsy with at least 2 to 3 mm margin. Do not perform punch biopsy
- Removal of all vulvar lumps with clear margins as they are potentially malignant; mesenchymal tumours may look benign
- Patients presenting with severe pain and burning sensation at introitus and vestibule will need prompt referral to vulva clinic to rule out erosive vulvar disease
- All pigmented lesions including white crusty lesions of vulva should be biopsied

Topical corticosteroids

- Main stay of treatment for dermatoses.
- Ointments are stronger than cream, less irritating, have fewer allergens and a longer duration of action
- Steroids are anti-inflammatory and control symptoms
- Maintenance steroids are always low potency and for intermittent use
- Vulvar mucous membrane (vulvar trigone and inner labia minora) is steroid-resistant. Inter-labial sulcus, labiocrural fold and thighs will thin easily and develop striae
- Ultra-potent steroids should be used for shorter duration under close supervision
- Prescribe systemic steroids rather than topical steroids for painful ulcers and erosions as initial treatment when indicated

Side effects of corticosteroids:

- Hypertension
- May worsen diabetic control
- Secondary infection — candidiasis.
- Glaucoma
- Atrophy/striae
- *Caution* — systemic absorption from vagina is high

ALTERNATIVES TO CORTICOSTEROIDS — calcineurin inhibitors

- Main use is for maintenance of steroid responsive dermatoses
- These are topical immunosuppressants, non-steroidal, and do not cause atrophy
- Pimecrolimus 1% cream (Elidel). Equivalent to a mild topical steroid
- Tacrolimus 0.03 and 0.1% ointment (protopic). Equivalent to a moderate to strong topical steroid

Side effects of calcineurin inhibitors

- Burning, stinging sensation
- Worsening of HSV, HPV, tinea infections
- *Caution* — reports of skin cancers and lymphoma with systemic calcineurin inhibitors used in organ transplant patients

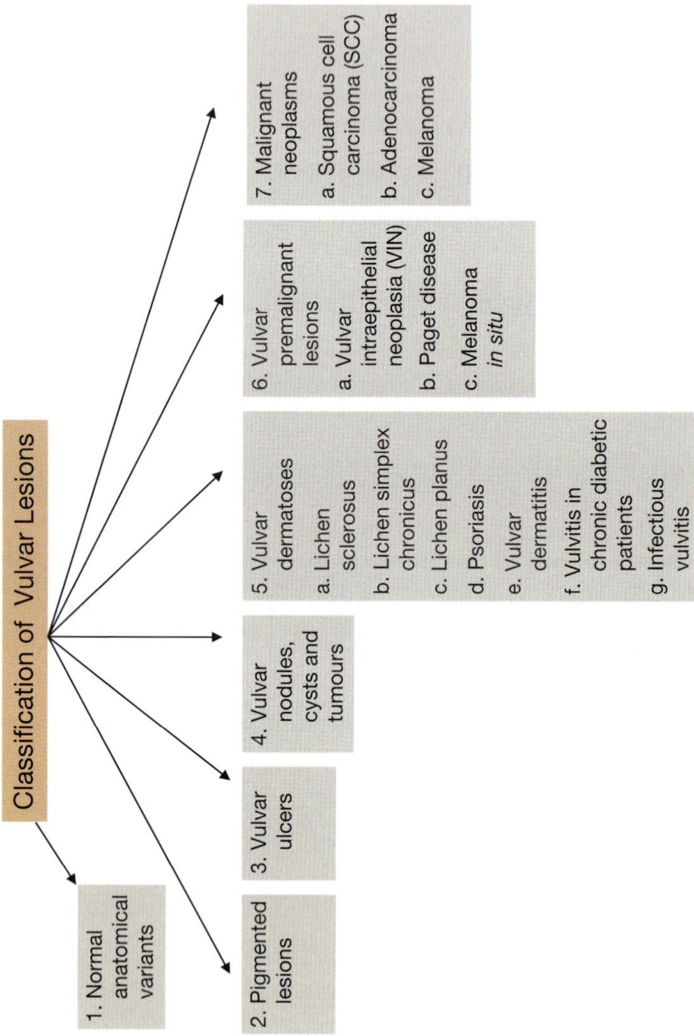
Classification of Vulvar Lesions
1. Normal anatomical variants
2. Pigmented lesions
3. Vulvar ulcers
4. Vulvar nodules, cysts and tumours
5. Vulvar dermatoses
a. Lichen sclerosus
b. Lichen simplex chronicus
c. Lichen planus
d. Psoriasis
e. Vulvar dermatitis
f. Vulvitis in chronic diabetic patients
g. Infectious vulvitis
6. Vulvar premalignant lesions
a. Vulvar intraepithelial neoplasia (VIN)
b. Paget disease
c. Melanoma *in situ*
7. Malignant neoplasms
a. Squamous cell carcinoma (SCC)
b. Adenocarcinoma
c. Melanoma

Pictures of various vulvar lesions

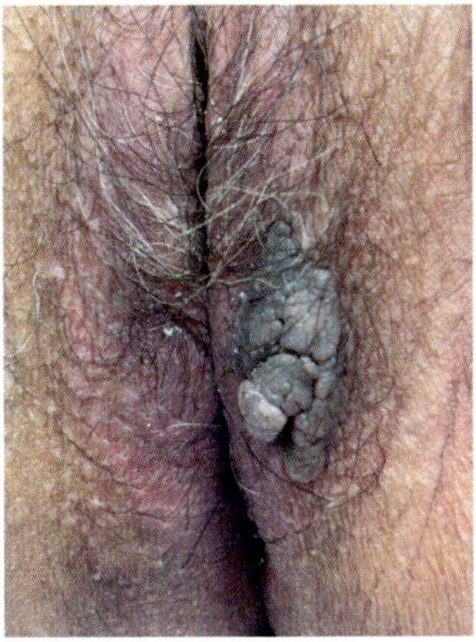

Figure 1. Seborrhoeic keratosis.

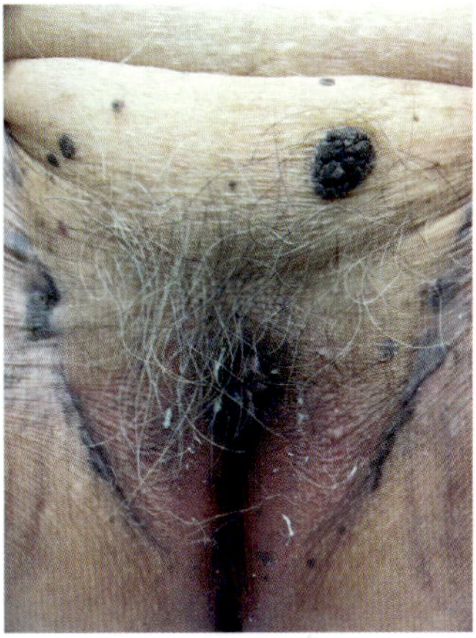

Figure 2. Extensive seborrhoeic keratosis.

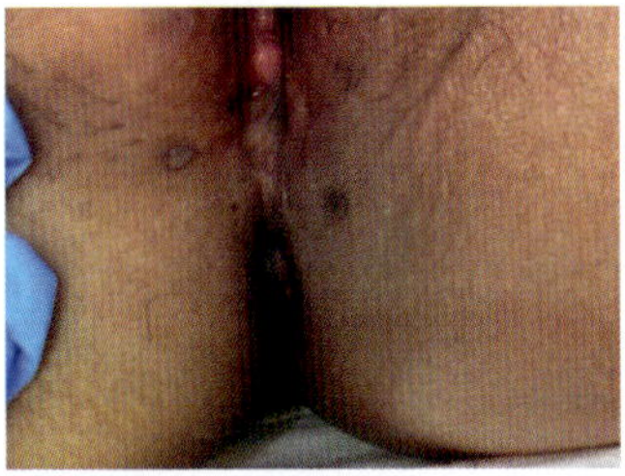

Figure 3. Flat pigmented warts. Need biopsy to rule out malignancy.

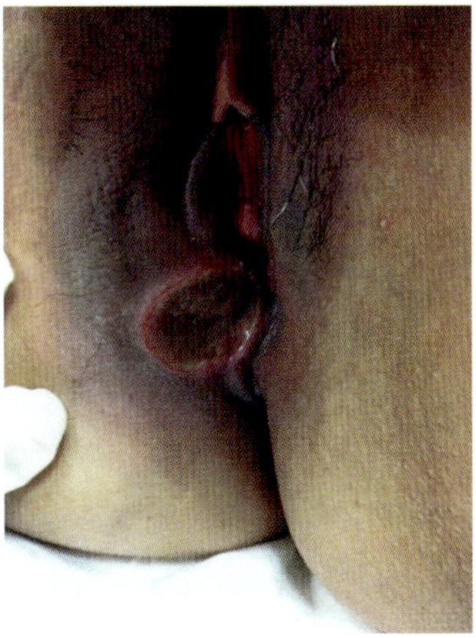

Figure 4. Aphthous ulcer.

Pictures of various vulvar lesions

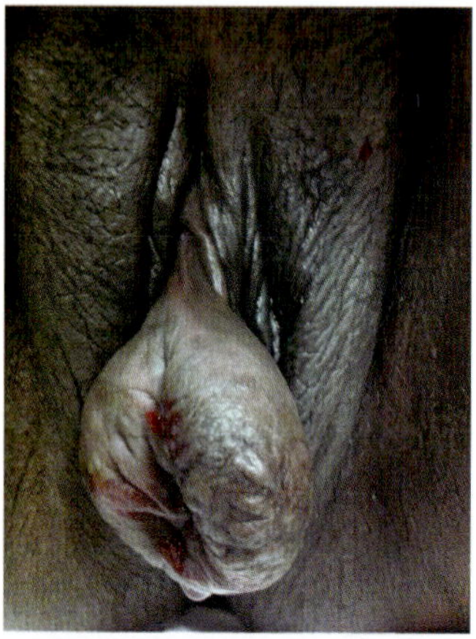

Figure 5. Infected pedunculated lipoma.

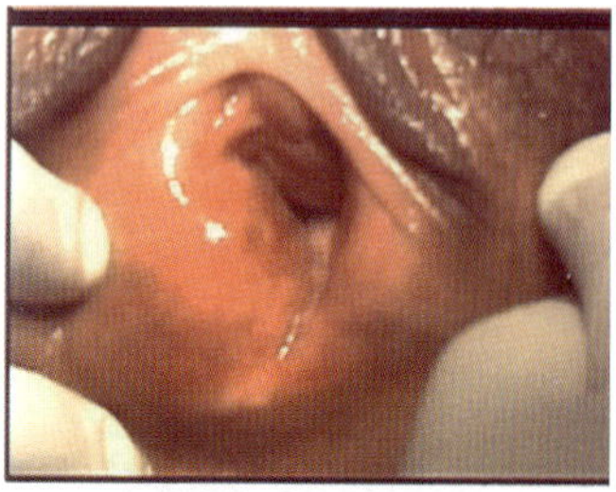

Figure 6. Right Bartholin cyst.

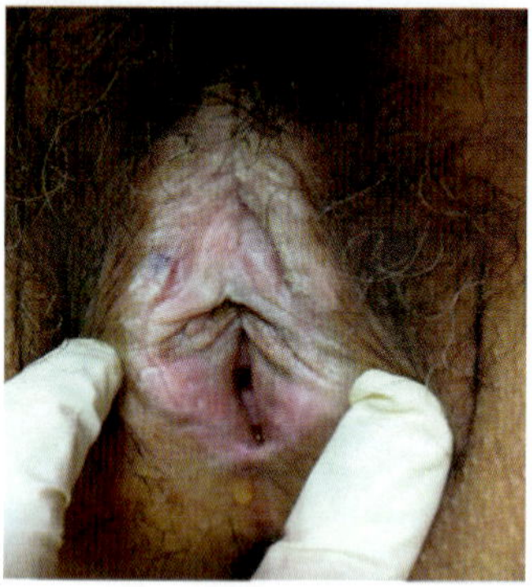

Figure 7. Lichen sclerosus (LS).

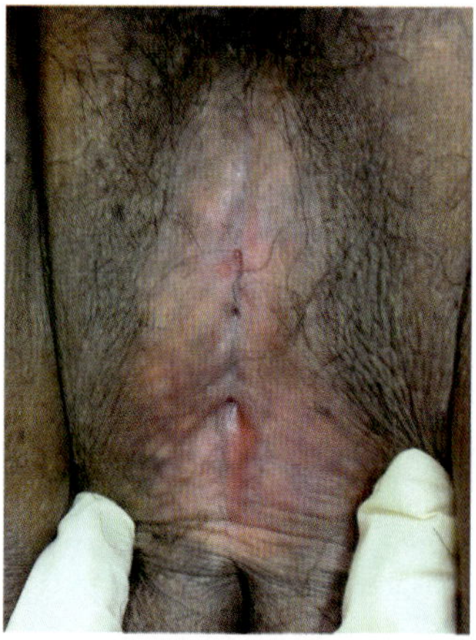

Figure 8. Lichen sclerosus (LS) with extensive scarring.

Pictures of various vulvar lesions

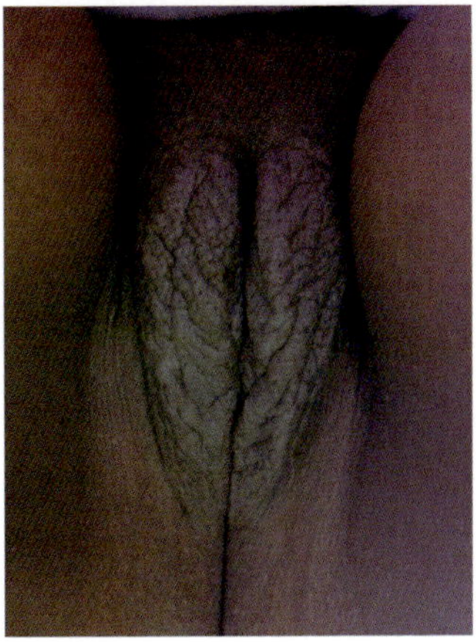

Figure 9. Lichen simplex chronicus (LSC).

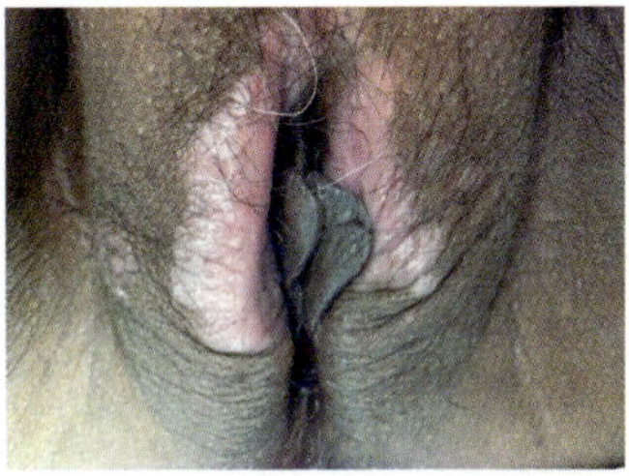

Figure 10. Lichen simplex chronicus with hypopigmentation.

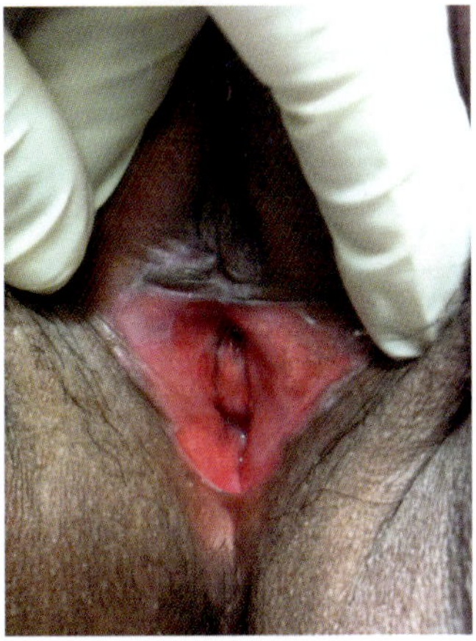

Figure 11. Erosive lichen planus.

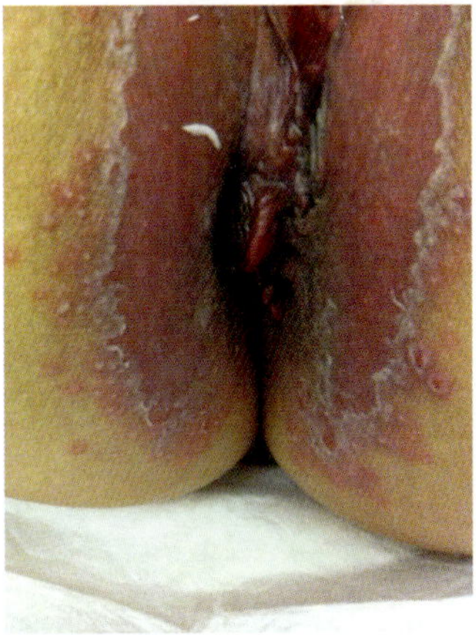

Figure 12. Contact dermatitis.

Pictures of various vulvar lesions

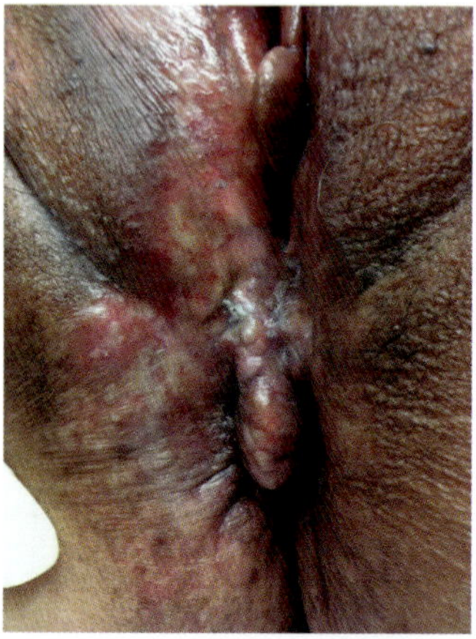

Figure 13. Radiation dermatitis.

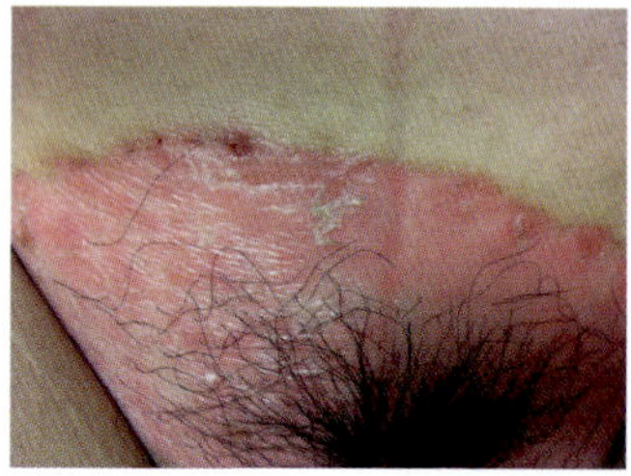

Figure 14. Psoriasis.

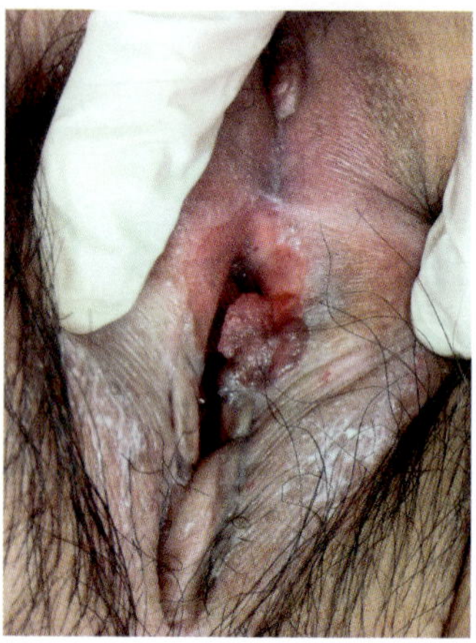

Figure 15. Vulvar intraepithelial neoplasia (VIN).

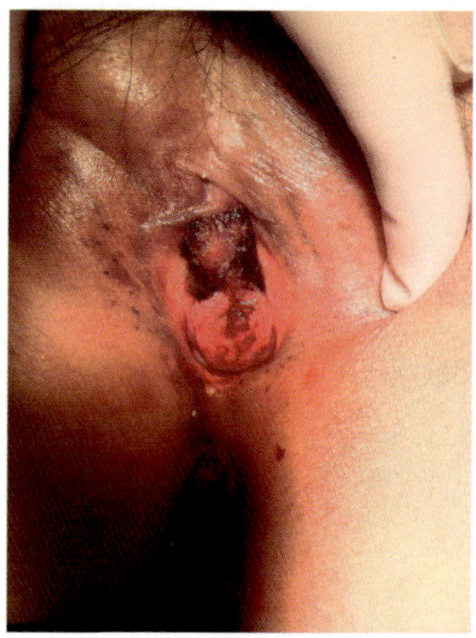

Figure 16. Vulvar cancer.

1. Normal anatomical variants. No treatment required

(a) *Vestibular papillomatosis*

30% of women
Few to hundreds of lesions
Asymptomatic, 2–10 mm lesions
Homogeneous, skin coloured, separate base,
Dome-shaped, cobblestone-like

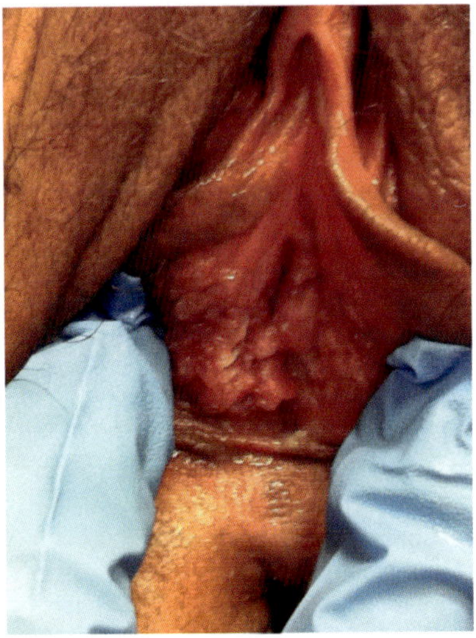

(b) *Sebaceous gland hyperplasia*

Fordyce spots
Enlarged ectopic sebaceous glands
Inner labia minora

Yellowish white
Asymptomatic, 1 to 2 mm lesions

2. Vulvar Pigmented Lesions

Genital tissue has a higher density of melanocytes than the rest of the body and is hormone dependent (pregnancy and with contraceptive use)

Condition	Location and Description of Lesion	Treatment
Physiological	Posterior introitus, the tips of the labia minora, labia majora, perineum, proximal medial thighs • Macular and symmetric, no change in texture from normal skin • Asymptomatic	• Reassurance
Acanthosis nigricans	Genitocrural folds and upper inner aspect of the thighs • Dark and velvety thickening of the skin	• Treat the primary cause such as diabetes, obesity
Pigmented basal cell carcinoma (BCC)	Common on labia majora • Ulcer, nodule or plaque • Brown/black	• Wide local excision (WLE)
Pigmented condylomata acuminata (anogenital warts)	Anywhere on the vulva • Biopsy required to rule out VIN if warts appear atypical	• Excision • Laser vapourisation • Liquid nitrogen • Imiquimod

(*Continued*)

(*Continued*)

Condition	Location and Description of Lesion	Treatment
Post inflammatory hyperpigmentation	Labia majora Secondary to scratching and excoriation	• Treat the primary cause
Melanoma	Anywhere on the vulva. • Large, irregularly pigmented and brown-shaped papules or nodule. Surface ulceration may be present	• Refer to oncologist
Seborrhoeic keratoses	Hair bearing areas, labia minora • They are flat-topped, sharply demarcated, brown or dark brown lesions with a stuck-on appearance	• No treatment required if asymptomatic • Excision with 2 to 3 mm margin if diagnosis is uncertain
Vulvar melanosis/lentiginosis	Modified mucous membrane of vulva • Brown black patchy hyperpigmentation	• No treatment required • Biopsy if diagnosis is uncertain
Vulvar intraepithelial neoplasia (VIN)	Any area on the vulva and perianal area • Red, brown or white flat topped papules and plaques	• VIN1 — no treatment required • VIN2 and VIN3 — refer to VIN management

3. Vulvar Ulcers

Diagnostically challenging
Ulcers should be differentiated from erosions

1. Erosions involve loss of epidermis only — appear deep red, weeping

Examples — herpes simplex (HSV), contact dermatitis, excoriated eczema

2. Ulcers involve loss of epidermis and dermis. Deeper. Yellowish base

Example — aphthous ulcer

Common Causes of Vulvar Ulcers

INFECTIVE

STI - refer to Chapter 55 on "STI"

Non–sexually transmitted

- Mycoplasma
- Herpes
- Hand foot mouth disease (HFMD)
- Candida
- Staphylococcus
- Streptococcus
- Tuberculosis
- Actinomycosis

INFLAMMATORY

- Aphthous ulcers
- Behcet disease
- Crohn disease
- Pemphigus vulgaris
- Pemphigoid
- Drug reactions —such as toxic epidermal necrosis (TEN) and erythema multiforme (EM)

NEOPLASTIC

- Vulvar intraepithelial neoplasia (VIN)
- Basal cell carcinoma (BCC)
- Squamous cell carcinoma (SCC)
- Extra-mammary Paget disease
- Melanoma
- Lymphoma
- Leukaemia

TRAUMATIC

- Genital mutilation
- Excoriations fissures ulceration secondary to itchy skin conditions

Management of Vulvar Ulcers

History

- Sexual history
- Geographic location of patient
- Pain and severity
- Ulcer development (vesicle-erosion-ulcer)
- Are there any associated skin, oral or ocular lesions?
- Is the lesion primary or recurrent?
- Any tender groin nodes or vaginal discharge?
- History of viral infections and fever
- Systemic symptoms (fever, headache, gastrointestinal tract or respiratory symptoms, myalgia)
- History of autoimmune disorders

Examination

Skin, oral mucosa, eyes
Lymphadenopathy (cervical/ inguinal/ femoral)
Size, shape, location of vulvar ulcer/ulcers
Examination of vagina and cervix

Laboratory Evaluation

- Full blood count
- Bacterial culture

(*Continued*)

- Serology for HSV, HIV, Syphilis
- Serology for EBV, CMV, Mycoplasma, antistreptolysin O titers (ASO) (based on clinical situation)
- ANA (autoimmune work up)
- Gastrointestinal tract (GIT) investigations for inflammatory bowel disease (based on clinical situation)

General principles of treatment

- General vulvar hygiene — patient education
- Sitz bath with warm water
- Zinc oxide barrier cream
- Topical anaesthetics
- Oral analgesics (NSAIDs) for mild pain
- Opioids for severe pain
- Oral fluconazole for secondary yeast infection
- Antibiotics for secondary bacterial infection

Specific treatment

- Antiviral: acyclovir if HSV likely diagnosis
- Steroids: consider topical corticosteroids for aphthous ulcers or Behçet disease.

(*Continued*)

(*Continued*)

- Antibiotics: if bacterial infection suspected
- Treatment of sexually transmited infections (CDC guidelines — refer to Chapter 55 on "STI")
- Immunosuppressants: (Behcet disease and inflammatory bowel disease and other rheumatological conditions suspected) under specialist supervision

Aphthous ulcers

- Diagnosis of exclusion
- Painful, deep ulcers
- History of recurrence
- Single or multiple
- Culture negative
- Biopsies non-specific
- Test for HIV

Note — in HIV patients with genital ulcers — 60% of genital ulcers are due to aphthous ulcers and 40% to HSV

Treatment of Aphthous Ulcers

- Steroids: topical, intralesional or oral
- Acute onset and painful lesions — Prednisolone 40–60 mg per day for 3–5 days and taper depending on response
- Pain relief

(*Continued*)

Recurrent and recalcitrant ulcers (under specialist supervision)

- Colchicine 0.6 mg bd to tds
- Dapsone 50–150 mg per day
- Colchicine plus dapsone together
- Thalidomide 100–150 mg per day

4. Vulvar Nodules, Cysts or Tumours

Condition	Location/ Description of Lesion	Treatment
Condyloma acuminatum (HPV 6,11)	Warty surface, variable size, shape and location. Colposcopy. Examine vagina, cervix. Pap smear	Imiquimod Excision, laser vapourisation, Liquid nitrogen
Molluscum contagiosum (Pox virus)	Umbilicated papules Commonly multiple Common in children	Self-limiting. Local excision, electrocautery, cryotherapy or laser therapy
Keratinocyte tumour: epidermal inclusion cyst, sebaceous cysts	Labia majora and minora. Other hair bearing areas, yellowish papules with a visible opening	Excision if symptomatic
Keratinocytic tumour: angiokeratoma	Purplish blue spots, bleeds on scratching	Excision/laser vapourisation if symptomatic
Keratinocyte tumour: seborrhoeic keratoses	Brown to black,warty stuck — on appearance Location — labia majora and labia minora	No treatment required. Excision if diagnosis is uncertain

(Continued)

Vulvar Nodules, Cysts or Tumours (*Continued*)

Condition	Location/ Description of Lesion	Treatment
Vulvar oedema	Lymphoedema or angioedema	Treatment directed towards cause
Mesenchymal cell origin: lipoma, leiomyoma, fibroma, granular cell tumour, granular cell myoblastoma	Variable size and consistency	Excision with 10 mm margin
Bartholin cyst	Within posterior vestibule. Variable size	Marsupialisation. Excision of gland for recurrences. Indurated cysts in postmenopausal women need excision even though asymptomatic (to rule out carcinoma)
Vulvar endometriosis	Biopsy of lesion to confirm histology Ultrasound pelvis to exclude endometriosis in pelvis Evaluate menstrual history	Offer excision of endometriosis if symptomatic
Fibroepithelial polyp	Pelvic examination	If asymptomatic and <1 cm, may offer conservative management If symptomatic or ≥1 cm, for excision

5. Vulvar Dermatoses

Lesion	Presentation	Investigation	Management
a) Lichen sclerosus (LS)	Long-standing intense pruritus *Colour changes* Hypopig-mentation, ivory white plaques *Architectural changes* • scarring and midline fusion • adhesions between labia majora and minora • buried clitoris Fissures and purpura Key hole distribution Involves perianal area Vagina is spared	• Keye's punch biopsy • Investigations to rule out (diabetes mellitus, thyroid dysfunction, Pernicious anaemia • Needs long-term follow up • Nodule, ulceration or hyperkeratotic (dense white or leukoplakia) areas need urgent biopsy (squamous cell carcinoma (SCC) — 5%)	• Ultra potent steroid ointment — Topical clobetasol propionate — 0.05% ointment daily for 1 month — alternate days for 1 month — twice weekly for 1 month — review patient in 3 months • Maintenance therapy with topical betamethasone valerate 0.05% — 0.1% twice or thrice a week recommended indefinitely • Night sedation • Vulva hygiene • Asymptomatic also need treatment

(*Continued*)

Vulvar Dermatoses (*Continued*)

Lesion	Presentation	Investigation	Management
b) Lichen simplex chronicus (LSC)	End-stage disorder due to chronic itch-scratch cycle. Relentless pruritus Symmetric, variable pigmentation Leathery or coarse texture Labia majora commonly involved Unilateral or bilateral	• Detailed history • Vulva biopsy to determine underlying problem (often more than one cause) *Common underlying causes* are atopic and contact eczema *Less common causes* Lichen sclerosus (LS), vulvar intraepithelial neoplasia (VIN), psoriasis, candida, diabetes Heat, stress and menstruation worsen LSC	• Mid to high potency steroids • Night sedation • Break itch-scratch cycle. • Stop irritation • Oral steroids may be required • Treat concurrent bacterial and fungal infection with oral medication • Sitz bath

(*Continued*)

Vulvar Dermatoses (*Continued*)

Lesion	Presentation	Investigation	Management
c) Lichen planus (LP)	Cutaneous or mucous membrane LP. Mucous membrane LP is erosive and more common. Vagina and vestibule involved Severe burning. Pain rather than itch is predominant. Oral mucosa, scalp, skin, nails and eye may be affected. Glossy red erosions and scarring, purulent vaginal discharge present.	• Refer vulva clinic as it is difficult to treat and cure • Look at mouth and skin for LP • Rule out drug induced erosions, bullous diseases such as pemphigus vulgaris and pemphigoid • Biopsy immuno-fluorescence if bullous diseases suspected.	• Super potent corticosteroids • Resistant cases need systemic steroids (Prednisolone 40–60 mg a day, taper dose accordingly. • Methotrexate 7.5 to 15mg PO or SC • Cyclosporin 3–4mg/kg per day • Vaginal steroids for vaginal involvement • Vaginal dilatation for adhesions. • Treatment of oral ulcers with topical steroids • Systemic immuno-suppressive medication (used under specialist supervision only) • Surgery for scarring in selected cases.

(*Continued*)

Vulvar Dermatoses (*Continued*)

Lesion	Presentation	Investigation	Management
d) Vulvar dermatitis	Convex surfaces such as labia majora and mons are involved. Erythema, oedema, blisters, scaling, excoriations.	• Examine skin surfaces • Biopsy to rule out Paget disease	• Avoid allergens and irritants • Steroid ointments and emollients • Oral anti-histamine to relieve pruritus • Vulva hygiene
Atopic dermatitis	Search other crural folds, scalp, umbilicus, extremities		
Irritant contact dermatitis	Symmetric and extending into areas of "irritant" contact.		
Allergic contact dermatitis	Same as above		
e) Psoriasis	Erythema with silvery scales and well-defined margins. Scalp, nails and flexures of the body may be involved.	• Biopsy • Elbows and knees (often affected) • Greater scaling in extragenital regions.	Refer to dermatologist

(*Continued*)

Vulvar Dermatoses (*Continued*)

Lesion	Presentation	Investigation	Management
f) Vulvitis in chronic diabetic patients	Macerated vulva Vulvovaginal candidiasis, folliculitis	Biopsy suspicious lesions	• Optimise diabetes • Vulva hygiene • Use steroids with caution
g) Infectious vulvitis	Commonly candida Consider dermatophytes (tinea cruris)	• VP3 (swab for candida/ trichomonas/ gardnerella) • Culture for resistant strains	Refer to Chapter 53 on "Vaginal Discharge and Recurrent Vulvo-Vaginal Candidiasis"

6. Vulvar premalignant lesions

a) Vulvar intraepithelial neoplasia (VIN)

b) Paget disease

c) Melanoma *in situ*

Lichen planus and lichen sclerosus are associated with the risk of squamous cell carcinoma (SCC) — 4 to 6% of cases.

Vulvar premalignant lesions (*Continued*)

a. ***Vulvar intraepithelial neoplasia (VIN)***

- New classification (2004 ISSVD oncology sub-committee based on morphology and histology)

▪ VIN usual type — Include baseloid type or warty

▪ VIN differentiated type — associated with lichen sclerosus

▪ Unclassified — features that do not fit the above 2 types

1. VIN usual type — low risk of progression to SCC (5%)
   - Incidence increasing
   - Young women
   - HPV-related
   - Associated with immunosuppression
   - Cigarette smoking
   - Multifocal/multicentric (HPV16,18,31)
   - Synchronous VAIN, CIN common
2. VIN differentiated type — high progression to SCC (30%)
   - 5% of VIN
   - Postmenopausal women

(*Continued*)

Vulvar premalignant lesions (*Continued*)

- Associated with lichen sclerosus (LS)
- HPV negative
- Unifocal lesions

Symptoms of VIN

- Lumps
- Burning and itch / irritation. May be asymptomatic

Signs of VIN

- Red, brown or white lesion
- Warty, moist, eroded or ulcerated
- Mostly non-hair bearing areas

Differential diagnosis of VIN

- Flat warts
- Seborrhoeic keratoses
- Vulvar dermatoses

Diagnosis of VIN

- Physical examination
- Biopsy (gold standard)
- Vaginal examination

(*Continued*)

Vulvar premalignant lesions (*Continued*)

- Cytology/colposcopy
- Perianal examination

Management of VIN
General advice — Stop smoking

(1) *Usual VIN*

- Excision
- Ablation (laser vapourisation (multifocal and extensive lesions) (3 mm depth hair bearing area; 2 mm depth non-hair bearing area)
- Immunomodulators (side effects—ulceration, erythema)

(2) *Differentiated VIN*

- Depends on location and extent of disease
- Wide local excision (WLE) 1 cm margin
- Skinning vulvectomy
- Long-term follow up is required

b. ***Extra-mammary Paget disease***

Mammary Paget disease — on the nipple and areola, where its presence signifies an underlying adenocarcinoma of the breast

Extra-mammary — genital, perianal and axillary regions

Paget disease

Extra-mammary Paget disease — vulva

1. *Primary extra-mammary Paget disease* is epidermotropic carcinoma arising within the epidermis or epidermal appendages — no underlying carcinoma (most common)
2. *Secondary extra-mammary Paget disease* is visceral carcinoma (anorectal, bladder or urethra) that is epidermotropic to the skin
   - 25% underlying adenocarcinoma
   - Most common in elderly, postmenopausal women
   - Labia majora and mons are commonly involved

Symptoms of extra-mammary Paget disease

- Pruritus
- Soreness
- Bleeding

(*Continued*)

***Extra-mammary Paget disease* (*Continued*)**

Signs of extra-mammary Paget disease

- Crusting lesion, eczematous (do not respond to topical steroids)
- Clear demarcation

Tip
Red and white lesions

Red sea with white islands (areas of ulceration and hyperkeratosis)

Diagnosis — biopsy lesion

Management of extra-mammary Paget disease

Investigations to detect associated adenocarcinoma (location dependent)

- Pap smear/mammogram/cystoscopy/oesophago-gastroduodenoscopy (OGD)/colonoscopy

Treatment of extra-mammary Paget disease

- Wide local excision full thickness skin to the subcutaneous fat, with 2 to 3 cm margin
- 5% imiquimod cream 2 to 3 times a week

Terminology and classification of vulvar pain from the International Society for the Study of Vulvovaginal Disease ISSVD 2003

A. **Vulvar pain related to a specific disorder**
   1. Infectious (candidiasis, herpes)
   2. Inflammatory (lichen planus, immunobullous disorders)
   3. Neoplastic (Paget disease, squamous cell carcinoma)
   4. Neurologic (herpes neuralgia, spinal nerve compression)

B. **Vulvodynia**
   1. Generalised
      a. Provoked (sexual, nonsexual, or both)
      b. Unprovoked
      c. Mixed (provoked and unprovoked)
   2. Localised (including vestibulodynia, clitorodynia, hemivulvodynia)
      a. Provoked (sexual, nonsexual, or both)
      b. Unprovoked
      c. Mixed (provoked and unprovoked)

- Vulvodynia, in which the vulva appears normal, other than occasional erythema, which is most prominent at the duct openings

As for vulvar pain, there are two major forms:

- **Hyperalgesia** (a low threshold for pain)
- **Allodynia** (pain in response to light touch)

Management (often difficult and multidisciplinary)

- Treat abnormal visible condition present (infections, dermatoses, premalignant or malignant conditions, etc.)
- Vulvar care measures
- Topical medications — emollients, anaesthetics and corticosteroids
- Oral medications — tricyclic antidepressants
- Biofeedback/physical therapy
- Pelvic floor exercises
- Low oxalate diet, calcium and citrate supplementation
- Cognitive behavioural therapy
- Sexual counselling

Common Vaginal Lesions

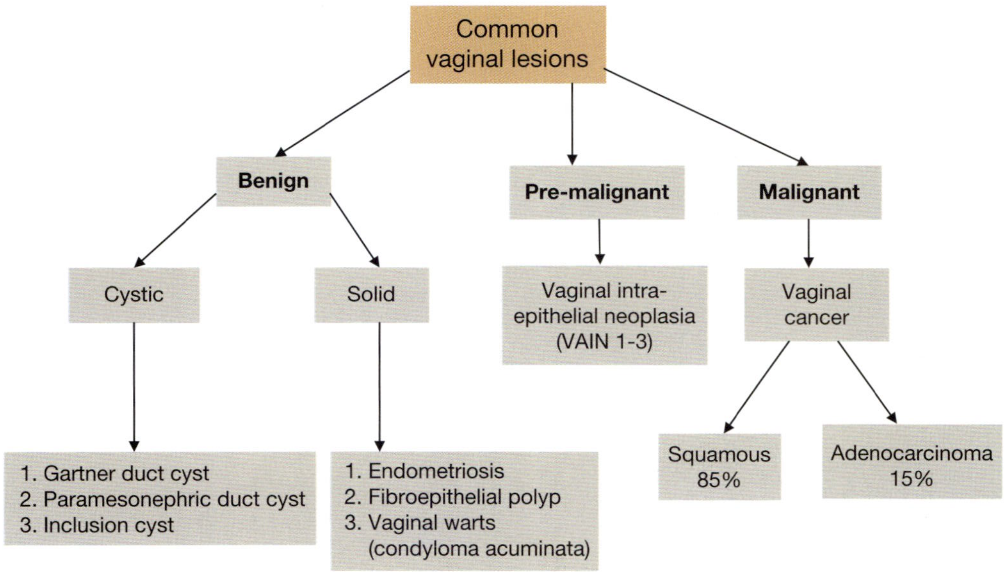

Common Vaginal Lesions (*Continued*)

Vaginal lesions	Investigations	Management
Gartner duct cyst (from remnant of mesonephric ducts) Usually asymptomatic < 1 cm but can enlarge	Pelvic examination Biopsy of cyst if looks suspicious to rule out malignancy	If asymptomatic, offer conservative management with routine examination to follow up cyst. If symptomatic, offer excision of cyst.
Paramesonephric duct cyst	Pelvic examination Biopsy of cyst if looks suspicious to rule out malignancy	
Inclusion cyst	Pelvic examination Biopsy of cyst if looks suspicious to rule out malignancy	
Vaginal endometriosis	Biopsy of lesion to confirm histology Ultrasound scan of pelvis to exclude endometriosis in pelvis Evaluate menstrual history	
Fibroepithelial polyp	Pelvic examination	
Vaginal warts (condyloma acuminata)	Colposcopy: to rule out warts affecting cervix and vagina Ensure Pap smear done	Depending on number, size and location of warts, offer: — Excision — Laser vapourisation — Topical imiquimod

(*Continued*)

Common Vaginal Lesions (*Continued*)

Vaginal lesions	Investigations	Management
VAIN *Risk factors* Radiation therapy Smoking History of CIN or VIN Immunosuppression	Colposcopy: need to assess vagina and cervix as well Ensure Pap smear done	*VAIN 1*: Offer expectant management with repeat colposcopy in 6 months *VAIN 2–3*: Depending on number/size and location of lesion offer : — Excision — Laser vapourisation — Topical imiquimod
Vaginal cancer (rare) * Refer to Chapter 40 on "Approach to Gynaecological Cancers"	Colposcopy Biopsy of vaginal tumour for histology	Refer Gynae-oncologist Examination under anaesthesia, cystoscopy *Early stages* Surgery or radiation therapy Surgery: Total hysterectomy Partial/radical vaginectomy, Inguinal/ pelvic lymph node dissection +/- vaginal reconstruction *Advanced stages* Radiation therapy May need chemotherapy as adjuvant treatment

Chapter 45

POSTMENOPAUSAL BLEEDING (PMB)

Definition of PMB

Any uterine bleeding in a menopausal woman (other than the expected cyclic bleeding that occurs in women taking sequential postmenopausal hormone therapy).

Menopause is one year of amenorrhoea after the final menstrual period.

Causes of PMB

- Atrophic vaginitis
- Polyps/fibroids (endometrial/endocervical)
- Endometritis (e.g. endometrial tuberculosis)
- Endometrial hyperplasia
- Carcinoma (endometrium/cervix/vagina/vulva/ovary/fallopian tube)

- Iatrogenic (drug-induced)
  - hormone replacement therapy
  - anticoagulants
- Others
  - Foreign body (e.g. pessary)
  - Hydrometra, pyometra, hematometra

Management of Postmenopausal Bleeding (PMB)

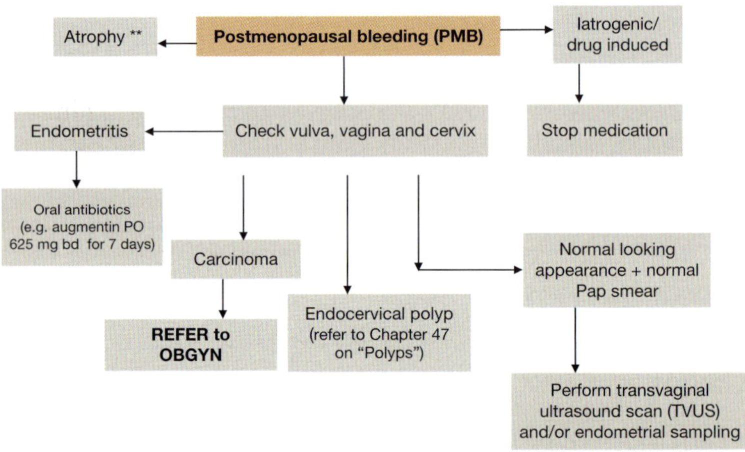

TVUS — Endometrial Thickness (mm)	Sensitivity for Detection of Endometrial Cancer	Specificity for Detection of Endometrial Cancer
4 mm	96%	53%
5 mm	96%	61%

Ultrasound measurement of endometrial thickness alone cannot be used reliably to exclude cancer.

Endometrial sampling methods:

1. Pipelle
2. Explora
3. Hysteroscopy and endometrial sampling/dilatation and curettage

(Note: Pipelle device is an endometrial sampling technique for obtaining an adequate and representative endometrial sample. It should be reserved for those patients with a low risk of endometrial cancer, hyperplasia and polyps. Any failure to obtain an adequate endometrial sample using pipelle would necessitate a full endometrial curettage.)

Management of PMB depends on the cause

a) If endometrial cancer — refer to oncology.

b) If no endometrial cancer and histology confirms atrophy — treat atrophy (as outlined below).

Treatment of Atrophy of genital tract

** Low dose vaginal oestrogen (≤50 μg oestradiol or ≤0.3 mg conjugated oestrogen). Preparations include:

1) Vaginal oestradiol tablet (Vagifem®) — 25 μg/10 μg.

2) Conjugated oestrogen cream (Premarin®) — 1 g contains 0.625 mg of conjugated oestrogen. Dose is 0.5–2 g of cream administered intravaginally.
3) Oestradiol cream (Estrace®) — 1 g contains 100 mcg of oestradiol. Dose is 1 g of cream daily.

These low dose oestrogen preparations are administered daily for one week, followed by twice weekly for maintenance.

Tamoxifen and PMB

Tamoxifen users have a 3–6-fold increased incidence of endometrial cancer due to its weak oestrogenic effect on the endometrium. Refer to OBGYN for urgent assessment of the endometrium if patients have PMB.

Chapter 46

THICKENED ENDOMETRIUM

- Management should depend on clinical symptoms.
- If increased endometrial thickness (ET) is persistent and patient is symptomatic, refer to OBGYN for further evaluation.

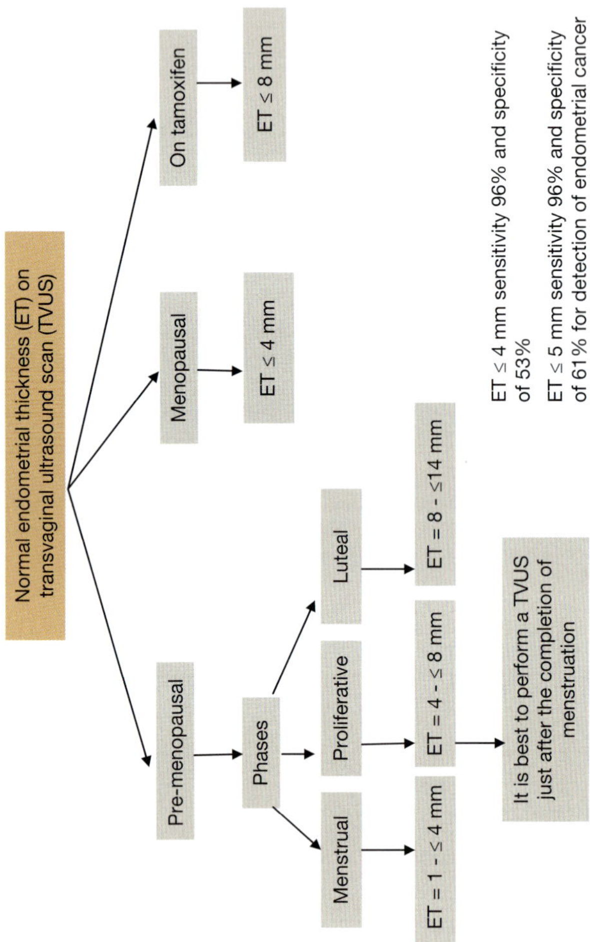
Normal endometrial thickness (ET) on transvaginal ultrasound scan (TVUS)
Pre-menopausal
Menopausal
On tamoxifen
ET ≤ 4 mm
ET ≤ 8 mm
Phases
Menstrual
Proliferative
Luteal
ET = 1 - ≤ 4 mm
ET = 4 - ≤ 8 mm
ET = 8 - ≤14 mm
It is best to perform a TVUS just after the completion of menstruation
ET ≤ 4 mm sensitivity 96% and specificity of 53%
ET ≤ 5 mm sensitivity 96% and specificity of 61% for detection of endometrial cancer

Causes of Thickened ET on Transvaginal Ultrasound Scan (TVUS)	Investigation (Ix)	Management (Mx)
1. Luteal phase	Ensure normal menstrual history Repeat ultrasound (TVUS) pelvis during or just after menses	Reassure if endometrial thickness is normal
2. Early pregnancy	Urine pregnancy test (UPT)	If UPT positive, for dating/viability ultrasound scan
3. Early pregnancy complications: (a) Miscarriage	Serum beta-HCG trending	If symptomatic (vaginal bleeding, abdominal pain), for evacuation of uterus by suction curettage If asymptomatic, may offer expectant management with oral antibiotic coverage, follow-up appointment in 1–2 weeks to review symptoms
4. Early pregnancy complications: (b) Ectopic pregnancy	Serum beta-HCG trending	Refer to gynaecologist Please refer to Chapter 12 on "Ectopic Pregnancy"

(*Continued*)

(*Continued*)

Causes of Thickened ET on Transvaginal Ultrasound Scan (TVUS)	Investigation (Ix)	Management (Mx)
5. Early pregnancy complications: (c) Molar pregnancy	Serum βhcg FBC, T+S, U/E/Cr, LFT, PT/PTT, TFT, CXR, (only if required) Histology of products of conception (POC)	Evacuation of uterus by surgical suction curettage, by an experienced surgeon Will need follow-up βhcg trending until negative Advise not to get pregnant until follow-up is complete
6. Retained products of conception (RPOC): (a) Incomplete miscarriage (b) Post-termination of pregnancy (c) Post-delivery	ET ≥15 mm Hyperechoic/hypoechoic material within endometrium with vascularity Irregular interface between endometrium and myometrium	If symptomatic (vaginal bleeding, abdominal pain, fever), for evacuation of uterus by suction curettage If asymptomatic, may offer expectant management with oral antibiotics; follow-up appointment in 1–2 weeks to review symptoms
7. Endometrial polyp	If polyp <1 cm and asymptomatic, offer repeat TVUS in 3 to 6 months (just after menses) to follow-up size of polyp If polyp ≥1 cm, refer to Chapter 47 on "Polyps"	Diagnostic hysteroscopy, dilatation & curettage, polypectomy Incidence of polyp recurrence: 10–30%

(*Continued*)

(*Continued*)

Causes of Thickened ET on Transvaginal Ultrasound Scan (TVUS)	Investigation (Ix)	Management (Mx)
8. Submucosal fibroid	If asymptomatic, offer repeat TVUS (just after menses) to follow-up size of fibroid If heavy menses, needs treatment.	If fibroid ≤5 cm, for transcervical resection of myoma (TCRM) If fibroid >5 cm, offer GnRH agonist to reduce size of fibroid, re-scan for size, and then offer (TCRM) if appropriate size Success rate of TCRM: ~80% Complications of TCRM: (a) Cervical trauma (b) Uterine perforation, with possible bowel injury (c) Fluid overload (if negative volume) (d) Bleeding (e) Infection Incidence of fibroid recurrence post-TCRM: • 15–30% over 10 years • 50% of those with incomplete resection will require repeat surgery within 2 years

(*Continued*)

(Continued)

Causes of Thickened ET on Transvaginal Ultrasound Scan (TVUS)	Investigation (Ix)	Management (Mx)
9. Endometrial hyperplasia High risk groups: • Older age group >35 • Irregular menses (i.e. Polycystic ovarian syndrome) • Unopposed oestrogen exposure • Obesity • Smoking • Diabetes mellitus, hypertension • Family history of hereditary non-polyposis colorectal cancer • Nulliparity • Early menarche • Late menopause • Tamoxifen	Diagnostic hysteroscopy, dilatation & curettage for histology	If histology: (a) Normal: — Reassurance — Offer repeat TVUS to follow-up ET (b) Simple hyperplasia without atypia: — risk of progressing to cancer < 1% (c) Simple hyperplasia with atypia: — risk of progressing to cancer < 3% (d) Complex hyperplasia without atypia: — risk of progressing to cancer < 10% (e) Complex hyperplasia with atypia — risk of progressing to cancer 25–30% — 30% risk of co-existing endometrial cancer — Mx for (b), (c), (d), (e):

(Continued)

(*Continued*)

Causes of Thickened ET on Transvaginal Ultrasound Scan (TVUS)	Investigation (Ix)	Management (Mx)
	Side effects of progesterone: — Bloatedness — Weight gain — Mood disturbances — Acne — Drowsiness — Irregular spotting	High-dose progesterone treatment × 6 months *Endometrial hyperplasia without atypia*: Cyclical PO Provera 10 mg bd × 14 days for 6 months *Endometrial hyperplasia with atypia*: Continuous PO Provera 20 mg bd × 6 months — Reassess histology after completion of progesterone treatment or — Definitive surgery: hysterectomy — Surgery preferable for (c), (d), (e), especially if completed family

(*Continued*)

(Continued)

Causes of Thickened ET on Transvaginal Ultrasound Scan (TVUS)	Investigation (Ix)	Management (Mx)
10. Endometrial cancer High risk groups: similar to that for endometrial hyperplasia Refer to Chapter 40 on "Approach to Gynaecological Cancers"	Diagnostic hysteroscopy, dilatation & curettage for histology	Refer to Gynae-Oncology team Preoperative work up: — CT scan of abdomen/pelvis — FBC, U/E/Cr, LFT, PT/PTT, T+S, Ca-125 (if indicated by atypical presentation or histology), CXR Staging laparotomy, total hysterectomy, bilateral salpingo-oophorectomy, pelvic lymph node dissection Depending on stage/grade/histology of disease, may require adjuvant therapy (i.e. radiotherapy, chemotherapy), hormonal treatment

(Continued)

(*Continued*)

Causes of Thickened ET on Transvaginal Ultrasound Scan (TVUS)	Investigation (Ix)	Management (Mx)
11. On tamoxifen	Assess for any abnormal vaginal bleeding or post-menopausal bleeding Assess risk factors for endometrial cancer (as stated above)	*If symptomatic* (abnormal vaginal bleeding/ postmenopausal bleeding): — TVUS — D+C and hysteroscopy for endometrial biopsy *If asymptomatic*: — No role for routine screening if low risk for endometrial cancer — If high risk for endometrial cancer/ ET $>$ 8 mm, refer to gynaecologist for further evaluation

Chapter 47

POLYPS (CERVICAL/ ENDOMETRIAL)

Cervical Polyps

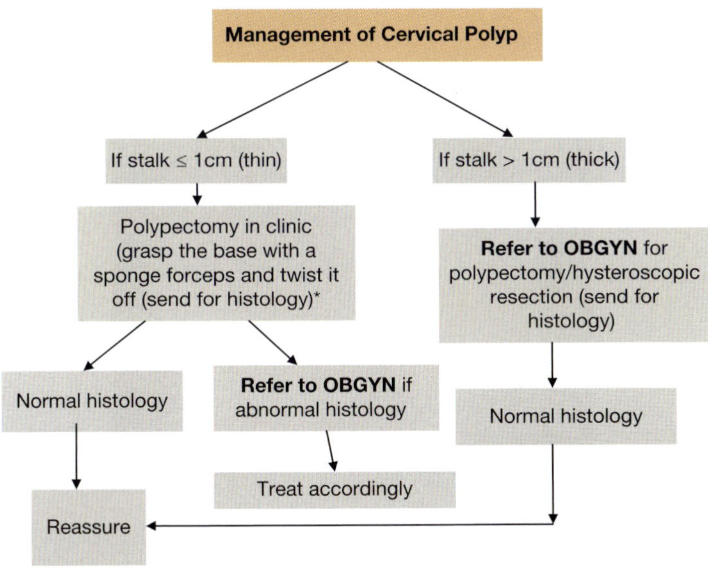

*Apply Monsels solution to secure haemostasis post procedure

Cervical Polyps

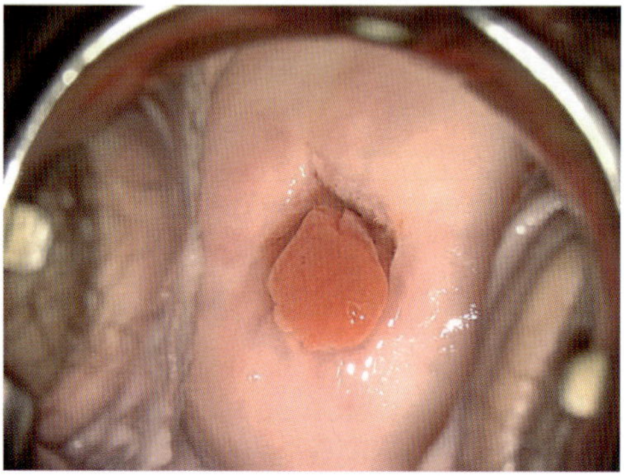

Figure 1. Pedunculated cervical polyp.

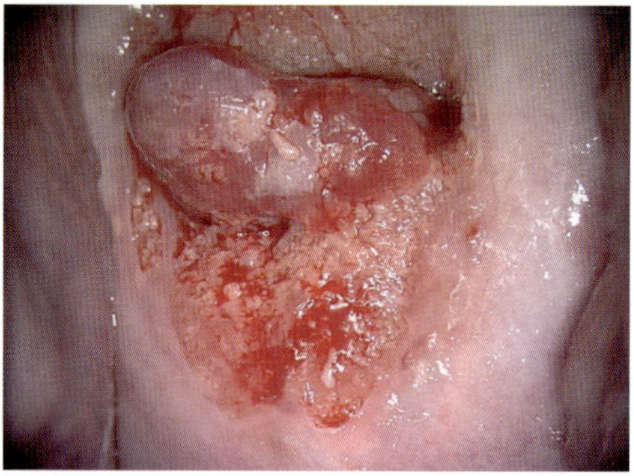

Figure 2. Broad based polyp.

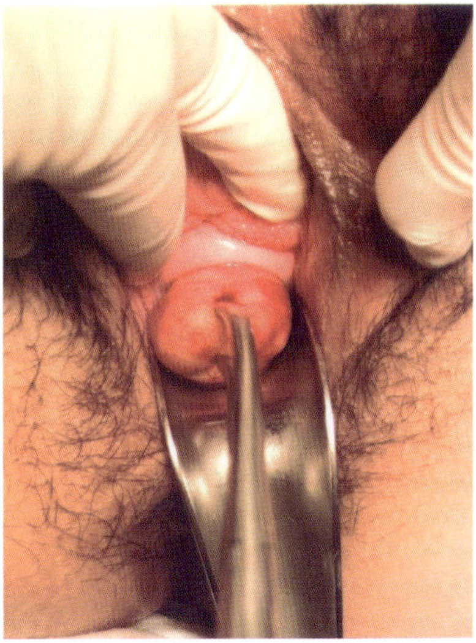

Figure 3. Large fibroid polyp protruding through cervical os.

Endometrial Polyps

- They are hyperplastic overgrowth of endometrial glands and stroma.

- **Risk factors**
  - Tamoxifen
  - Obesity
  - Hormone therapy (oestrogen ± progesterone)

- **Clinical presentation of endometrial polyps**
  - Discovered incidentally on ultrasound, hysteroscopy or on speculum examination (may prolapse at external cervical os)
  - Abnormal uterine bleeding (AUB)

- **Diagnosis of endometrial polyps**
  - Transvaginal ultrasound scan (TVUS)
  - Saline infusion sonogram (SIS)
  - Diagnostic hysteroscopy

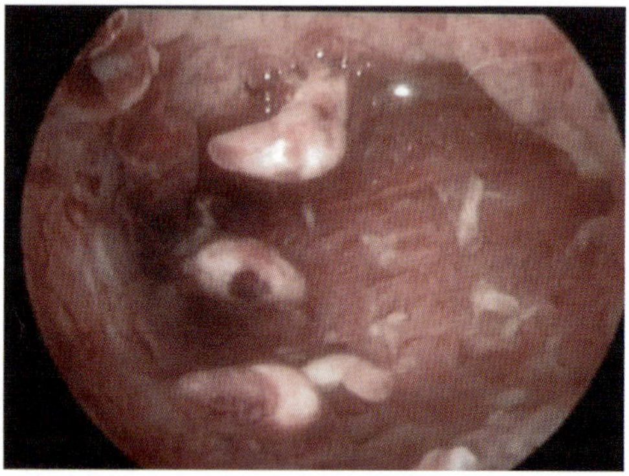

Figure 4. Hysteroscopic picture of endometrial polyps.

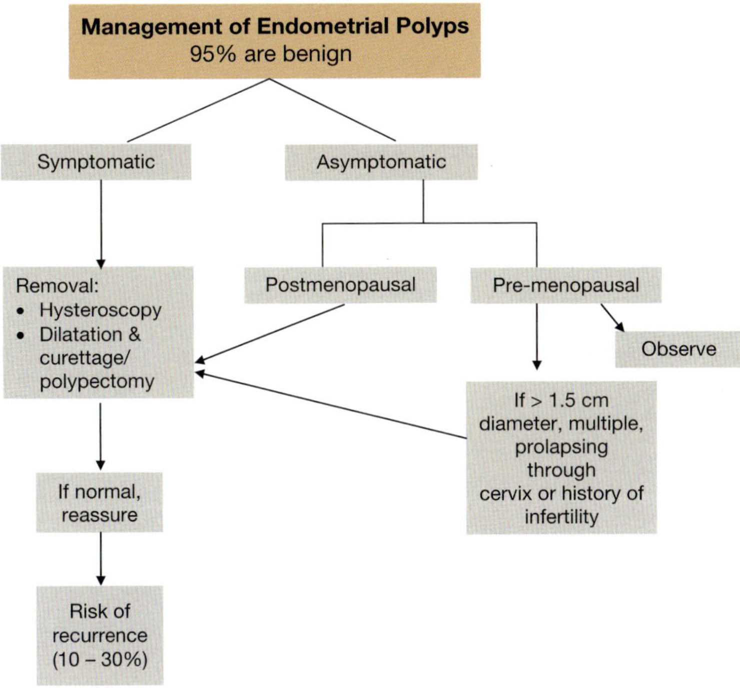
Management of Endometrial Polyps
95% are benign
Symptomatic
Asymptomatic
Removal:
• Hysteroscopy
• Dilatation & curettage/ polypectomy
Postmenopausal
Pre-menopausal
Observe
If > 1.5 cm diameter, multiple, prolapsing through cervix or history of infertility
If normal, reassure
Risk of recurrence (10 – 30%)

Chapter 48

FIBROIDS

Fibroids are benign smooth muscle tumours of the uterus and are present in 30% of women in the reproductive age group. They grow in response to oestrogen and progesterone, and may even shrink after menopause.

Exact Aetiology

This is not clearly understood.

Location of Fibroids

1. Intramural
2. Submucosal/Fibroid polyp
3. Subserosal/Pedunculated
4. Cervical

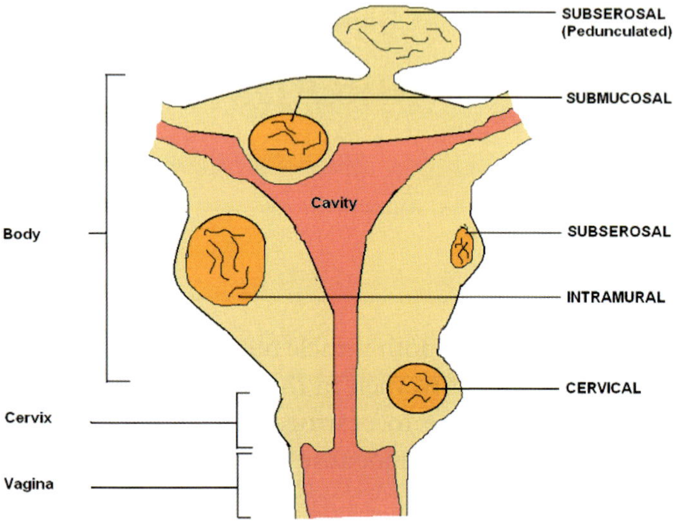

Figure 1. Different locations of uterine fibroids.

Risk Factors

1. Race — black women have a 2–3-fold increased risk as compared with white women
2. Early menarche — <10 years old
3. Nulliparity
4. Obesity
5. Polycystic ovarian syndrome (PCOS)
6. Hypertension
7. Diabetes mellitus

Fibroids can be asymptomatic (majority) or symptomatic.

Symptoms include:

1. Heavy menstrual bleeding (HMB)
2. Pain
   - usually due to degeneration, torsion or associated adenomyosis
   - dysmenorrhoea, usually associated with adenomyosis, heavy menstrual flow or passage of clots
3. Pelvic pressure and pain
   - urinary frequency, difficulty passing urine and acute retention of urine with fibroid causing direct pressure on the bladder/bladder outlet
   - hydronephrosis/hydroureter can rarely occur with obstruction of the distal ureter
   - constipation can occur with external pressure on the rectum
4. Reproduction
   - difficulty in conceiving and higher risk of miscarriage (in patients with submucosal fibroids or intramural fibroids with a submucosal component that distort the endometrial cavity)
   - possible adverse pregnancy outcomes, e.g. miscarriage, abruptio placentae, placenta praevia, preterm labour, malpresentation

Physical Examination

An enlarged, palpable uterus per abdomen or on bimanual palpation. Size is usually described in weeks, corresponding to uterine size during pregnancy.

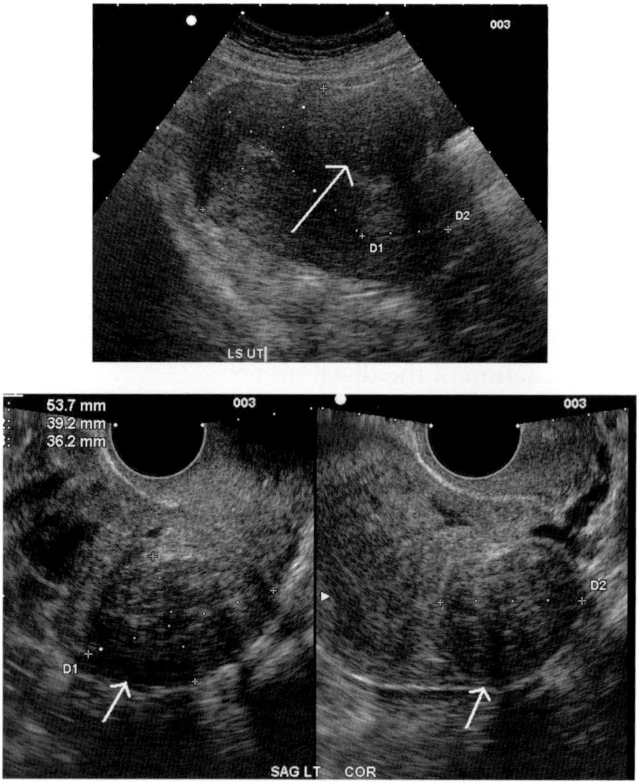

Figure 2. Ultrasound images of fibroids as shown.

Investigations:

1. Full blood count to check for anaemia
2. Ultrasound scan of pelvis
   - highly sensitive to detect fibroids
3. Magnetic resonance imaging (MRI) pelvis
   - useful for differentiating leiomyomas from leiomyosarcomas

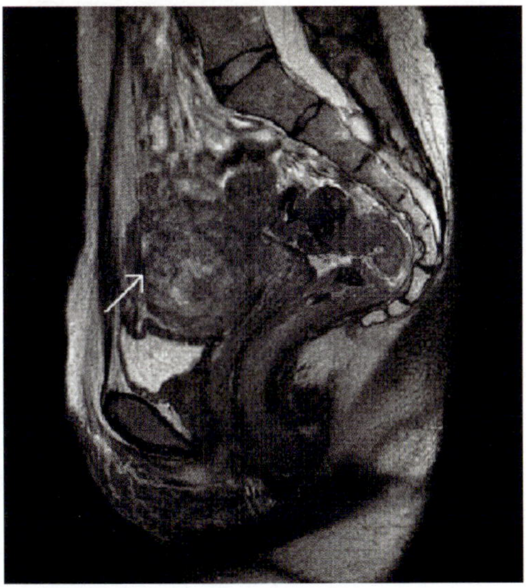

Figure 3. MRI images of a large intramural fibroid as indicated.

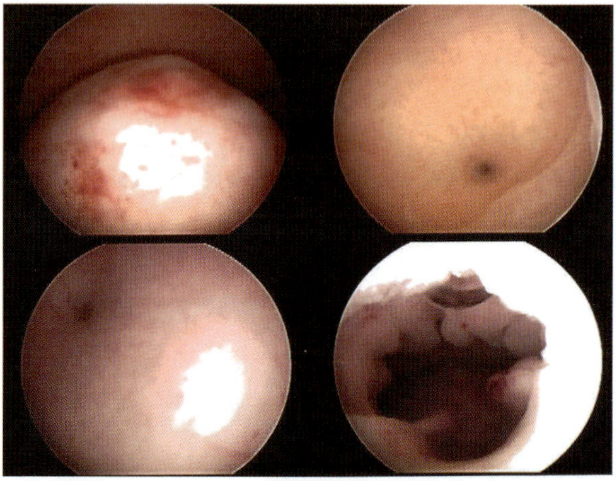

Figure 4. Hysteroscopic picture of a submucosal fibroid.

Management of fibroids:

In women with abnormal uterine bleeding, it is important to exclude an underlying endometrial pathology.

1. Conservative

- Fibroids are benign tumours, and can be managed expectantly if asymptomatic
- Surveillance with follow-up ultrasound scans
- **Tranexamic acid and NSAIDs** both decrease menstrual flow. Tranexamic acid is an anti-fibrinolytic. NSAIDs act by decreasing prostaglandin production. The most effective NSAID is mefenamic acid.

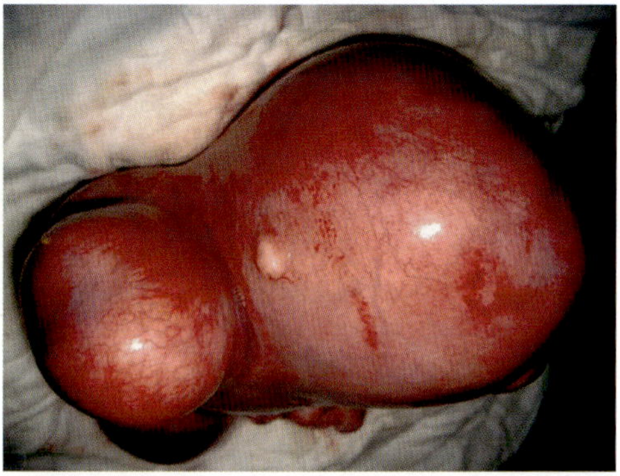

Figure 5. Uterus irregularly enlarged with multiple fibroids.

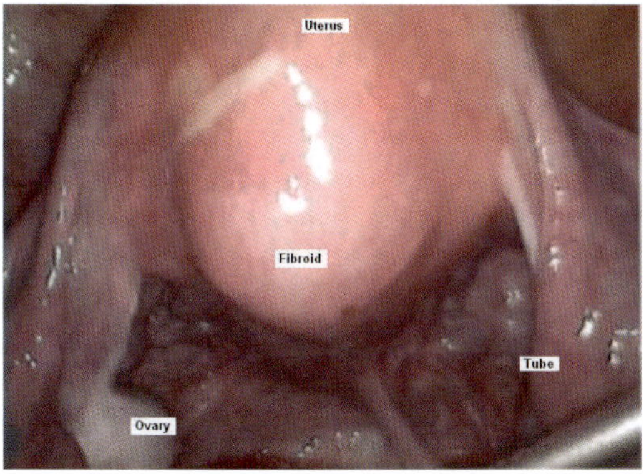

Figure 6. Laparoscopic picture of an intramural fibroid.

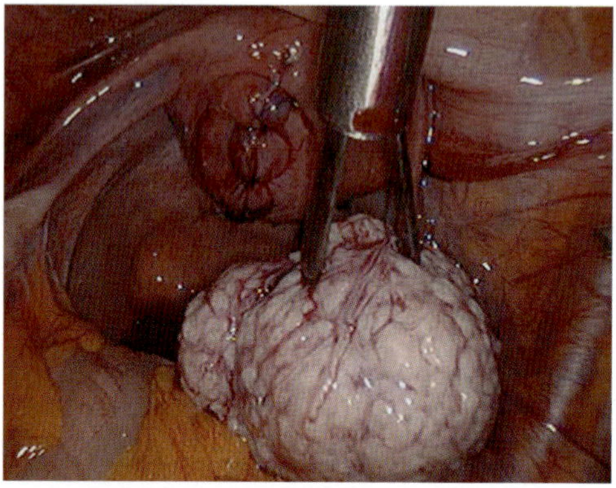

Figure 7. Laparoscopic myomectomy.

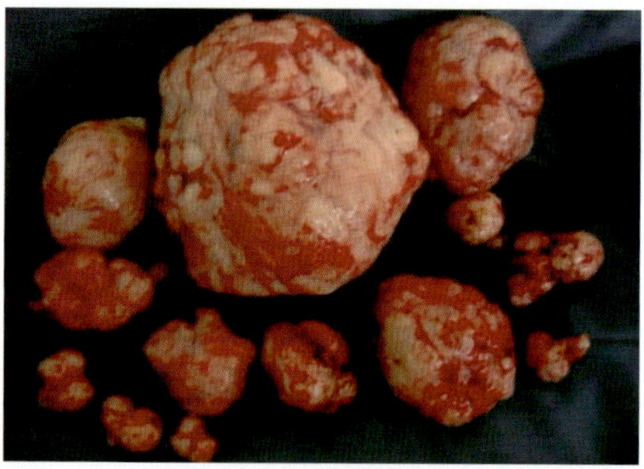

Figure 8. Multiple uterine fibroids removed via myomectomy (laparotomy).

- **GnRH agonists** induce a menopausal state and are very effective for short-term relief of symptoms and preoperative preparation. They cause fibroids to shrink by up to 50% of their volume within 3 months, but re-growth usually occurs within 12 weeks of stopping treatment. Their use should not be continued beyond 6 months as there are concerns about reduced bone mineral density.

2. Surgery

- **Hysterectomy** is a definitive treatment.
- **Myomectomy** is ideal for patients who desire future fertility and/or wish to retain their uterus. There is a risk of uterine rupture in subsequent pregnancies after myomectomy.
- There are 3 approaches to myomectomy: laparotomy, laparoscopy and hysteroscopy.
- Hysteroscopic removal of fibroids is indicated for submucosal fibroids (≤ 5 cm).
- The laparoscopic approach is preferred over laparotomy for intramural/subserosal fibroids because of less pain, faster recovery post-operatively and lower morbidity. However, not all patients are suitable for laparoscopic myomectomy. Laparoscopic myomectomy in patients with large fibroids, multiple fibroids or previous surgery may be technically difficult and a laparotomy may be more suitable.
- Patients should wait for 3 to 6 months after myomectomy before trying to conceive.

- There is a 15% recurrence rate for fibroids following myomectomy. 10% of women who have had myomectomy may need hysterectomy within the next 5 to 10 years.

3. Magnetic resonance-guided focused-ultrasound surgery (MRgFUS)

- Non-invasive technique that utilises ultrasound waves to focus on the fibroid tissue and cause thermal destruction.
- Outpatient procedure and is available in KK Hospital.
- As there is inadequate data on impact on fertility, patients who desire fertility should consider alternative treatment modalities.
- The disadvantage is that there is no histological diagnosis.

4. Uterine artery embolisation (UAE)

- Minimally invasive interventional radiology technique where a catheter is passed via the femoral artery to achieve embolisation of the uterine artery. The blood supply to the fibroids is diminished, leading to decreased size and symptomatic relief.
- May need future intervention. In a study of 2112 women who underwent UAE, 15% had a hysterectomy or myomectomy within 3 years after UAE.
    - As there is inadequate data on impact on fertility, patients who desire fertility should consider alternative treatment modalities.

Fertility and Fibroids

- Fibroids estimated to account for only 1–2% of patients with subfertility, hence other causes should be excluded before considering fibroids as the cause of subfertility.
- Submucosal and intramural fibroids with intracavitary component distort the endometrial cavity and interfere with implantation. Patients with such fibroids have decreased spontaneous pregnancy rates, decreased IVF pregnancy rates and increased risk of spontaneous miscarriages. Subserosal fibroids do not impact on fertility.
- Myomectomy has been shown to improve pregnancy rates by 2-fold in patients with submucosal fibroids.

Pregnancy and Fibroids

- Most pregnant patients with fibroids do not have any complications.
- Complications are more common in patients with large fibroids, i.e. >5 cm.

Potential complications of fibroids in pregnancy include:

(1) Pain
  - — most common complication, usually due to red degeneration
  - — other cause is torsion of pedunculated fibroid

(2) Pregnancy loss
    — Fibroids may interfere with circulation to the placenta causing pregnancy loss/affect implantation
(3) Increase in size
    — 20–30% of fibroids increase in size during pregnancy, especially large fibroids (>5 cm) and this occurs usually in the first trimester
(4) Antepartum haemorrhage (APH)
(5) Preterm labour
(6) Placental abnormalities
    — Placental abruption and praevia may be more common
(7) Malpresentation
    — May cause breech presentation/transverse lie
(8) Poor progress in labour
(9) Caesarean delivery
    — Occurs more commonly if fibroids are found in the lower uterine segment
(10) Postpartum haemorrhage (PPH)

Myomectomy during pregnancy

- Myomectomy is generally contraindicated during pregnancy, due to risk of severe haemorrhage and pregnancy loss.

- Patients who have undergone previous myomectomy have a higher chance of uterine rupture in subsequent pregnancy. Those who have undergone open myomectomy are thought to have a lower risk of uterine rupture as compared with laparoscopic myomectomy. This is due to better suturing and closure of the myometrial defect in open surgery.
- There is no high quality data comparing rates of rupture in open versus laparoscopic myomectomy. Risk of pre-labour uterine rupture is very low (0.002%) in patients with open surgery, based on small case series. On the other hand, there are case reports of uterine rupture in patients as early as 17 weeks gestation who have had a previous laparoscopic myomectomy. In one of the largest studies following pregnancies after laparoscopic myomectomies, only 1 rupture was reported in 386 pregnancies. Thus, risk of rupture is highly dependent on the surgeon's technique.
- If the endometrial cavity is breached during myomectomy, there is a higher chance of uterine rupture, so Caesarean section should be done for subsequent pregnancies.

Uterine Sarcoma

- Rare tumour, extremely poor prognosis. It is difficult to differentiate between leiomyoma and sarcoma clinically.
- Sarcomas are generally thought to arise de novo and not from sarcomatous change in leiomyomas.
- The mean age of diagnosis is 60.

Risk factors of uterine sarcoma

Age, postmenopausal status, pelvic irradiation, long-term tamoxifen use, childhood retinoblastoma, hereditary leiomyomatosis and renal cell carcinoma syndrome.

Symptoms of uterine sarcoma

Abnormal uterine bleeding (AUB), pelvic pain, pelvic mass, foul-smelling vaginal discharge.

- Warning sign: rapidly enlarging uterine mass in a postmenopausal woman
- MRI scan can be helpful in differentiating leiomyoma from leiomyosarcoma. Some features specific to leiomyosarcoma are absence of calcifications and ill-defined margins
- Diagnosis is based on histology
- Rapid growth in a fibroid may not indicate sarcomatous change

Treatment of uterine sarcoma

- Staging laparotomy (total abdominal hysterectomy and bilateral salpingoophorectomy) followed by radiation/chemotherapy.

Chapter 49

ENDOMETRIOSIS AND ADENOMYOSIS

Endometriosis

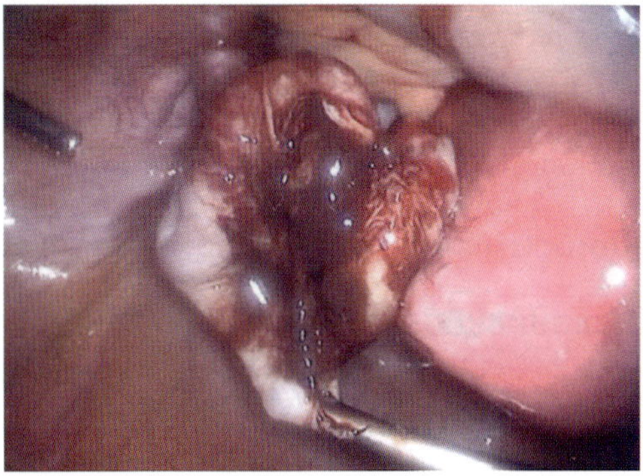

Figure 1. Endometriotic cyst of the ovary.

Definition of endometriosis

Presence of endometrial-like tissue outside the uterus and includes a chronic inflammatory reaction.

Symptoms of endometriosis

- Severe dysmenorrhoea
- Deep dyspareunia
- Chronic pelvic pain (CPP)
- Cyclical or perimenstrual symptoms, such as bowel or bladder symptoms (dyschezia/constipation/bloating/diarrhoea/haematuria)
- Subfertility
- Low back pain

Signs of endometriosis

On vaginal examination:

- Pelvic tenderness/fixed, retroverted uterus/tender uterosacral ligaments
- Endometriotic ovarian cysts

The diagnosis is more certain if deeply infiltrating nodules are palpated on the uterosacral ligaments or in the Pouch of Douglas and/or visible lesions are seen in the vagina or on the cervix.

Investigations for Endometriosis:

1. *Laparoscopy is the gold standard*

Appearance of lesions on laparoscopy

- Superficial powder-burn or gunshot lesions on the ovaries, serosal surfaces, and peritoneum, especially the posterior cul-de-sac, uterosacral ligaments and ovarian fossa. The lesions are black, dark-brown or bluish puckered lesions, nodules or small cysts containing old haemorrhage surrounded by a variable extent of fibrosis.
- Lesions can have a variety of shapes and colours, including clear, red, blue-black, yellow, brown, white or mixed. The lesions may be microscopic or macroscopic or appear as a peritoneal window.
- Endometriomas typically contain thick fluid, are densely adherent to the surrounding structures, e.g. peritoneum, tubes and bowel. Deeply infiltrating endometriotic nodules extend >5 mm beneath the peritoneum and may involve the uterosacral ligaments, vagina, bowel, bladder or ureters.

Positive histology confirms the diagnosis of endometriosis; negative histology does not exclude it.

Visual inspection is usually adequate but histological confirmation of at least one lesion is ideal. In cases of ovarian endometrioma (>5 cm) and in deeply infiltrating disease, histology should be obtained to identify endometriosis and to exclude malignancy (endometriosis is associated with ovarian clear cell carcinoma).

2. *Imaging studies*

Lack adequate resolution for visualising adhesions and superficial peritoneal/ovarian implants.

(a) *Transvaginal Ultrasound Scan* (TVUS): useful in the diagnosis of an endometrioma, and may be helpful in the diagnosis of rectovaginal, bladder, or ureteral disease
(b) *Magnetic Resonance Imaging* (MRI): limited role

3. *Serum CA 125 — elevated (greater than* 35 U/mL)

Serum CA 125 is not a specific marker of endometriosis (refer to Chapter 71 on "Ovarian Tumour Markers").

Differential diagnosis of endometriosis

- Pelvic inflammatory disease/adenomyosis/irritable bowel syndrome/interstitial cystitis/ovarian neoplasms.

Treatment of endometriosis

(1) Endometriosis associated pain
(2) Endometriosis associated subfertility

1. Endometriosis Associated Pain

Empirical treatment

Medical treatment of endometriosis-associated pain

- counselling
- adequate analgesia
- progestogens
- combined oral contraceptive pills (COCP)
- gonadotrophin-releasing hormone (GnRH) agonist (drug is more expensive and associated with more side effects and concerns about bone density)
- Visanne® (refer to Chapter 37 on "Dysmenorrhoea")
- LNG-intrauterine device (Mirena®)

Duration of therapy
The combined oral contraceptive and Depo-Provera can be used long term but the use of danazol and GnRH agonists is usually restricted to 6 months.

Visanne® can be used for longer than six months.

Management of suspected endometriomas

Guidelines for the management of suspected ovarian malignancy should be followed in cases of ovarian endometrioma.

Surgical treatment of endometriosis-associated pain

Indications for surgical intervention:

(a) Severe acute symptoms
(b) No response to medical treatment
(c) Advanced disease suspicious of malignancy

- To diagnose and remove endometriosis surgically
- Ablation of endometriotic lesions reduces endometriosis-associated pain
- Laparoscopic uterine nerve ablation (LUNA) by itself does not reduce endometriosis-associated pain
- If a hysterectomy is performed, all visible endometriotic tissue should be removed at the same time. Bilateral salpingo-oophorectomy may result in improved pain relief and a reduced chance of future recurrences

Combination of medical and surgical treatment in selected cases.

2. Endometriosis Associated Subfertility

- Suppression of ovarian function to improve fertility in minimal to mild endometriosis is not effective and should not be offered for this indication alone. There is no evidence of its effectiveness in severe disease.
- Ablation of endometriotic lesions and adhesiolysis to improve fertility in minimal to mild endometriosis is effective.

- Laparoscopic cystectomy for ovarian endometriomas is better than drainage and coagulation.
- Postoperative hormonal treatment has no beneficial effect on pregnancy rates after surgery.
- Tubal flushing appears to improve pregnancy rates in women with endometriosis-associated infertility.

Assisted reproduction in endometriosis

Treatment with SO-IUI (super ovulation intrauterine insemination) improves fertility in minimal to mild endometriosis.

IVF is an appropriate treatment, especially if tubal function is compromised, if there is associated male factor infertility, and/or other treatments have failed.

Laparoscopic ovarian cystectomy is recommended for endometriomas ≥5 cm in diameter.

Treatment with a GnRH agonist for 3–6 months before IVF in women with endometriosis increases the rate of clinical pregnancy.

Alternative therapies in treatment of endometriosis associated pain include:

- Diet — no guidelines but decreased risk with high intake of green vegetables
- Acupuncture/TENS/reflexology
- Vitamin B1, Vitamin E, magnesium
- Herbal medications/Traditional Chinese Medicine (TCM)

Adenomyosis

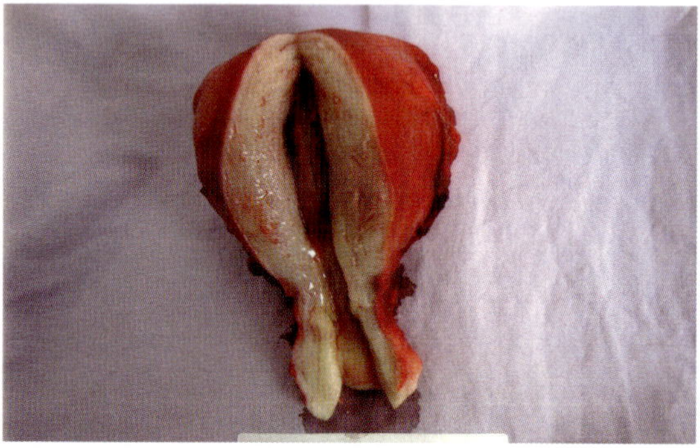

Figure 2. Cut-section of uterus showing adenomyosis.

Definition of Adenomyosis

Adenomyosis is a benign, common gynaecological condition defined histologically (usually on a hysterectomy specimen) as the presence of endometrial-like glands and stroma in the myometrium.

Symptoms of Adenomyosis

Heavy menstrual bleeding (HMB) ± dysmenorrhoea

Differential Diagnosis of Adenomyosis

Uterine fibroids, endometriosis and HMB due to ovulatory or endometrial dysregulation

Investigations of Adenomyosis

1. ***Transvaginal Ultrasound Scan (TVUS) — 70% sensitivity/specificity***

Criteria used — enlarged globular, regular uterus with no fibroids, myometrial cystic areas and decreased myometrial echogenicity

2. ***Magnetic Resonance Imaging: (MRI) — 85% sensitivity/specificity***

Higher diagnostic capability, irrespective of the presence or absence of uterine fibroids

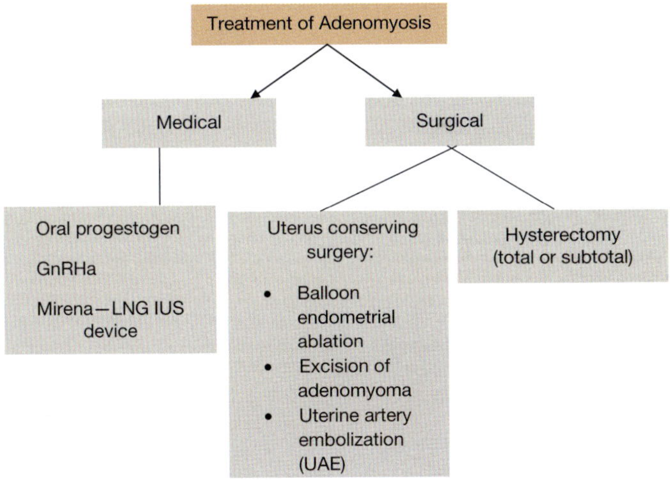

Chapter 50

OVARIAN CYST

Types of Adnexal Masses and Management of Ovarian Cysts in Women

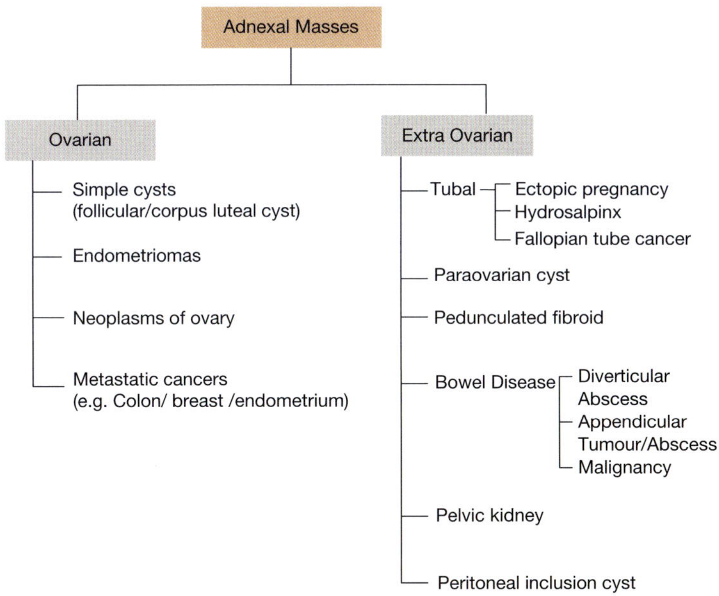

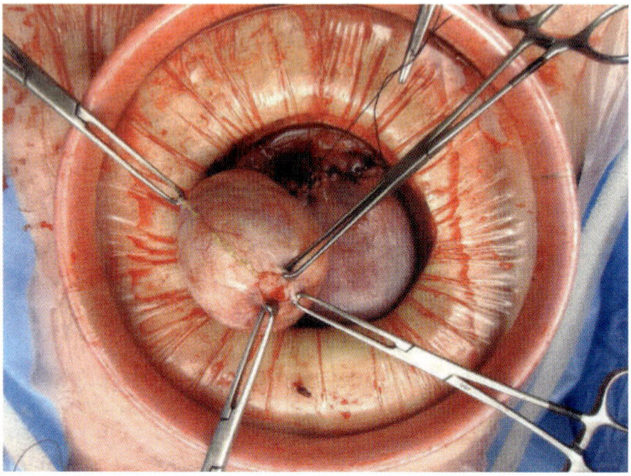

Figure 1. Ovarian cyst.

Ultrasound findings suspicious of malignancy include:

1. Solid component (nodules/papillary structures)
2. Thick septations (>2–3 mm)
3. Ascites
4. Peritoneal masses
5. Enlarged nodes
6. Colour Doppler demonstrating flow in the solid components
7. Bilateral tumours
8. Large tumours (≥ 10 cm)

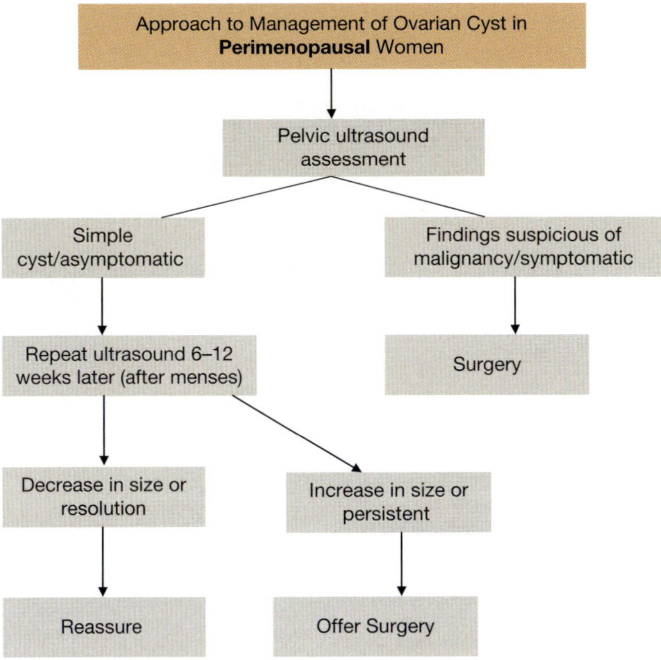
Approach to Management of Ovarian Cyst in **Perimenopausal** Women
Pelvic ultrasound assessment
Simple cyst/asymptomatic
Findings suspicious of malignancy/symptomatic
Repeat ultrasound 6–12 weeks later (after menses)
Surgery
Decrease in size or resolution
Increase in size or persistent
Reassure
Offer Surgery

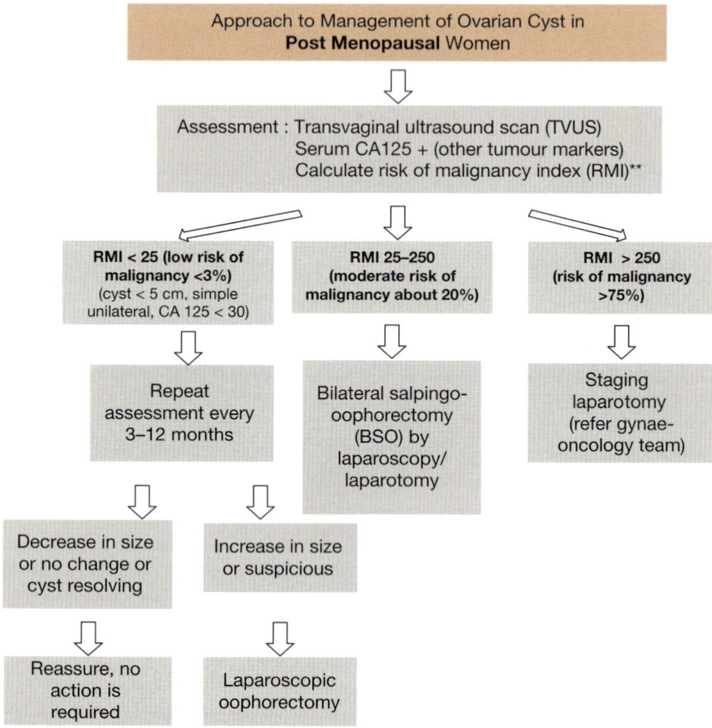

**Calculating the risk of malignancy index (RMI)
RMI = U × M × CA125
U = 0 (for ultrasound score of 0); **U** = 1 (for ultrasound score of 1); **U** = 3 (for ultrasound score of 2–5)
Ultrasound scans are scored one point for each of the following characteristics: multilocular cyst; evidence of solid areas; evidence of metastases; presence of ascites; bilateral lesions
M = 3 for all postmenopausal women dealt with by this guideline
CA125 is serum CA125 measurement in u/mL

Refer to gynae-oncology team:

If other patient characteristics are suspicious of malignancy in postmenopausal women with ovarian cyst. These include:

(1) Physical examination revealing a pelvic mass, fixed uterus, groin or cervical lymphadenopathy , ascites.
(2) Hereditary breast/ovarian cancer syndrome or history of ovarian cancer in a first degree relative.
(3) Atypical glandular cells on cervical cytology in a woman with negative findings on evaluation of cervix and endometrium.

Pregnancy with Adnexal Mass

Mostly are incidental findings at routine prenatal diagnoses. Majority are physiological or benign.

Causes of adnexal masses in women with an intrauterine pregnancy

a) *Ovarian*

Simple cyst

Haemorrhagic cyst

Hyperstimulated ovaries following fertility treatment

Corpus Luteal cyst

Endometrioma

Epithelial tumours, Germ Cell Tumour,

Dysgerminomas, Sex cord-stromal tumours

b) *Tubal*

Hydrosalpinx

c) *Leiomyoma*

d) *Non-gynaecological*

Mesenteric cyst

Pelvic kidney

Role of ovarian tumour markers in pregnancy

- Limited

(Serum alpha foetoprotein, βhcg, inhibin are elevated due to placental synthesis and CA125 is elevated due to decidual cell production in a normal pregnancy)

Complications of adnexal mass in pregnancy

Cyst rupture
Cyst haemorrhage
Torsion (up to 5%)
Obstructed labour
Foetal malpresentation

Management of adnexal mass in pregnancy

1. Expectant
2. Surgical

1. *Expectant management*:

50 to 70% of adnexal masses resolve during pregnancy. Risk factors for persistence are size >5 cm and complex morphology on transvaginal ultrasonography (TVUS).

Approximately 10% of adnexal masses that persist during pregnancy are malignant. A substantial portion of these are epithelial low malignant potential tumours or germ cell tumours. Both tumours have typically favourable prognosis.

Risk of ovarian torsion occurs most frequently in the first trimester, occasionally in the second and rarely in the third. Repeat pelvic ultrasound 6 to 12 weeks' postpartum.

The reported rate of complications with expectant management is <2%.

2. ***Surgical management — usually planned during second trimester of pregnancy***

Indications include:

- Suspected malignancy
- An acute complication e.g. torsion or rupture
- The size of the tumour likely to cause obstetric complication such as obstructed labour.

Chapter 51

PELVIC ORGAN PROLAPSE (POP)

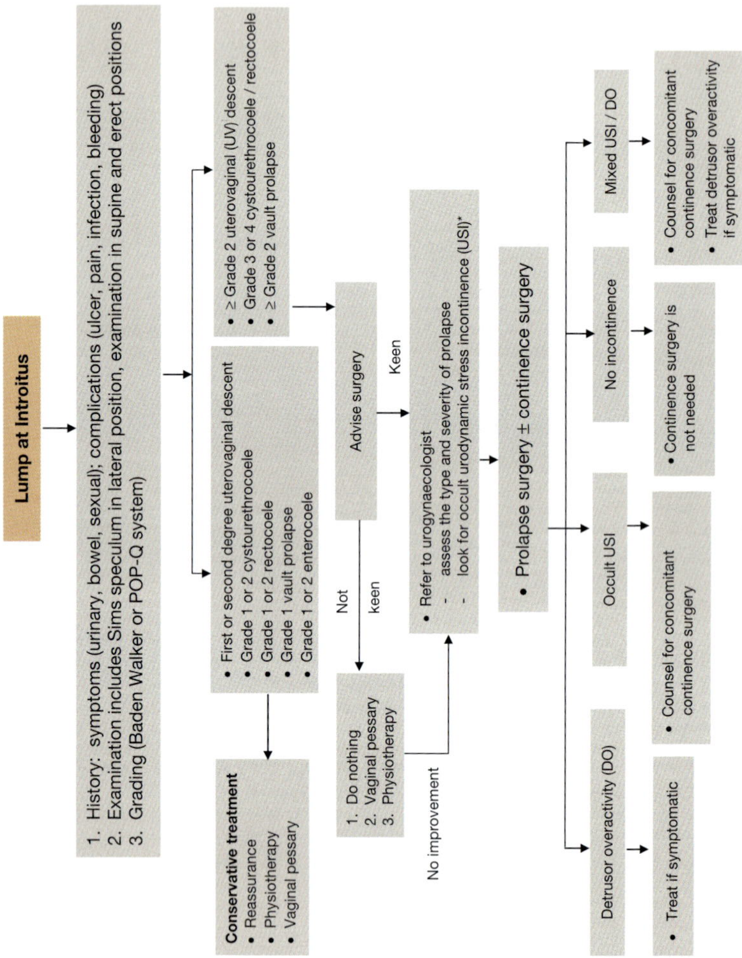
Lump at Introitus
1. History: symptoms (urinary, bowel, sexual); complications (ulcer, pain, infection, bleeding)
2. Examination includes Sims speculum in lateral position, examination in supine and erect positions
3. Grading (Baden Walker or POP-Q system)
• First or second degree uterovaginal descent
• Grade 1 or 2 cystourethrocoele
• Grade 1 or 2 rectocoele
• Grade 1 vault prolapse
• Grade 1 or 2 enterocoele
• ≥ Grade 2 uterovaginal (UV) descent
• Grade 3 or 4 cystourethrocoele / rectocoele
• ≥ Grade 2 vault prolapse
Conservative treatment
• Reassurance
• Physiotherapy
• Vaginal pessary
Advise surgery
Not keen
Keen
1. Do nothing
2. Vaginal pessary
3. Physiotherapy
No improvement
• Refer to urogynaecologist
- assess the type and severity of prolapse
- look for occult urodynamic stress incontinence (USI)*
• Prolapse surgery ± continence surgery
Detrusor overactivity (DO)
Occult USI
No incontinence
Mixed USI / DO
• Treat if symptomatic
• Counsel for concomitant continence surgery
• Continence surgery is not needed
• Counsel for concomitant continence surgery
• Treat detrusor overactivity if symptomatic

Types of Pelvic Organ Prolapse Surgery

Pelvic Organ Prolapse Surgery
(Isolation or in Combination)

- **Grade 2 Uterovaginal prolapse** →
  - Vaginal hysterectomy (VH) ± bilateral salpingo-oophorectomy (BSO)
  - Manchester operation
  - Sacrospinous hysteropexy
- **Grade 3 or 4 Uterovaginal prolapse** →
  - VH ± BSO & Sacrospinous ligament fixation ✶
  - Open or laparoscopic hysterectomy ± BSO & Sacrocolpopexy
  - Manchester operation
  - Sacrospinous hysteropexy
- **≥ Grade 2 vault prolapse** →
  - Sacrospinous ligament fixation✶
  - Open or laparoscopic sacrocolpopexy
- **Grade 2 or 3 cystourethrocoele** →
  - Anterior repair
- **Grade 4 cystourethrocoele** →
  - Anterior repair✶ ± gynaemesh
  - Anterior prolift✶
  - Paravaginal cystocoele repair
- **≥ Grade 2 rectocoele** →
  - Posterior repair ± mesh✶ ± sacrospinous ligament fixation
  - Posterior Prolift✶
- **Grade 2 enterocoele** →
  - High ligation of enterocoele

✶Vaginal route is preferred over abdominal and laparoscopic routes.

✶Combinations of surgery to prevent recurrence of pelvic organ prolapse with follow up required, especially if mesh is used.

Chapter 52

VOIDING AND URINARY DISORDERS

Urinary Incontinence

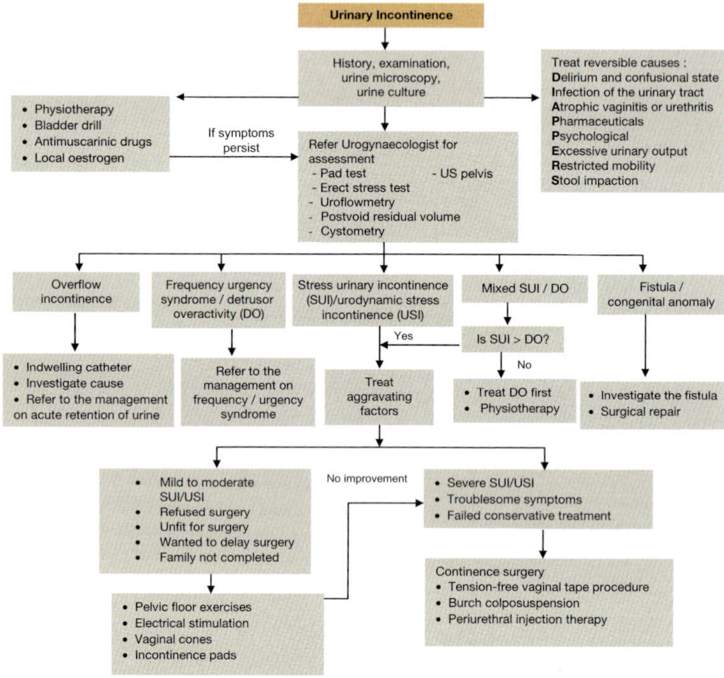

Note 1. If a patient has secondary uterovaginal prolapse and requires Burch colposuspension, counsel for hysterectomy as well.
2. Route of hysterectomy and continence surgery preferably to be the same.

Detrusor Overactivity (DO)

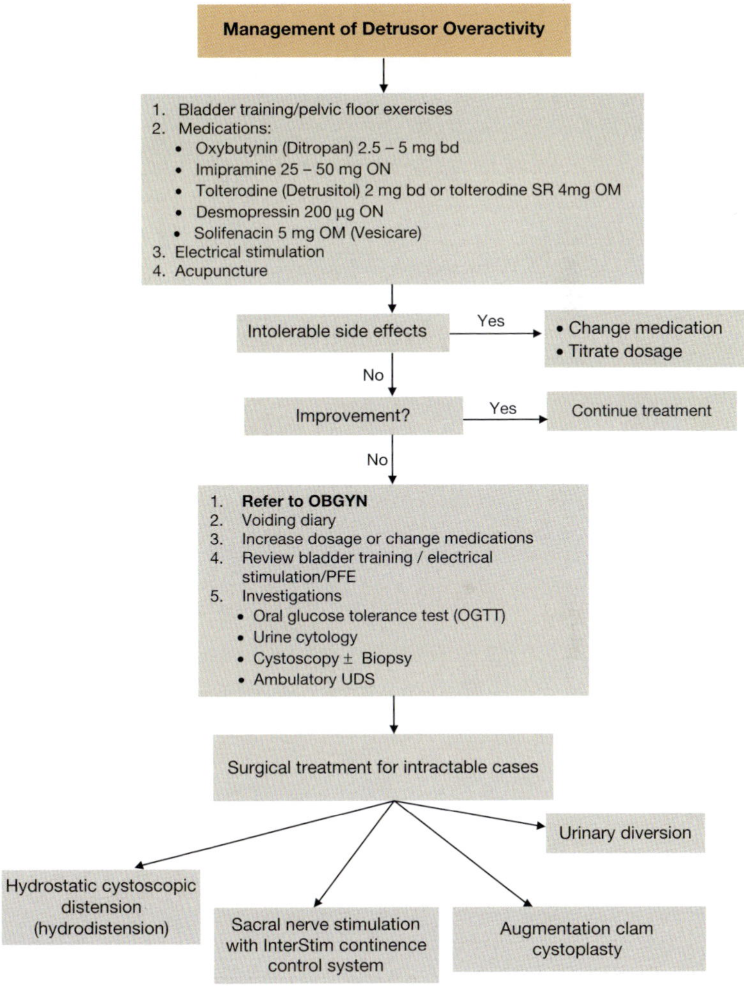

Frequency/Urgency Syndrome

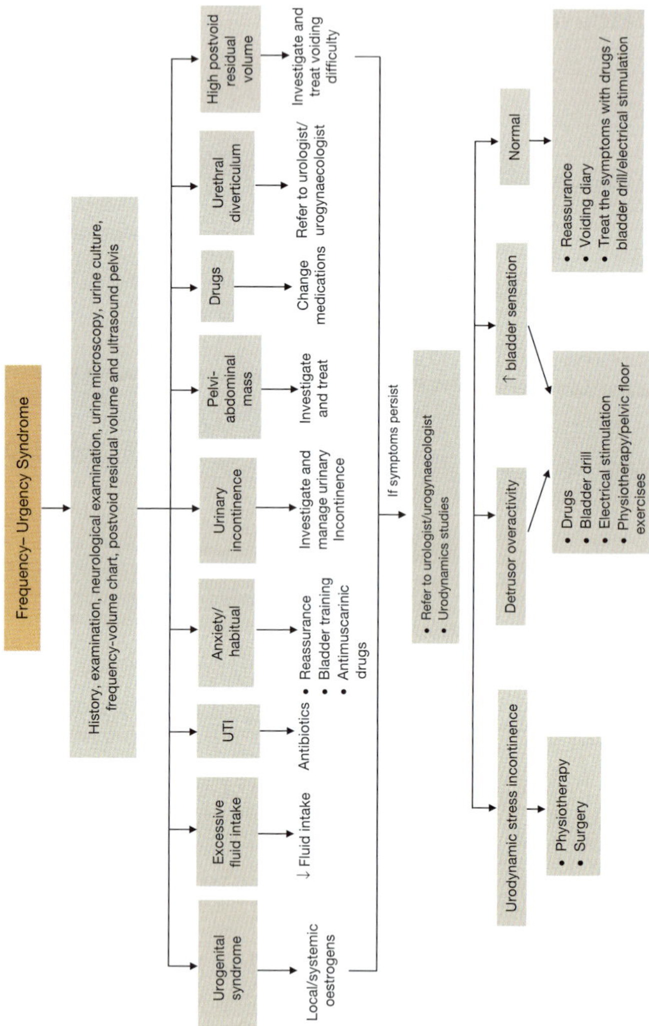

Simple Urinary Tract Infection (UTI)

Symptoms of Simple Urinary Tract Infection (UTI)*

- Dysuria, Frequency, Nocturia, Urgency
- Haematuria

↓

Urine microscopy
Urine culture

↓

Negative

↓

Symptomatic treatment

↓

Look for other causes e.g. urethritis – urethral culture for mycoplasma/gonococcus/ chlamydia. Treat accordingly

Positive

↓

First line

1. Nitrofurantoin 50 mg QDS x 5 days
2. Trimethoprim-sulfamethoxazole (Bactrim) 160mg/800 mg PO bd x 5 days
3. Cephalexin 250 mg PO tds x 5 days
4. Ciprofloxacin 250 mg PO bd x 5 days

Alternatives:

1. Fosfomycin (3 om) 1 satchet as single dose
2. Cefuroxime 250 mg PO bd x 5 days
3. Amoxycillin-clavulanate (Augmentin) 625 mg bd x 5 days
4. Ampicillin-sulbactam (Unasyn) 375 mg bd x 5 days
5. Choose antibiotics according to culture and sensitivity result

↓

Repeat urine microscopy in 2 weeks

↓

- Symptoms resolved
- Normal urine microscopy

↓

Routine follow up

Symptoms persist or urine microscopy still abnormal:

- Repeat urine culture and treat according to sensitivity

↓

Repeat urine microscopy in 2 weeks

↓

Symptoms resolved
Urine microscopy normal

No → Investigate and treat as for recurrent UTI

Yes ↓

Routine follow up

* Simple UTI is defined as an isolated UTI or UTIs occurring less than 3 times a year

Recurrent Urinary Tract Infection (UTI)

Recurrent UTI Ω

↓

Look for high risk factors and treat accordingly

- Immunocompromised patients
- Diabetic patients
- Patients on steroids
- Cancer patients
- Advanced age
- Inefficient bladder emptying (e.g. neuropathic bladder, post operation, drug-induced voiding difficulties)
- Indwelling catheter
- Recurrent vulvovaginitis
- Post menopause

↓

Investigations

- Urine microscopy, culture, acid-fast bacillus
- Urine for cytology
- Postvoid residual volume
- Ultrasound of kidneys
  KUB/intravenous urogram
- Cystoscopy
- CT urogram

↓

- Treat UTI
- Initiating antibiotic prophylaxis — such as nitrofurantoin 50–100 mg on a monthly rotation for 3 to 6 months
- Stat dose Nitrofurantoin 100 mg or Bactrim 2 tablets after each sexual intercourse if related to sex
- Increase fluid intake
- Void frequently especially after intercourse
- Perineal hygiene education

- If upper tract abnormality: calculi or tumour, refer to urologist
- If lower tract abnormality, refer to urogynaecologist/ urologist

Ω Recurrent UTI is defined as UTI occurring 3 or more times a year, which can be caused by the same or different organisms

Acute Retention of Urine

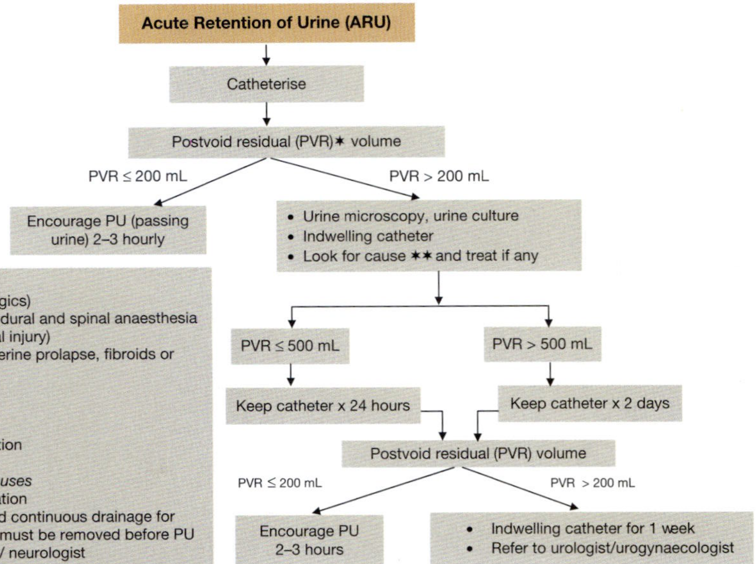

✶✶ *Causes of ARU*

1. Drugs (e.g. anticholinergics)
2. Postoperative ARU, epidural and spinal anaesthesia
3. Neurological (e.g. spinal injury)
4. Gynaecological (e.g. uterine prolapse, fibroids or cystocoele)
5. Urinary tract infection
6. Constipation
7. Urethral stricture
8. Urethritis/ herpes infection

Treatment for the above causes

1. Stop or change medication
2. Adequate analgesia and continuous drainage for 1–2 days Vaginal pack must be removed before PU
3. Refer to neurosurgeon / neurologist
4. **Refer to OBGYN** for assessment/ surgery
5. Treat with antibiotics
6. Laxatives
7. Refer urologist for urethral dilatation
8. Antibiotics, analgesics, acyclovir

✶ The significance of PVR varies with the total volume voided.

Microscopic Haematuria (MH)

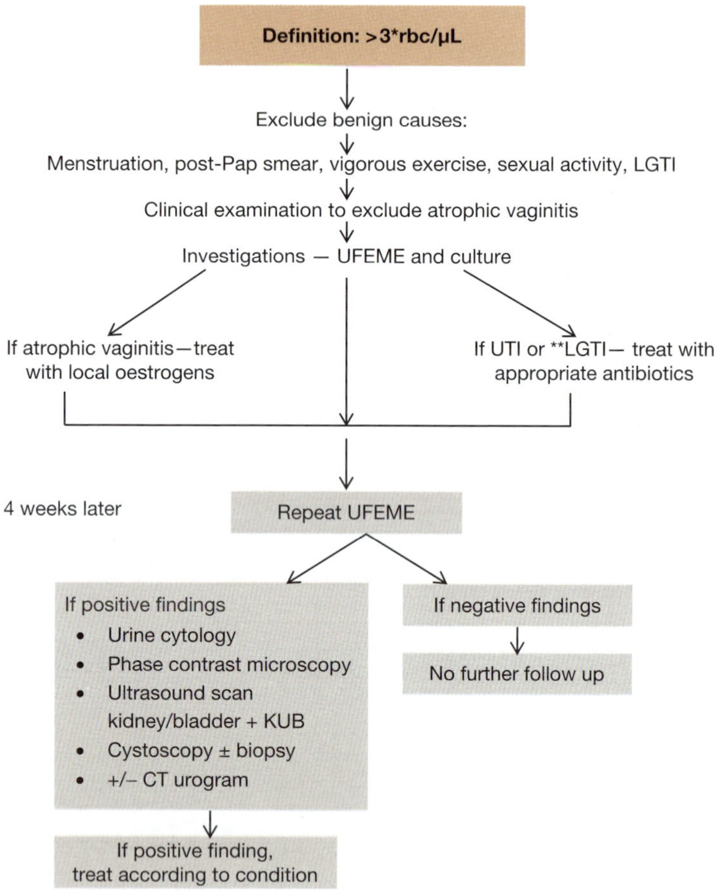

*rbc – red blood cells
**LGTI – lower genital tract infection

Chapter 53

VAGINAL DISCHARGE AND RECURRENT VULVOVAGINAL CANDIDIASIS

Causes of Vaginal Discharge

1. Physiologic
   - Cyclical hormones — oral contraceptive pills, menses
   - Pregnancy
2. Pathologic
   - Infective causes — Bacterial Vaginosis, Trichomoniasis, Candidiasis, Chlamydia, *Neisseria gonorrhoea*
   - Cancer — endometrial, cervical, vaginal
   - Atrophic vaginitis
   - Local causes — intrauterine contraceptive device, tampon, polyp, fistula

Management of Vaginal Discharge

Symptoms and clinical appearance of vaginal discharge are variable and do not permit accurate determination of a specific infective cause in most cases.

History	
Discharge	Previous episodes, onset, duration, amount, odour, colour
Associated symptoms	• Itch • Pain • Postcoital bleeding

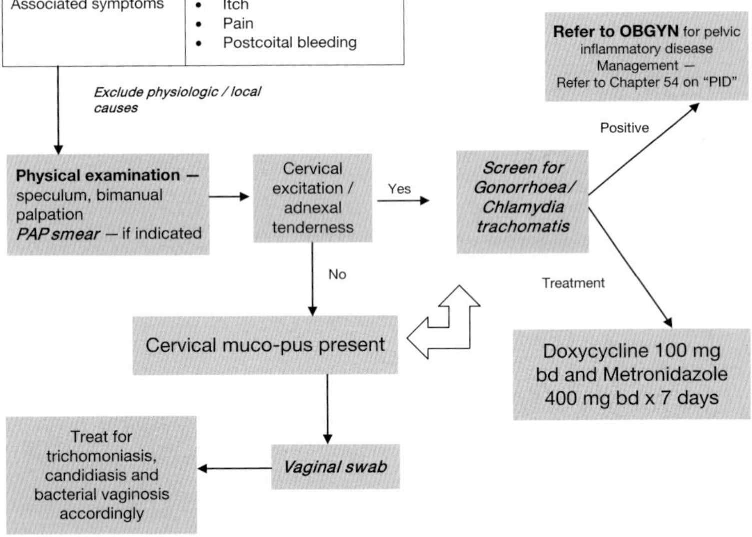

Treatment of Vaginal Discharge

General treatment

Educate and counsel to reduce anxiety, perineal hygiene and avoidance of triggers and use of soaps.

Specific treatment

Trichomoniasis

- Oral metronidazole (400 mg bd × 7 days or 2 g × one single dose)
- Sex partners should be treated on epidemiological grounds

Trichomoniasis in pregnancy

- Trichomoniasis has been associated with adverse pregnancy outcomes (premature rupture of membranes, preterm delivery and low birth weight)
- Although oral metronidazole in pregnancy has not been shown to be teratogenic or mutagenic, it should be used with caution in the first trimester.

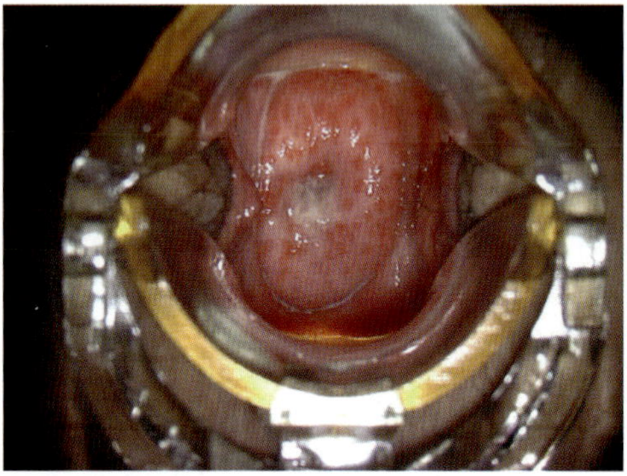

Figure 1. Strawberry cervix — characteristic of *Trichomonas cervicitis.*

Treatment of Uncomplicated Acute Vulvovaginal Candidiasis (VVC)

- Butoconazole-sustained released (SR) gel 2% (5g) intra-vaginally × single application or
- Clotrimazole (Canestan) vaginal pessary 200 mg ON × 3 days or
- Miconazole nitrate vaginal pessary 200 mg ON × 3 days or
- Isoconazole vaginal pessary 600 mg × single dose or
- Nystatin vaginal pessary 100,000 U daily × 7 days or
- Fluconazole 150 mg orally single dose or
- Itraconazole 200 mg orally once a day × 3 days

Treatment of Recurrent Vulvovaginal Candidiasis (VVC)

Induction regime

- Topical imidazole therapy 7–14 days according to symptomatic response
- Fluconazole 150 mg orally every 3 days for 3 doses

Maintenance regime

- Clotrimazole pessary 500 mg intravaginally once a week or 200 mg intravaginally twice weekly for 6 months or
- Fluconazole 150 mg orally weekly for 6 months

Vulvovaginal candidiasis (VVC) in pregnancy

Only topical azole therapy should be given for 7–14 days. *No* oral azoles as they are potentially teratogenic.

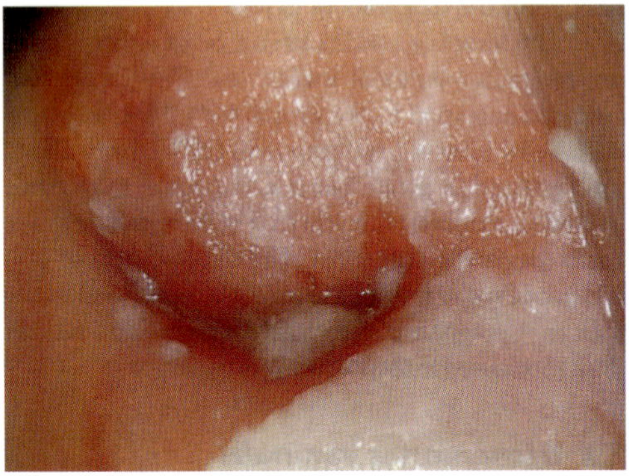

Figure 2. Cervicovaginal candidiasis.

Treatment of Bacterial Vaginosis

- Oral metronidazole 400 mg bd × 7 days
- Oral clindamycin 300 mg bd × 7 days
- Oral tinidazole 2 g single dose

Treatment of Bacterial Vaginosis in Pregnancy

High risk pregnant women (previous preterm delivery)

- Metronidazole 400 mg orally bd for 7 days (avoid oral metronidazole in the first trimester)
- Clindamycin 300 mg bd for 7 days (use in first half of pregnancy as its use is associated with low birth-weight and neonatal infections from 16 to 32 weeks)

Low risk symptomatic pregnant women

Metronidazole gel 0.75% one full applicator (5 g) intravaginally bd for 5 days

- No clinical counterpart is recognised in males
- Screening and treatment of male partner has not been shown to be beneficial

Treatment of Atrophic Vaginitis

- Local oestrogen cream (premarin cream 1 g ON × 2 weeks followed by 2 times a week for 3 months)

When should investigations be done for vaginal discharge?

If the patient:

1) Is at high risk of STI (i.e. <25 years old, change of new sexual partner or has >1 sexual partner in the last year)
2) Complains of fever or abdominal pain to suggest upper genital tract infection (UGTI)
3) Has failed previous medical treatment.

(*Continued*)

(*Continued*)

4) Is postnatal, post-abortal or has recent miscarriage
5) Has recent intrauterine contraceptive device insertion in the past 2 months

It is reasonable to treat empirically a patient with vaginal discharge without investigations if a thorough sexual history and physical examination reveals that she is at low risk of sexually transmitted infections (STI), has no signs to suggest upper genital tract infection (UGTI) and she can return for a follow-up if the symptoms do not resolve.

Treatment of Chlamydia Trachomatis

- Doxycycline 100 mg orally bd × 7 days
- Azithromycin 1 g orally single dose
- Tetracycline orally 500 mg qds × 7 days
- Erythromycin base or stearate 500 mg orally qds × 7 days

Treatment of *Chlamydia Trachomatis* Infection in Pregnancy

- Erythromycin base or stearate 500 mg orally qds × 7 days
- Erythromycin ethylsuccinate 800 mg orally qds × 7 days

- Amoxicillin 500 mg orally tds × 7 days
- Azithromycin 1 g orally single dose

Treatment of *Neisseria Gonorrhoea*

- Ceftriaxone 250 mg intramuscular injection × one dose
- Spectinomycin 2 g intramuscular injection × one dose
- Cefuroxime 1 g orally single dose with probenecid 1 g orally single dose

Treatment of Gonococcal Infection in Pregnancy

- Cephalosporins are safe and effective in pregnancy
- Spectinomycin can be administered to pregnant women who are unable to tolerate cephalosporins

Simultaneous treatment for chlamydia infection with erythromycin stearate or base 500 mg orally qds × 7 days

Follow-Up after initial treatment of STI

- Culture for test-of-cure 14 days after treatment for *Neisseria gonorrhoea* or *Chlamydia trachomatis*
- All male sex partners within 60 days should be evaluated and treated for *Neisseria gonorrhoea* or *Chlamydia trachomatis*

Chapter 54

PELVIC INFLAMMATORY DISEASE (PID)

Pelvic inflammatory disease (PID) refers to acute infection of the upper genital tract in a woman, involving any or all of the uterus including the cervix, fallopian tubes and the ovaries. This can be accompanied by involvement of the neighbouring pelvic organs resulting in endometritis, salpingitis, oophoritis, peritonitis, peri-hepatitis (Fitz-Hugh-Curtis Syndrome) and tubo-ovarian abscess.

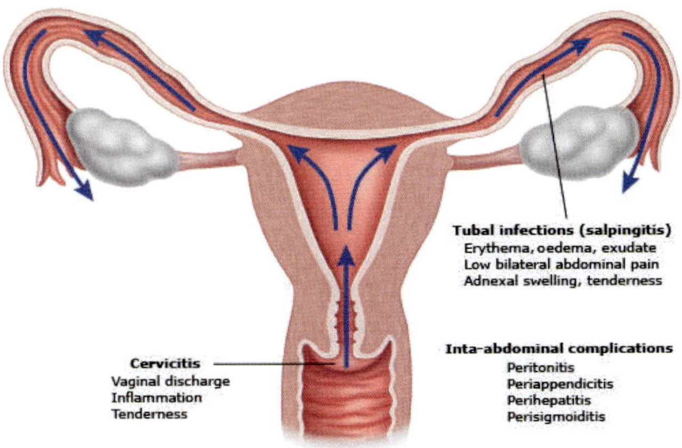

Pathogenesis of PID

- Sexually transmitted infection
  - *Neisseria gonorrhoea*
  - *Chlamydia trachomatis*
- Normal vaginal flora of healthy women
  - Streptococci
  - Staphylococci
  - Enterobacteriaceae (e.g. Klebsiella, *Escherichia coli*, Proteus)
  - Anaerobes, e.g. bacterial vaginosis
- Postoperative pelvic abscess
- Pregnancy-related pelvic infection
- Pelvic infection secondary to spread of a primary infection
  - Appendicitis
  - Diverticulitis
  - Tuberculous peritonitis
  - Actinomyosis

Clinical Features of PID

- PID represents a spectrum of clinical disease, which ranges from a continuum starting from asymptomatic to fatal intraabdominal sepsis

Pelvic Inflammatory Disease (PID)

SYMPTOMS
- Bilateral lower abdominal pain
- Intermenstrual bleeding (IMB)
- Postcoital bleeding (PCB)
- Breakthrough bleeding
- New onset vaginal discharge
- Fever and chills (50%)
- Deep dyspareunia
- Urethritis
- Proctitis

SIGNS
- Fever (>38°C)
- Rebound tenderness in lower abdomen
- Right upper quadrant tenderness (possible Fitz-Hugh Curtis in 10% of patients)
- Purulent endocervical discharge
- Cervical excitation
- Adnexal tenderness on bimanual examination ± mass

- Subclinical PID is common, so index of suspicion for clinical diagnosis of PID should be high, especially in adolescent women, even if they deny sexual activity — do swabs if necessary
- **Remember to exclude differential diagnosis of lower abdominal pain in a young woman:**
  - Ectopic pregnancy
  - Acute appendicitis
  - Endometriosis
  - Irritable bowel syndrome
  - Complications of an ovarian cyst, e.g. torsion, rupture
  - Urinary tract infection
  - Functional pain

A low threshold for empiric treatment for PID is recommended as the potential consequences of not treating PID are serious.

Fitz-Hugh Curtis Syndrome

- A form of peri-hepatitis associated with PID
- Results from infection of the liver capsule and peritoneal surfaces of the anterior upper right quadrant, with minimal stromal hepatic involvement
- Presents with sudden onset of severe right upper quadrant abdominal pain, with distinct pleuritic component, and hence can mask the diagnosis of PID
- May result in abnormal aminotransferases on liver function tests (LFT) in about 50% of patients

Risk factors for Sexually Transmitted Infection (STI)

- Age less than 25 years
- Young age at first coitus
- Multiple or new sexual partners in last 6 months
- Low educational and socioeconomic status

Factors that potentially facilitate PID

- History of PID
- Vaginal douching
- Bacterial vaginosis
- Intrauterine device contraception

HISTORY

Abdominal pain associated with

- Fever >38°C
- Abnormal vaginal discharge
- Intermenstrual bleeding (IMB)/ Postcoital bleeding (PCB)

Examination

- **Vitals**: fever, tachycardia, hypotension
- **Abdomen**: lower abdominal tenderness /right upper quadrant tenderness
- **Speculum**: strawberry cervix, mucopurulent discharge
- **Vaginal examination**: cervical excitation, adnexal tenderness/mass

Investigations

- Urinary pregnancy test: to exclude ectopic pregnancy
- FBC/CRP
- Endocervical swabs to test for chlamydia and gonorrhoea
- High vaginal swab to test for trichomonas, bacterial vaginosis and candida
- Ultrasound pelvis to look for tubo-ovarian abscess, pyosalpinx
- Other STI testing: HIV, syphilis, hepatitis B

Treatment

- **Mild PID**: **outpatient** management with oral antibiotics for 14 days
- **Moderate and severe PID: inpatient** monitoring with intravenous antibiotics
- Contact tracing
- Enforce compliance with medication and follow up
- Counselling regarding long-term sequelae

Investigations for PID

- **Urine**: urine pregnancy test to rule out pregnancy; urine can also be sent for chlamydia and gonorrhoea testing
- **Blood**: FBC, CRP; STI testing (HIV, hepatitis B and syphilis); blood cultures if septic
- **Endocervical swabs** to test for chlamydia and gonorrhoea
- **High vaginal swab** to test for trichomonas, bacterial vaginosis and candida
- **Ultrasound pelvis** to look for associated PID pathology, e.g. tubo-ovarian abscess and to exclude other genital tract pathology
- **Diagnostic laparoscopy**: 15–30% of cases may have no laparoscopic evidence of acute infection despite organisms being identified from swabs

Treatment of PID

- **Broad coverage with antibiotics. Surgical management** should be considered if clinical condition is severe or deteriorates despite adequate antibiotic therapy, e.g. pelvic abscess.
- **Indications for hospitalisation**
  - Lack of response or tolerance to oral medications
  - Non-adherence to therapy
  - Severe clinical illness, e.g. high fever, nausea, vomiting, severe abdominal pain

Severity of PID	Suggested Therapy		Duration
	First Line	Alternative (Allergy)	
MILD	PO doxycycline100 mg BD AND PO metronidazole 400 mg bd	PO azithromycin 2 g STAT	14 days
MODERATE	IM ceftriaxone 250 mg STAT AND PO doxycycline 100 mg BD	PO azithromycin 2 g STAT	14 days
SEVERE	IV ceftriaxone 1 g OM AND IV metronidazole 500 mg Q8H AND PO doxycycline 100 mg BD	IV clindamycin 900 mg Q8H AND IV gentamicin 5 mg/kg OM	14 days
PREGNANCY	IV augmentin 1.2 g Q8H AND IV azithromycin 500 mg OM	Consider ID referral	14 days

*Patients who improve clinically should be converted to oral therapy as soon as they can tolerate oral intake.

  - Complicated PID with pelvic abscess (including tubo-ovarian abscess)
  - Possible need for surgical intervention or diagnostic exploration for alternative aetiology, e.g. appendicitis
- Patient monitoring and counselling are crucial components in the overall management of the PID patient
- Should outpatient therapy be used, patient should be reviewed within 48–72 hours to ensure clinical improvement
- Medication **compliance** should also be enforced via patient education
- **Counselling** regarding the route of acquisition of sexually acquired infections should be done, with concomitant partner treatment and safe sex practices; long-term complications of PID should also be explained in detail
- Screening for other sexually transmitted infections should be offered (HIV, hepatitis B and syphilis)
- Contact tracing

Tubo-ovarian abscess (TOA)

- Occurs in about one-third of women who are hospitalised with a diagnosis of PID
- Serious and potentially life-threatening condition
- Requires aggressive medical or surgical treatment or else sepsis might ensue if rupture occurs

- Computed tomography (CT) may be useful when the pathology is associated with the gastrointestinal tract
- **Antibiotics** remain the mainstay of treatment for TOA
- Choice of antibiotic therapy alone or in combination with drainage or surgery depends on the clinical status of the patient and characteristics of the abscess

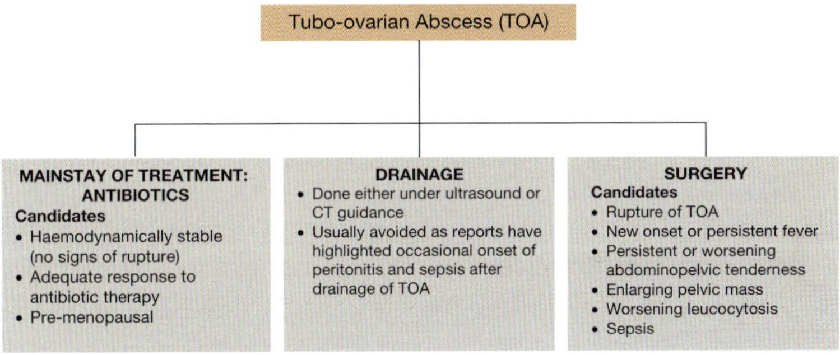

Long-term Complications of PID

- Recurrent PID
- **Hydrosalpinx** secondary to tubal damage
- **Chronic pelvic pain**: may affect up to one-third of patients with history of PID secondary to scarring and adhesions from inflammatory process
- **Infertility**: secondary to tubal damage
- **Ectopic pregnancy**: after 1, 2 and 3 episodes of PID, the risk of ectopic pregnancy is 5%, 15% and 30% accordingly

- **Ovarian cancer**: nearly two-fold increase in risk of ovarian cancer with the highest risk in women with multiple episodes of PID

Neisseria gonorrhoea

- Gram negative diplococci
- First identified cause of PID
- Rapid decline in incidence with the introduction of penicillin
- 15% of women with endocervical gonorrhoea develop PID

- **Clinical manifestations**
  - PID: accounts for 30–40% of overall PID
  - Cervicitis: 50% of infected women are asymptomatic
  - Urethritis
  - Anorectal infection and proctitis: usually asymptomatic
  - Oropharyngeal infection: usually asymptomatic colonisation; increased risk in pregnant women
- **Diagnosis**: culture; nucleic acid amplification test (NAAT)
- **Treatment**: PO ciprofloxacin 500 mg stat or PO ofloxacin 400 mg stat or IM cefotaxime 500 mg stat

Chlamydia trachomatis

- Obligate intracellular parasite
- Fewer acute manifestations and more significant long-term complications as compared with *Neisseria gonorrhoea*
- 15% of women with endocervical chlamydia develop PID
- **Clinical manifestations**:
    - PID: accounts for 30–40% of overall PID
    - Cervicitis: >70% of infected women are asymptomatic
    - Urethritis: often accompanies cervicitis
    - Fitz-Hugh Curtis syndrome: 5–15% of PID
- **Diagnosis**: nucleic acid amplification test (NAAT) is the "gold standard" method
- **Treatment**: PO Azithromycin 2 g stat or PO Doxycycline 100 mg BD for one week

Screening of young women

- Women at high risk for PID should be screened for chlamydia and gonorrhoea.

Chapter 55

SEXUALLY TRANSMITTED INFECTION (STI)

Organism Causing STI	STI	Causative Agent
Bacteria	Chlamydia	*Chlamydia trachomatis*
	Gonorrhoea	*Neisseria gonorrhoea*
	Chancroid	*Hemophilus ducreyi*
	Granuloma inguinale	*Calymmatobacterium granulomatis*
	Lymphogranuloma venerum (LGV)	*Chlamydia trachomatis*
	Syphilis	*Treponema pallidum*
Virus	Genital herpes	Herpes simplex virus (HSV 1 & 2)
	Genital warts	Human papilloma virus (HPV)
	HIV/AIDS	Human immunodeficiency virus (HIV)
	Molluscum contagiosum	Pox virus
	Hepatitis B/C	Hepatitis virus
Protozoan	Trichomoniasis	*Trichomonas vaginalis*

Risk Factors for STI

- Young age
- Unmarried
- New sex partners in the past two months
- Multiple sex partners
- History of prior STI
- Illicit drug use
- Contact with sex workers

Screening Approach for (STI)

1. Offer

Universal screening (testing and counselling) for HIV to all patients being evaluated for STI.

2. High risk (Gonorrhoea/Chlamydia)

Screen annually for gonorrhoea/chlamydia if risk factors are present.

3. High risk and pregnant

Screen for hepatitis B, syphilis, HIV, gonorrhoea, chlamydia and hepatitis C.

4. Antenatal screening for Herpes

Not recommended routinely for asymptomatic women.

Approach to Management of STI

History

a. Lesion history
b. Medical history
c. Sexual history: 5 "P"s (CDC)

   - Partners (sexual)
   - Prevention of pregnancy
   - Practices
   - Protection from STIs
   - Past history of STIs (sexual encounters)

Physical Examination

Differentials of genital ulcers

STI-related genital ulcers

- Genital herpes (HSV-1 or HSV-2)
- Primary syphilis
- Chancroid

- Granuloma inguinale
- Lymphogranuloma venerum (LGV)

Non STI related genital ulcers

- Bullous dermatoses
- Non bullous dermatoses
- Malignancy

STI-related Genital Ulcers

Aetiologic Agent	Genital Herpes	Primary Syphilis	Chancroid	Granuloma Inguinale (Donovanosis)	Lympho-granuloma Venerum (LGV)
Incubation period	2–14 days	10–90 days (average 21)	3–10 days (average 4–7)	50 days	5–21 days
Initial lesions	Papule — vesicle	Papule	Papule/ pustule	Extensive progressive granulation-like tissue with "beefy" red ulcer	Small, painless blister or sore
Presenting lesion	Vesicles	Chancre	Ulcer/bubo	Papules/ulcer	
Number	Multiple/coalesce Bilateral in primary Unilateral in recurrent	Usually one	Single/multiple	Single	Multiple
Diameter	1–2 mm	5–15 mm	Variable	Extensive	Small
Edges	Erythematous	Sharply demarcated elevated, round or oval	Undermined ragged irregular	Rolled	

(Continued)

(Continued)

Aetiologic Agent	Genital Herpes	Primary Syphilis	Chancroid	Granuloma Inguinale (Donovanosis)	Lympho-granuloma Venerum (LGV)
Depth	Superficial	Superficial deep	Excavated deep	Deep	Shallow
Base	Serous/ erythematous non-vascular	Smooth, clean non purulent non vascular	Necrotic generally purulent, grey or yellow exudate bleeds easily	"Beefy" red ulcer	
Pain	Common often with prodrome of tingling	Uncommon	Common severe	Single	Usually painless
Lymphaden-opathy	Present in primary Absent in recurrences	Firm, non-tender, bilateral	Tender suppurative, unilateral, fluctuant buboes	Absent	Tender inguinal/ femoral nodes (buboes — painful fluctuant suppurative nodes) ±Sinuses ±Strictures

Laboratory Investigations for STI

- Send swab for herpes PCR
- If chancroid/or other diagnoses suspected. Refer to Department of STI Control (DSC)
- Send blood sample (5 mL plain tube CMIA test to screen for syphilis → VDRL/TPPA)
- Offer HIV testing
- Usually empirical treatment recommended as 25% will have no laboratory confirmed diagnosis

Specific STI Investigations and Management

1. Genital herpes

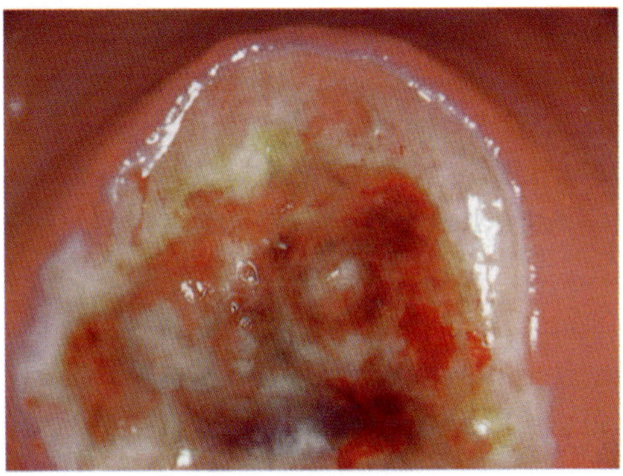

Figure 1. Herpes simplex ulcer of the cervix.

Investigations for genital Herpes

- Virus isolation in cell culture is sensitive and specific; viral typing is possible
- Herpes simplex virus (HSV) antigen detection by direct fluorescent — antibody (DFA) or enzyme immunoassay (EIA) techniques is economical and quick but insensitive; viral typing is not possible
- Polymerase chain reaction (PCR) detection of viral nucleic acid has highest sensitivity but expensive and is not widely available; viral typing is possible
- Tzanck test demonstrates giant cells from lesions but is not sensitive; only presumptive evidence of infection by a herpes virus
- Type specific serological tests (TSST) for HSV 1 & 2 — based on recombinant type-specific glycoproteins G1 and G2 have good sensitivity and specificity; useful in certain clinical situations, e.g. confirming a clinical diagnosis of genital herpes, counselling of sexual partners of infected persons and detection of unrecognised infection
- Older serological tests based on crude antigen extracts are inaccurate, cannot reliably differentiate HSV 1 and 2 and are of very little value in the management of genital herpes

Treatment of first episode of genital herpes:

- Acyclovir 200 mg orally 5 times a day × 7 to 10 days or
- Acyclovir 400 mg orally tds × 7 to 10 days or
- Valacyclovir 1 g orally bd × 7 to 10 days or
- Famciclovir 250 mg orally tds × 7 to 10 days
- For optimal benefit, the treatment should be started within 72 hours of onset of lesions, when new lesions continue to form or when symptoms and signs are severe. The duration of treatment depends on the clinical response

Treatment of recurrent genital herpes:

Episodic treatment

- Initiate during prodrome or within 1 day of attack
- Acyclovir 400 mg orally tds × 5 days or 800 mg tds × 2 days or 800 mg tds × 5 days
- Valacyclovir 500 mg orally bd × 5 days or 1 g qds × 5 days
- Famciclovir 125 mg orally bd × 5 days or 500 mg × 1 dose or 250 mg bd × 2 days

Suppressive treatment

- Reduces the number of recurrences and reduces transmission of HSV
- Acyclovir 400 mg orally bd or

- Valacyclovir 500 mg orally od or
- Famciclovir 250 mg orally bd
- 6 or more recurrences per year

Genital herpes in pregnancy (Refer to Chapter 17 on "Infections in Pregnancy")

Management of sexual contacts of genital herpes

- Sex partners of patients with genital herpes are likely to benefit from evaluation and counselling
- They should be questioned on history of typical and atypical genital lesions and encouraged to examine themselves for lesions and seek medical attention promptly if lesions appear
- Type-specific serological test (TSST) may be useful in counselling

2. Syphilis

Investigations for syphilis

Darkfield microscopy

To demonstrate *Treponema pallidum* in the secretions from the primary chancre or moist lesions of secondary syphilis

Serological tests

Non-treponemal tests — VDRL[a] or RPR[b] — screening tests, titres are useful for monitoring response to therapy

Treponemal tests — TPHA[c], TPPA[d], FTA-Abs[e], LIA[f], EIA[g] and rapid diagnostic tests are specific tests

Screen with

CMIA (a chemiluminescent immunoassay) on Abbott Architect analyser
Normal or *reactive* (abnormal)

- If reactive, samples tested for VDRL and TPPA[d] (treponema pallidum particle agglutination test — this is a test for treponema pallidum antibodies as well)

Interpretation and Management Guidelines of Tests for Syphilis

	VDRL positive	VDRL negative
TPPA positive	Active infection	Past infection
TPPA negative	False positive	No infection

---

[a] VDRL — Venereal Disease Research Laboratory
[b] RPR — Rapid plasma reagin
[c] TPHA — Treponema pallidum haemagglutination assay
[d] TPPA — Treponema pallidum particle agglutination assay
[e] FTA-Abs — Fluorescent treponemal antibody absorption
[f] LIA — Line immunoassay
[g] EIA — Enzyme immunoassay

Interpretation and Follow-up of Reverse Screening Results

Patient history	Test and result			Interpretation	Follow up
	EIA/ CMIA/MFI	RPR	TPPA		
Unknown history of syphilis	Non-Reactive	N/A	N/A	No serologic evidence of syphilis	None, unless clinically indicated (e.g., early syphilis)
Unknown history of syphilis	Reactive	Reactive	N/A	Untreated or recently treated syphilis	Treat as per CDC guidelines
Unknown history of syphilis	Reactive	Non-reactive	Non-reactive	Probable false-positive screening test	No follow up testing, unless clinically indicated
Unknown history of syphilis	Reactive	Non-reactive	Reactive	Possible syphilis (e.g., early or latent) or previously treated syphilis	Historical or clinical evaluation required
Known history of syphilis	Reactive	Non-reactive	Reactive or N/A	Past, successfully treated syphilis	None

CMIA, chemiluminescence immunoassay; EIA, enzyme immunoassay; MFI, multiplex flow immunoassay; N/A, not applicable; RPR, rapid plasma reagin; TPPA *Treponema pallidum* particle agglutination
http://www.cdc.gov/std/treetment/2010/

- Recommend re-testing in 2 weeks, i.e. request for TPPA

If both remain negative, then syphilis infection is excluded

Treatment of primary syphilis, secondary syphilis, latent syphilis of less than 1 year duration

- Benzathine penicillin G 2.4 million units I/M (intra-muscularly), weekly × one dose or
- Aqueous procaine penicillin G 600,000 units I/M daily × 10–14 days

For Penicillin-allergic patients

- Tetracycline 500 mg orally qds × 14 days or
- Doxycycline 100 mg orally bd × 14 days or
- Erythromycin 500 mg orally qds × 14 days or
- Ceftriaxone 500 mg I/M od × 10 days (limited data only) or
- Azithromycin 500 mg od × 10 days (limited data only)

Treatment of latent syphilis of more than 1 year duration or of unknown duration, late-benign syphilis, cardiovascular syphilis

- Benzathine penicillin G 2.4 million units I/M, weekly × 3 doses or
- Aqueous procaine penicillin G 600,000 units I/M daily × 14–21 days

For Penicillin-allergic patients

- Tetracycline 500 mg orally qds × 28 days or
- Doxycycline 100 mg orally bd × 28 days or
- Ceftriaxone 2 g I/M or IV od × 14 days or
- Erythromycin 500 mg orally od × 28 days

Treatment of neurosyphilis

- Aqueous procaine penicillin G 2.4 million units intramuscular (I/M) daily × 10–14 days with Probenecid 500 mg orally qds × 10 days followed by benzathine penicillin G 2.4 million units I/M weekly × 3 doses or
- Aqueous crystalline benzyl penicillin 3 to 4 million units IV every 4 hours (total: 18 to 24 million units a day) × 10–14 days followed by benzathine penicillin G 2.4 mega units I/M weekly × 3 doses

For Penicillin-allergic patients

- RAST tests, skin testing and de-sensitisation should be performed in consultation with an expert
- Penicillin is the drug of choice unless really contraindicated
- Tetracycline 500 mg orally qds × 28 days or
- Doxycycline 100 mg orally bd × 28 days or
- Ceftriaxone 2 g I/M or IV (intravenous) od × 14 days or
- Erythromycin base or stearate 500 mg orally qds × 28 days (least effective)

Follow Up

Refer to Department of STI Control (DSC Clinic)

- At 3, 6, 12, 18 and 24 months
- If VDRL titre increases/persistently high (>1 : 32) or develops symptoms and signs (treatment failure or infection)

Syphilis in pregnancy (Refer to Chapter 17 on "Infections in Pregnancy")

Management of sexual contacts of syphilis

- At risk partners are those who have been exposed within 3 months of symptoms for primary syphilis, 6 months for secondary syphilis and 1 year for early latent syphilis

- Treatment should be given to sexual contacts who were exposed 3 months prior to the diagnosis of primary, secondary or early latent syphilis or if follow up is uncertain.
- Sexual partners of late syphilis should be screened and evaluated for syphilis and treated on the basis of these findings

3. Chancroid

Investigations for chancroid

— Culture for *Hemophilus ducreyi* of smear from ulcer or aspirate from buboes
— Diagnosis is often based on typical clinical presentation and after exclusion of syphilis and HSV infection
— PCR detection

Treatment of chancroid

Therapy is typically given in whom diagnosis is suspected on clinical grounds

- Ceftriaxone 250 mg I/M single dose or
- Azithromycin 1 g oral single dose or
- Ciprofloxacin 500 mg bd × 3 days (contraindicated for pregnant and lactating women)

Management of sexual contacts of chancroid

- Sex partners should be screened and treated when indicated

4. Granuloma Inguinale (GI) — Rare

Investigations for Granuloma inguinale

Tissue biopsy — "Donovan" bodies in tissue samples
On Wright Giemsa stain, large mononuclear cells with intra-cytoplasmic cysts filled with deep purple gram negative Donovan bodies

Treatment of Granuloma inguinale (GI):

Treat for 3 weeks with antibiotics

- Azithromycin
- Tetracycline
- Erythromycin
- Ampicillin
- Cotrimoxazole

Management of Sexual Contacts of Granuloma Inguinale (GI):

Contact tracing within 60 days prior to onset of symptoms and treatment of sexual contacts

Screen for other STIs

5. Lymphogranuloma venerum (LGV) — Rare

Investigations for lymphogranuloma venerum (difficult diagnosis)

Nucleic acid amplification technique (NAAT)

Culture — yield low from ulcers/lymph node aspirates

Serology — Complement fixation (CF)/microimmunofluorescence (MIF)

Skin testing — Frei skin test (low sensitivity and specificity — no longer used)

Treatment of Lymphogranuloma venerum (LGV)

Treat for 3 weeks with antibiotics

- Doxycycline
- Azithromycin
- Erythromycin

Management of Sexual contacts of lymphogranuloma venerum (LGV)

Contact tracing and treatment of sexual contacts

Screen for other STIs

6. Genital warts

1. Genital warts are the commonest cause of growths on the anogenital region
2. 90% of warts are caused by HPV 6 or 11
3. Incubation period — 1 to 6 months
4. Transmission approximately 60% between partners
5. Asymptomatic or painful, pruritic, papular genital lesions
6. Multifocal — usually 5 to 15; in areas of trauma during sex, about 1–10 mm diameter; may coalesce especially in immunosuppressed or diabetic patients

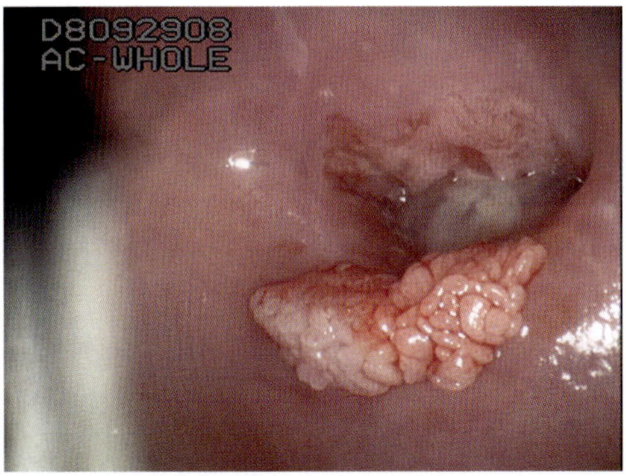

Figure 2. Wart or condyloma on the cervix.

7. May be coinfected with oncogenic "high-risk" HPV, e.g. types 16 and 18 Oncogenic HPV — mostly give rise to subclinical lesions, intraepithelial neoplasia (IN) and anogenital cancer
8. Consider other differentials: condylomata lata, seborrhoeic warts, squamous cell carcinoma, molluscum contagiosum and angiofibromas
9. Skin biopsy — for atypical cases (bowenoid papulosis, ulceration, dermal induration, pigmented lesions, cases not responding to treatment or worsening during treatment, immunocompromised/postmenopausal)
10. Subclinical mucosal warts can be identified as they turn white (acetowhite) on after application of 5% acetic acid for 3 minutes
11. Regular Pap smear as per standard Pap smear screening guidelines
12. HPV DNA testing not recommended as it does not alter management
13. Advise condom use and screening of partners in the last six months
14. Asymptomatic or subclinical genital HPV is self limiting
15. Common — about 50% get it at least once in a lifetime

16. In absence of lesions, treatment is not recommended
17. Pre-exposure HPV vaccination is recommended (refer to Chapter 43 on "HPV Vaccine and HPV Testing")

Treatment of Genital Warts

A. *Vulval, perineal and perianal warts*

Home therapy

1. Podophyllotoxin (0.15% cream) bd × 3 days a week, rest 4–7 days
   — contraindicated in pregnancy (teratogenic)
   — women of childbearing age must use contraception
   — 4 weeks' treatment

2. Imiquimod (5% cream) e.g. Aldara®
   — 3× a week at bedtime, washed off next morning, until clearance or for 16 weeks
   — No studies in pregnant women

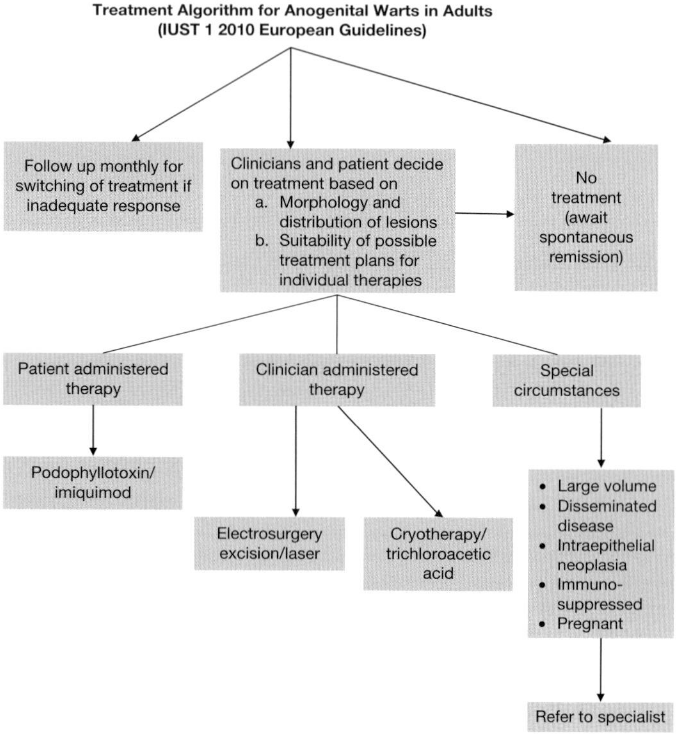

Office therapy

1. Cryotherapy — liquid nitrogen weekly
2. Trichloroacetic acid (50%–80%) weekly, one application for 8–10 weeks
3. Electrosurgery (1–6 treatment sessions)
4. CO_2 laser
5. Scissors excision (1–2 excision sessions)

B. *Vaginal or cervical warts*

1. CO_2 laser
2. Electrosurgery
3. Trichloroacetic acid

    - Dysplasia must be excluded before starting treatment
    - Cervical cytology and colposcopy (if necessary) are advised

Interferon alpha and beta as adjuvants to surgery in problematic cases

Adverse effects of treatment for genital warts

- Hypo/hyperpigmentation
- Depressed/hypertrophic scarring
- Chronic pain syndrome (hyperesthesia/vulvodynia)
- Systemic effects from podophyllotoxin

Genital warts in pregnancy (Refer to Chapter 17 on "Infections in Pregnancy")

Management of sexual contacts

- All regular contacts should be examined and clinical warts treated

Only surgical treatment has primary clearance rates of about 100%. Recurrence — after all therapies often 20%–30% or more.Side effects of treatments — local skin reactions, pain, itch, burns, erosion.

Role of HPV Vaccine

- Effective in primary prevention of HPV infection (for warts — use Gardasil®)
- Use for treatment of anogenital warts or prevention of recurrent disease is not recommended

7. Human Immunodeficiency Virus (HIV) infection

There were 469 newly reported HIV infections in Singapore in 2012 — the total number of HIV infected Singapore residents is 5775 as at end 2012. As of 31 Dec 2012, 2814 persons are asymptomatic carriers, 1379 have or have had AIDS-related illness and 1582 had died.

The Ministry of Health (MOH) and Health Promotion Board (HPB) urge individuals to protect themselves from HIV infection and its effects by following the principles of "ABCD"

(A) Abstinence

(B) Being faithful

(C) Correct and consistent use of condoms, and

(D) Early detection

Human immunodeficiency virus (HIV) is transmitted through sexual intercourse with an infected person, or through contaminated syringes and needles, transfusion of infected blood and blood products, and from infected mothers to babies.

HIV-1 accounts for almost all the global infections except for a small number of infections by HIV-2 that originate in West Africa.

HIV-1 is divided into subtypes A to K (the M subtypes) and O. N is the newest subtype reported.

Clinical features of HIV infection

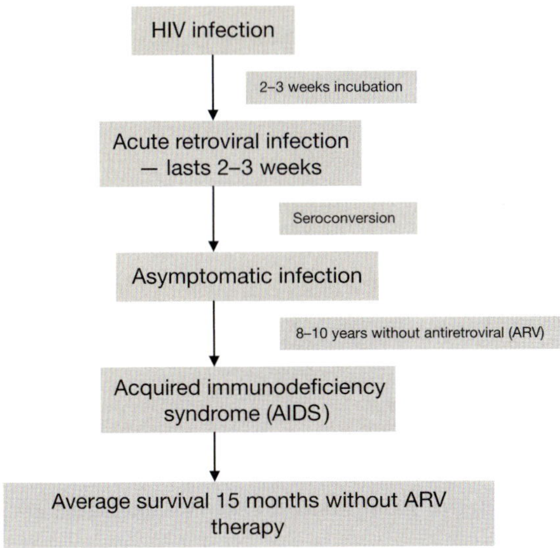

Opportunistic diseases associated with AIDS include:

1. *Bacterial* diseases, e.g tuberculosis
2. *Protozoal* diseases, e.g. *Pneumocystis carinii* pneumonia (PCP), toxoplasmosis
3. *Fungal* diseases, e.g. candidiasis
4. *Viral* diseases, e.g. CMV, herpes simplex and herpes zoster
5. HIV-associated malignancies, e.g. Kaposi sarcoma, lymphoma and squamous cell carcinoma

Investigations for HIV

a. *Screening tests*

- Enzyme-linked immunoassay (EIA) technique to detect anti-HIV antibodies
- A positive screening test must be confirmed due to false-positive EIA result
- There is a window period which is the time delay from infection to positive EIA
- This averages 3–4 weeks but practically all will seroconvert by 3 months

b. *Confirmatory tests*

- Western blot (WB) technique
- Persons who are EIA positive but WB negative are negative for HIV

- When the EIA test is positive but the WB does not fulfil the required number of bands, the test is considered to be indeterminate
- Indeterminate test may be seen during seroconversion, late-stage HIV infection, cross-reacting antibodies, infection with the O strain or HIV-2 and HIV vaccine recipients. Repeat testing is recommended after 3 months
- Using both EIA and WB tests, the sensitivity and specificity exceed 99.9%

Treatment of HIV

Refer to Centre for Disease Control (CDC) for treatment

HIV In Pregnancy (refer to Chapter 17 on "Infections in Pregnancy")

Prevention of STIs

(i) Vaccines

Immunisations are available for prevention of hepatitis A, hepatitis B and HPV

No vaccines are available for HIV and hepatitis C

(ii) Use of barrier — condoms

Though the amount of protection provided is difficult to establish, CDC and WHO have both recommended condoms as an essential component in public health strategies to prevent STIs

(iii) Counselling

Behavioural interventions/partner notification/empiric therapy in victims of sexual assault (including HIV post-exposure prophylaxis)/strategies to improve sexual health

(iv) Suppressive therapy

e.g. for genital HSV with valacyclovir

(v) Prevention of vertical transmission of STI (mother to foetus)

- Breastfeeding is contraindicated for HIV positive mothers
- In women with hepatitis B — hepatitis B immunoglobulin is administered to neonates within 12 hours of delivery. First dose of HBV vaccine is administered within 7 days of delivery; second dose at one month; and third dose at six months
- Caesarean section is recommended for all women:
  - — presenting with first episode of genital herpes at the time of labour or within six weeks of expected date of delivery

— with HIV on zidovudine monotherapy, on HAART with viral load >50 copies or co-existent hepatitis C infection.

— If pelvic outlet is obstructed by genital warts or if vaginal delivery would result in excessive bleeding.

Chapter 56

ORAL HORMONAL CONTRACEPTION

Combined Oral Contraceptive (COC) Pill

COC pill

Contraceptive usage
Failure 0.2–3 per
100 woman-years

Non-contraceptive benefits

Alleviation of

- Abnormal uterine bleeding (AUB)
- Dysmenorrhoea
- Chronic pelvic pain (CPP)
- Hirsutism and polycystic ovary syndrome (PCOS)
- Premenstrual syndrome (PMS)
- Premenstrual dysphoric disorder (PMDD)
- Endometriosis
- Benign breast disease
- Acne (if contraception required)

Reduction in

- Risk of colorectal cancer
- Risk of ovarian and endometrial cancer that continues several decades after stopping COC pill (50% reduction)
- *Regulation* of menstrual cycles
- *Manipulation* of timing of menstruation

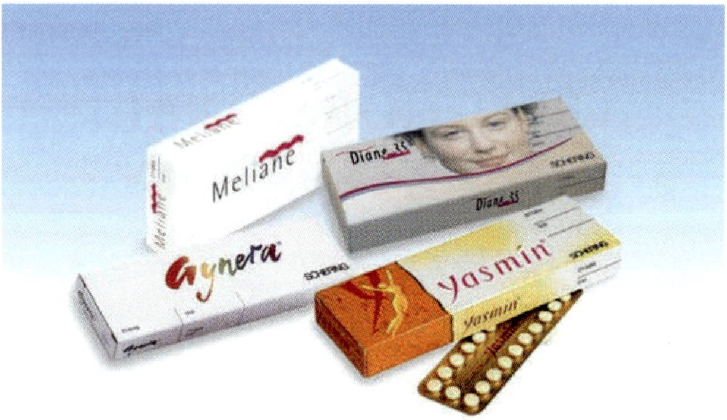

Figure 1. Various combined oral contraceptive pills.

Mode of action of COC

- Suppresses ovulation
- Reduces sperm penetrability by thickening the cervical mucous
- Alters endometrium and reduces the likelihood of implantation

COC pills		
Type	**Composition in each Pill**	**Remarks**
1st generation		
(Not used)	e.g. COC containing progestogens like: Norethisterone, Norethindrone, Ethynodiolacetate, Lynestrenol	
2nd generation		
NORDETTE/ MICROGYNON	Ethinyl oestradiol 30 μg and levonorgestrel 150 μg	Less thrombogenic side effect than 3rd and 4th generation progestins
3rd generation	contains progestogen, desogestrel or gestodene	
MELIANE	Ethinyl oestradiol 20 μg and 0.075 mg gestodene	Less androgenic side effect Lowest oestrogen content
GYNERA	Ethinyl oestradiol 30 μg and 0.075 mg gestodene	Less androgenic side effect
4th generation		
YASMIN	Ethinyl oestradiol 30 μg and 3 mg drospirenone	Drospirenone is a novel progestogen with anti-mineralocortioid properties • No reported clinically significant changes in potassium concentration • Counteracts water retention-related weight gain

Table 1: Different combined oral contraceptive preparations

COC pills		
Type	Composition in each Pill	Remarks
		Favourable effect on skin condition Reduces severity of premenstrual symptoms (PMS)
YAZ	Ethinyl oestradiol 20 μg and 3 mg drospirenone	Novel regimen ("24 / 4" i.e. 24 days of active pills and 4 days of placebo pills) with shortened pill-free interval. This secures the benefits of a lower daily oestrogen dose while maintaining a lower breakthrough bleeding pattern. Indicated for treatment of severe premenstrual syndrome (PMS) or premenstrual dysphoric disorder (PMDD) with significant improvements in physical, mood and behavioural symptoms Treats moderate acne vulgaris
Others		
DIANE 35	Ethinyl oestradiol 35 μg and 2 mg cyproterone acetate	Anti-androgenic properties: • Treatment of acne • Treatment of hirsutism in polycystic ovarian syndrome (PCOS)

Table 1: (*Continued*)

Side Effects of COC pill

- Breakthrough bleeding
- Amenorrhoea
- Leukorrhoea
- Mastalgia
- Nausea/vomiting/bloating
- Melasma
- Gallstone formation

Health Risks Associated with COC pill

Venous thromboembolism (deep vein thrombosis and pulmonary embolism)

- COC pills with desogestrel, gestodene and cyproterone are associated with higher risk of thromboembolism than those containing levonorgestrel, norethisterone and norgestimate

Small increase in absolute risk of ischaemic stroke/breast cancer/cervical cancer

Contraindications to COC pill use

Absolute Contraindications to COC Pill Use	Relative Contraindications to COC Pill Use
Past or present cardiovascular disease	
Family history <45 years old with abnormal lipid profile or haemostatic profile. Poorly controlled diabetes/or diabetic complications, e.g. retinopathy. BP consistently >160/95 mmHg Smokes >40 cigarettes/day. Smokers > 35 years old BMI >35	Family history >45 years old with normal lipid and haemostatic profiles. Well controlled, short duration DM. Systolic BP 135–160 mmHg, diastolic BP 85–95 mmHg. Smokes 5–40 cigarettes/day. BMI 30–35
Focal or crescendo migraine or migraine requiring ergotamine treatment	Uncomplicated migraine
Active liver disease. Recurrent cholestatic jaundice or cholestatic jaundice occurring in pregnancy. Dubin-Johnson or Rotor syndrome. Liver adenoma/carcinoma. Gallstones Porphyrias	Long-term partial immobilisation, e.g. patients using a wheelchair Hyperprolactinaemia Chronic systemic diseases (UK Medical Eligibility Criteria for Contraceptive Use)
Medical condition affected by sex steroids, e.g. chorea, pemphigoid gestationis	Very severe depression
Pregnancy	Some malabsorption conditions
Undiagnosed genital tract bleeding	Conditions requiring drug treatment which may interact with COC pill use
Oestrogen dependent tumours, e.g. breast cancer	

Management of Missed Pills for 21-day Regimen — COC

Definition of a missed pill

A "missed pill" is a combined oral contraceptive (COC) pill that is completely omitted from being taken (i.e. 48 hours have elapsed since the last COC pill was taken).

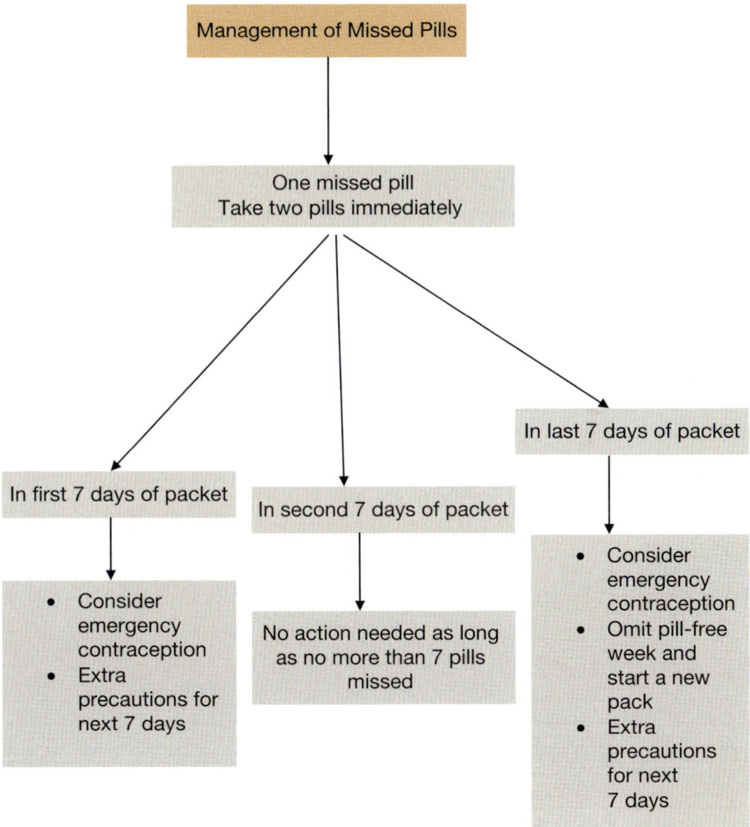

Advice to patients for missed pills

1) If pills are missed in weeks 1, 2 or 3 of pack:

The patient should be advised to take the last missed pill as soon as possible and continue with the usual pill-taking schedule. Depending on when she remembers, she may take two pills at different times (the moment of remembering and her regular time), or two pills at the same time.

2) If pills are missed in week 3 or 4 of pack:

The patient should be advised to finish the active pills in the current pack and then immediately start a new pack (omitting the pill-free interval or discarding any inactive pills).

(For users of 24/4 or 26/2 COCs):

If inactive pills are missed in week 4, she should throw away the missed inactive pills and continue the usual pill-taking schedule.

3) If more than SEVEN pills are missed:

Advise the patients to restart COC on day two of next menses as if she had not used the pills before.

4) Assess for loss of contraception

Loss of contraception is most likely when more than two pills (for 20 μg ethinyl oestradiol pills) and three pills (for 30 μg ethinyl oestradiol pills) are missed. (REMEMBER: "Two for twenty and three for thirty".)

a. **Advise additional protection** such as condoms or abstinence, until the woman has taken her COC for 7 days in a row if contraception is unreliable.
b. If the patient has had unprotected intercourse, consider **emergency contraception**.

Note:

- It takes **SEVEN** consecutive pills to ensure that ovulation has been suppressed.
- Follicular activity may resume at the end of a 7-day break in some women.

Progestin Only Pill (POP)

- Useful for older pre-menopausal women who wish to avoid risks from exogenous oestrogen and lactating mothers
- Pre-requisite criteria: motivated woman who can maintain reliable and timely pill-taking
- Can start on day 1–2 of menses or same day after abortion or miscarriage
- Failure 0.4–4 per 100 woman-years

Mode of action of POP

- Decrease sperm permeability by altering the cervical mucous
- Reduce endometrial receptivity to implantation

Advantage of POP

- Lighter, shorter, less painful periods.

Disadvantage of POP

- Woman may have irregular pattern of bleeding
- Short effect of each pill which lasts only 24 hours
- Requires the woman to take the pill at the same time everyday
- If the pill is delayed by >3 hours, extra protection is needed for the next 7 days

Side Effects of POP

- Irregular periods
- Tender breasts
- Nausea, headache, dizziness
- Mood changes
- Weight gain

Contraindications of POP:

- Sensitivity to progesterone
- Unreliable pill taker
- Pregnancy
- Undiagnosed vaginal bleeding
- Previous ectopic pregnancy
- During follow up of a hydatidiform mole

Chapter 57

NON-ORAL CONTRACEPTION/ CONTRACEPTION FOR LACTATING MOTHERS

Barrier Method

- Includes condom, femidom or diaphragm
- Has the added *advantage* of protection against sexually transmitted infections (STIs)
- *Disadvantage*: highly operator-dependent, disrupts sexual intercourse as a condom has to be put on prior to penetration and has to be removed immediately after ejaculation
- Failure rate 2–15 per 100 woman-years
- Diaphragm has to be left in place for 8 hours after intercourse
- Spermicides can be used together with condom or diaphragm to increase the efficacy

Depot Provera (Progestin-Only Injectables)

- Depot medroxyprogesterone acetate (DMPA) 150 mg
- Intramuscular injection every 12 weeks
- *Mode of action*:
  a) suppresses hypothalamic-pituitary axis with inhibition of ovulation
  b) change in cervical mucous and tubal mobility (alters sperm transport inhibit fertilisation)
- First injection on day 1–5 of menses or on day of last combined oral contraceptive pill or at 6 weeks after childbirth
- Failure 0.4 per 100 woman-years
- *Common side effects*: Irregular menstrual cycles, amenorrhoea, headache, breast tenderness, mood changes and weight gain. Long-term use is associated with osteoporosis (though reversible).
- *Return of fertility:* does not impact endocrine function permanently. However, return of fertility may be delayed up to 18 months after the last injection.
- *Non contraceptive benefits of Depot Provera include* alleviation of :
  - Endometriosis
  - Heavy menstrual bleeding (correction of anaemia)
  - Dysmenorrhoea

- Decreased risk of PID (due to changes in cervical mucous/decreased menstrual flow)
- Prevention of haemorrhagic corpus luteal cysts in women on anticoagulants

Evra Patch

- One patch (0.75 mg ethinyloestradiol and 6 mg norelgestromin) applied each week for 3 weeks and patch-free for one week.
- Timing of application:
  - If no hormonal contraception is used in the past month — day 1 of menses/any other day of the cycle — use spermicide or barrier contraception for the following 7 days
  - After first trimester miscarriage or abortion — apply within first five days
  - After second trimester miscarriage or abortion — apply 4 weeks later (spermicide or barrier for following 7 days)
- If accidentally removed or detached for < 24 hours — reapply the patch
- If detached > 24 hours — apply a new patch and use additional contraception for 7 consecutive days
- *Risks*: venous thromboembolism/migraine/depression

- Failure rate <1%
- *Side effects*: unscheduled bleeding/headache/nausea/allergy or irritation due to the patch/breast tenderness/mood changes
- *Contraindications*: history of thromboembolism/an oestrogen-dependent tumour/abnormal liver function/pregnancy/undiagnosed vaginal bleeding

Implanon® Nxt Implants

- Single rod, biodegradable, radiopaque and subdermal
- Contains 68 mg etonorgestrel
- Provides protection for 3 years

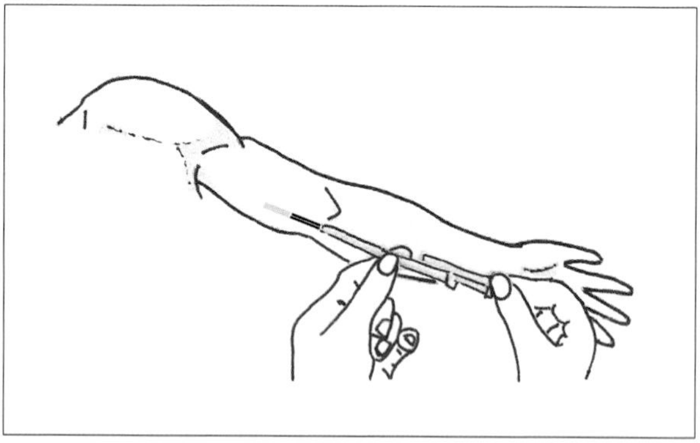

Figure 1: Implanon insertion.

- Mode of action: suppresses hypothalamic-pituitary axis with inhibition of ovulation and change in cervical mucous and tubal motility
- Simple insertion subdermally in the medial aspect of arm and easy removal under local anaesthesia
- *Timing of insertion*

  Day 1–5 of menstrual cycle (exclude pregnancy before insertion)

  After miscarriage/abortion — insert immediately within first five days

  Postpartum within 21 days.

  Breastfeeding: insert anytime (ensure not pregnant)
- Highly effective; failure 0.07 per 100 woman-years
- *Common side effects*: irregular menstrual cycles, amenorrhoea, headache, breast tenderness, mood changes and weight gain
- *Problems*: infection, haematoma, local irritation or rash, allergic reaction, expulsion.
  - During removal — rods that are deeply placed and not palpable under skin, perform X-ray/ultrasound to locate it prior to removal
- *Return to fertility*: more than 90% of women ovulate within 3 to 4 weeks of removal

Intrauterine Contraceptive Device (IUCD)

- *Mode of action*: exact mechanism unknown. Proposed theories — inhibition of sperm transport/inhibition of fertilisation and implantation
- Types — copper containing IUCDs or levonorgestrel containing IUCD (Mirena)
- Examples are Nova T and Multiload IUCD
- Provides protection of 3 to 5 years depending on the type of IUCD
- Used only in parous women and suitable for breastfeeding mothers
- *Contraindications*:

  Pregnancy

  Severe distortion of uterine cavity due to fibroids/uterine anomaly

  Acute/recurrent pelvic infection

  Known copper allergy (for copper containing IUCDs)

  Acute liver disease/tumour; suspected breast carcinoma
- *Removal*: on expiry of the device at any time during menstrual cycle or at menopause
- *Immediate risks*: uterine perforation, vasovagal response
- Failure 0.1–0.5 per 100 woman-years.
- *Common side effects*: pelvic infection (usually occurs within first 3 weeks of insertion), heavy menses and pelvic pain
- Problems — Refer to Chapter 60 on "IUCDs and Dilemmas"

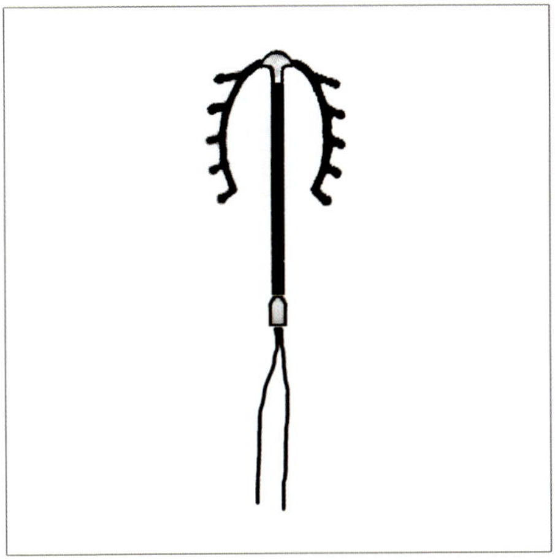

Figure 2: Multiload copper IUCD.

- Follow up: after 1 to 3 months or earlier if symptoms like severe abdominal pain/fever/heavy menstrual bleeding/foul smelling vaginal discharge/suspected expulsion or pregnancy

Levonorgestrel Intrauterine System (Mirena IUCD)

- *Mode of action*: contraceptive effect by achieving endometrial glandular and stromal atrophy
- Contains 52 mg reservoir of levonorgestrel (LNG) in Nova T-shaped device, releases 20 µg of LNG daily
- Low local hormonal effect in the endometrium which provides shorter and lighter menses and reduces dysmenorrhoea
- Low systemic circulation of hormone

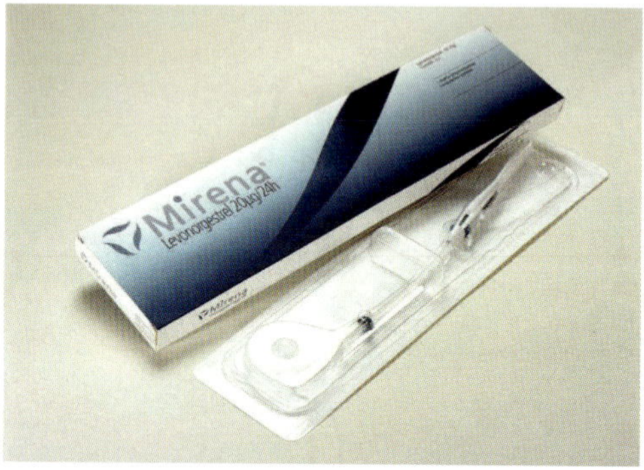

Figure 3: Mirena intrauterine system

- Best inserted during menses
- Provides protection for 5 years
- Approved for breastfeeding mothers. To be inserted 6 weeks postpartum
- Failure 0.16 per 100 woman-years; risk of ectopic pregnancy 0.02 per 100 woman-years
- *Common side effects*: 20% of women have intermittent per-vaginal spotting in 1st 6 months and 20% of women are amenorrhoeic after 1 year
- 5–10% may experience headache, migraine, depressed mood
- *Contraindications*: pregnancy, serious/acute pelvic inflammatory disease (PID), unexplained bleeding from genital tract (suggestive of cancer), liver disease, current or past history of breast cancer, history of stroke/thromboembolism, severe migraines

Mesigyna/Norigynon (Monthly Combined Injectables)

- Monthly injections containing both a progestin and an oestrogen
- Mesigyna/Norigynon contains 50 mg of norethisterone and 5 mg oestradiol valerate.
- Compared with progestin-only injectables, combined injectables disturb vaginal bleeding patterns less and allow earlier return to ovulation after women discontinue use
- Failure 0.1–0.4 per 100 woman-years.
- *Common side effects*: irregular menstrual cycles, headache, breast tenderness and giddiness
- *Contraindications*: pregnancy, hypersensitivity, undiagnosed genital tract bleeding, active liver disease, thrombosis or thromboembolic disorders

Nuva Ring

Contraception: 15 μg of ethinyl oestradiol and etonogestrel 0.12 mg/day

- *Vaginal* : one ring left in place for 3 weeks and removed for one week
  A new ring inserted 7 days after the last is removed
- *Timing of insertion*:
  - If no hormonal contraception is used in the past month — day 1 of menses (use spermicide or barrier contraception for the following 7 days).

- After the first trimester miscarriage or abortion — insert within first 5 days
- After the second trimester miscarriage or abortion — insert 4 weeks later (spermicide or barrier for following 7 days).

- If accidently removed within the 3 weeks — rinse with lukewarm water and reinsert within 3 hours.
- If removed for longer than 1 week, rule out pregnancy prior to insertion and use barrier or spermicide 7 days following insertion.
- *Contraindications*: pregnancy, hypersensitivity, undiagnosed genital tract bleeding, active liver disease, thrombosis or thromboembolic disorders.
- *Risks*: Venous thromboembolism/migraine/depression.
- Failure rate <1%.
- *Side effects*: headache/nausea/weight gain/mood changes/chloasma/breakthrough bleeding.

Permanent Sterilisation

Tubal ligation

- Irreversibility of fertility
- *Timing*: postpartum, post-abortion or interval ligation of fallopian tubes
- Includes Filshie clip application, Falope ring (silastic band) application, Pomeroy method (ligation and resection of segment of fallopian tubes)

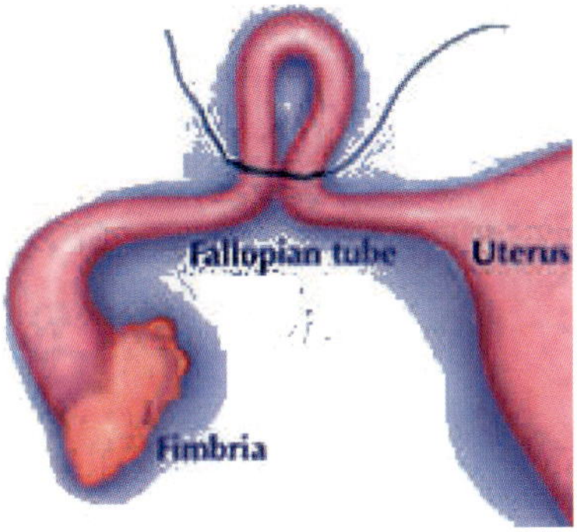

Figure 4: Pomeroy method of fallopian tube ligation

- Laparoscopic for interval ligation or via mini-laparotomy for postpartum sterilisation
- Disadvantages: Regret, failure, cannalisation can be difficult if required later.
- Discuss alternative reversible contraception and male vasectomy prior to female tubal ligation.
- Essure procedure (hysteroscopic insertion of micro-insert into each fallopian tube). Use alternative contraception for three months post-procedure. Do check hysterosalpingogram (HSG) day 7 to 10 of cycle

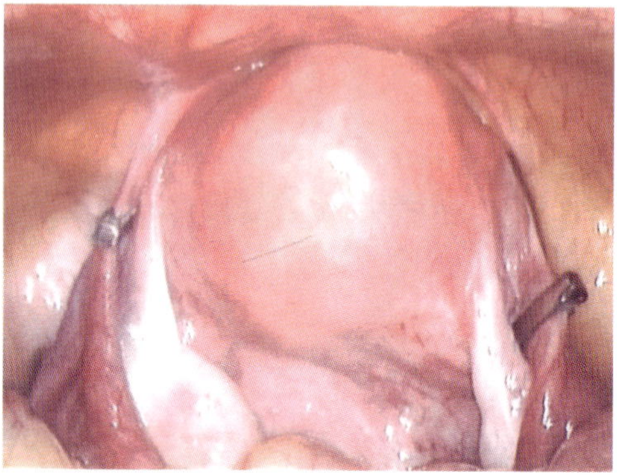

Figure 5: Laparoscopic picture of tubal ligation with Filshie clips

Vasectomy

- Most reliable of all birth control methods
- Irreversibility of fertility for men
- Involves an operation where the vas deferens are cut or tied so that the sperms are not released during ejaculation
- Can be done under local anaesthesia
- No hormonal side-effects
- Failure rate 1 in 2000 (0.05%)
- Not immediately effective, needs up to 20 ejaculations before 2 negative seminal analysis of spermatozoa

Contraception for Lactating Mothers

- Lactational amenorrhoea method (LAM)
  - For mothers who are fully breastfeeding and have continuing amenorrhoea in the first 6 months postpartum
  - 1–2 % failure rate
- Progestin-only pills (POP)
- MIRENA intra-uterine system (after 6 weeks postpartum)
- Intrauterine contraceptive device (after 6 weeks postpartum)
- Barrier method
- Tubal ligation
- Vasectomy (for male partner)

Chapter 58

CHOICE OF CONTRACEPTION

The Faculty of Sexual and Reproductive Healthcare in The United Kingdom categorised the choice of contraceptives based on personal characteristics and reproductive history.

Key: Combined hormonal contraception e.g. oral contraceptive pill/patch/vaginal ring (CHC), Progestogen only pill (POP), Depot medroxyprogesterone acetate (DMPA), Progestogen implant (IMP), Copper Intrauterine Device (Cu-IUD), Levonorgestrel Intrauterine Device (LNG-IUD), Barrier methods e.g. condom/diaphragm/spermicide (CD)

Contraceptive Choice Based on Personal Characteristics and Reproductive History

Personal Characteristics and Reproductive History	**Best Choice** *UK Category 1* No restriction for the use	**Alternative** *UK Category 2* Advantages generally outweigh the theoretical or proven risks	**Not Recommended** *UK Category 3* Theoretical or proven risks generally outweigh the advantages. Not recommended unless other more appropriate methods not available or acceptable *UK Category 4* Unacceptable risks	**Additional Information**
Age	POP, IMP, CHC in patients aged <40 DMPA in patients 18–45 years Cu-IUD and LNG-IUD in patients aged >20 years Barrier method—all ages	CHC in patients ≥40 years old DMPA in patients <18 and >45 years Cu- IUD and LNG-IUD in patients aged ≤ 20 (concerned about risk of expulsion from nulliparity and STIs from sexual behaviour in younger age group)		The risk for cardiovascular disease increases with age and might increase with CHC use. In the absence of other adverse clinical conditions, CHCs can be used until menopause Women lose BMD while using DMPA but regain BMD after discontinuation

(*Continued*)

(*Continued*)

Personal Character-istics and Reproductive History	**Best Choice** *UK Category 1* No restriction for the use	**Alternative** *UK Category 2* Advantages generally outweigh the theoretical or proven risks	**Not Recommended** *UK Category 3* Theoretical or proven risks generally outweigh the advantages. Not recommended unless other more appropriate methods not available or acceptable *UK Category 4* Unacceptable risks	**Additional Information**
Postpartum Breastfeeding • <6 weeks postpartum	CD, POP, IMP	DMPA	CHC	No significant negative effect of progestin only contraception on breastfeeding Theoretical concerns about effects of CHCs on breast milk production are greater in the early postpartum period when milk flow is being established
• >6 weeks to <6 months	Above +DMPA, Cu-IUD, LNG-IUD	CHC (if stopped breastfeeding)	CHC (if full breastfeeding)	
• >6 months	Above +CHC			

(*Continued*)

(*Continued*)

Personal Character-istics and Reproductive History	**Best Choice** *UK Category 1* No restriction for the use	**Alternative** *UK Category 2* Advantages generally outweigh the theoretical or proven risks	**Not Recommended** *UK Category 3* Theoretical or proven risks generally outweigh the advantages. Not recommended unless other more appropriate methods not available or acceptable *UK Category 4* Unacceptable risks	**Additional Information**
Non breastfeeding • <21 days	CD, POP, DMPA, IMP		CHC, Cu-IUD, LNG-IUD	Concern exists about the association between CHC use and risk for thrombosis Blood coagulation and fibrinolysis are essentially normalised by 3 weeks postpartum
• >21 days	Above +CHC		Cu-IUD, LNG-IUD	
• >6 weeks	Above +Cu-IUD and LNG-IUD			
Past-ectopic pregnancy	All methods can be used		None	All methods protect against pregnancy in general, including ectopic gestation

(*Continued*)

(Continued)

Personal Characteristics and Reproductive History	Best Choice *UK Category 1* No restriction for the use	Alternative *UK Category 2* Advantages generally outweigh the theoretical or proven risks	Not Recommended *UK Category 3* Theoretical or proven risks generally outweigh the advantages. Not recommended unless other more appropriate methods not available or acceptable *UK Category 4* Unacceptable risks	Additional Information
Post-abortion • First trimester	All methods			Women who started taking COCs immediately after the first trimester medical or surgical abortion did not experience more side effects or adverse vaginal bleeding outcomes or clinically significant changes in coagulation parameters than did women who used a placebo, an IUD, a non-hormonal contraceptive method, or delayed COC initiation
• Second trimester	CHC, POP, DMPA, IMP, CD	Cu-IUD and LNG-IUD		
• Immediately post-septic abortion	CHC, POP, DMPA, IMP, CD	Expulsion was greater when an IUD was inserted after a second trimester abortion than when inserted after a first trimester abortion Safety or expulsion for post-abortion insertion of an LNG-IUD did not differ from that of a Cu-IUD	Cu-IUD and LNG-IUD	

(Continued)

(*Continued*)

Personal Character-istics and Reproductive History	**Best Choice** *UK Category 1* No restriction for the use	**Alternative** *UK Category 2* Advantages generally outweigh the theoretical or proven risks	**Not Recommended** *UK Category 3* Theoretical or proven risks generally outweigh the advantages. Not recommended unless other more appropriate methods not available or acceptable *UK Category 4* Unacceptable risks	**Additional Information**
Obesity • BMI ≥30–34 kg/m^2	POP, DMPA, IMP, Cu-IUD, LNG-IUD, CD	CHC		Obese women who use CHC are more likely than non users to experience venous thromboembolism (VTE). The effectiveness of the patch decreased among women who weighed >90 kg; however, no association was found between pregnancy risk and BMI
• BMI ≥35 kg/m^2	POP, DMPA, IMP, Cu-IUD, LNG-IUD, CD		CHC not advised	

(*Continued*)

(Continued)

Personal Characteristics and Reproductive History	**Best Choice** *UK Category 1* No restriction for the use	**Alternative** *UK Category 2* Advantages generally outweigh the theoretical or proven risks	**Not Recommended** *UK Category 3* Theoretical or proven risks generally outweigh the advantages. Not recommended unless other more appropriate methods not available or acceptable *UK Category 4* Unacceptable risks	**Additional Information**
Smoking WHO study showed significant increased risks of myocardial infarction in female smokers > 35 years who use the CHC	POP, DMPA, IMP, Cu-IUD, LNG-IUD, CD	CHC can be used in patients <35 years or ex-smokers who have stopped for at least a year	CHC should be denied to smokers ≥35 years old	

Chapter 59

CONTRACEPTION IN PATIENTS WITH MEDICAL CONDITIONS AND DRUG INTERACTIONS

The Faculty of Sexual and Reproductive Healthcare in the United Kingdom categorised the risk of using contraception into 4 categories and had published guidelines for the use of different contraceptive methods in the presence of different medical conditions.

Key: Combined hormonal contraception e.g. oral contraceptive pill/patch/ vaginal ring (CHC), Progestogen only pill (POP), Depot medroxyprogesterone acetate (DMPA), Progestogen implant (IMP), Copper Intrauterine Device (Cu-IUD), Levonorgestrel Intrauterine Device (LNG-IUD), Barrier methods e.g. condom/diaphragm/spermicide (CD)

Medical Condition	**Best Choice** *UK Category 1* No restriction for the use	**Alternative** *UK Category 2* Advantages generally outweigh the theoretical or proven risks	**Not Recommended** *UK Category 3* Theoretical or proven risks generally outweigh the advantages. Not recommended unless other more appropriate methods not available or acceptable *UK Category 4* Unacceptable risks	**Additional Information**
Hypertension BP >140/90 mmHg Known risk factor for cardiovascular disease and cerebrovascular accidents	POP IMP Cu-IUD LNG-IUD CD	DMPA	CHC users were at higher risk than non-users for stroke, acute myocardial infarction, and peripheral arterial disease	DMPA is associated with a slight increased risk of cardiovascular events. Use is not recommended if there is existing vascular disease

(*Continued*)

(Continued)

Medical Condition	**Best Choice** *UK Category 1* No restriction for the use	**Alternative** *UK Category 2* Advantages generally outweigh the theoretical or proven risks	**Not Recommended** *UK Category 3* Theoretical or proven risks generally outweigh the advantages. Not recommended unless other more appropriate methods not available or acceptable *UK Category 4* Unacceptable risks	Additional Information
Diabetes Mellitus • Good glycemic control prior to getting pregnant will lower the risks of congenital abnormalities so effective contraception is crucial to prevent unplanned pregnancies • Evaluation of blood pressure and weight, and baseline fasting lipids and investigations to exclude retinopathy, vascular and renal complications	Cu-IUD (no increased pelvic infection rates compared to non-diabetics) CD	*Well controlled diabetes* with no renal, vascular and retinal disease: CHC POP IMP DMPA LNG-IUD	Underlying renal or vascular complications: CHC and DMPA should be avoided	POP and DMPA increase insulin resistance while progestogen implants have minimal effect. Oestrogen has no effect on insulin resistance

(Continued)

(*Continued*)

Medical Condition	**Best Choice** *UK Category 1* No restriction for the use	**Alternative** *UK Category 2* Advantages generally outweigh the theoretical or proven risks	**Not Recommended** *UK Category 3* Theoretical or proven risks generally outweigh the advantages. Not recommended unless other more appropriate methods not available or acceptable *UK Category 4* Unacceptable risks	**Additional Information**
Thrombophilia/ venous thromboembolism (VTE) *Thrombophilias* include thrombo-genic mutations like Factor V Leiden, prothrombin mutation, protein C, protein S and antithrombin deficiencies *VTE risk assessment:* • Personal history • Family history • Surgery • Prolonged immobilisation	Cu-IUD CD	POP, DMPA, IMP, LNG-IUD (progestogen containing contraceptives) are category 2 in patients with a personal or family history of VTE, current VTE on anticoagulants, with known thrombogenic mutations or undergoing major surgery with prolonged immobilisation	CHC increases the VTE risk through the effect of oestrogen on clotting factors. 3rd generation progestogen (desogestrel, e.g. *Mercilon*® or gestodene e.g. *Meliane*®) is associated with a 2 fold increase compared to a combined pill containing levonorgestrel (e.g. Microgynon®)	• Among women with thrombogenic mutations, COC users had a 2-to 20-fold higher risk for thrombosis than did non-users • All methods can be used in patients with superficial venous thrombosis, e.g. varicose veins

(*Continued*)

(Continued)

Medical Condition	**Best Choice** *UK Category 1* No restriction for the use	**Alternative** *UK Category 2* Advantages generally outweigh the theoretical or proven risks	**Not Recommended** *UK Category 3* Theoretical or proven risks generally outweigh the advantages. Not recommended unless other more appropriate methods not available or acceptable *UK Category 4* Unacceptable risks	**Additional Information**
Current and history of ischaemic heart disease (IHD) and stroke	Cu-IUD CD	POP, IMP, LNG-IUD may be initiated in never before users. But users should be advised to stop if the patient develops IHD or stroke while on the above methods	CHC, DMPA	
Hyperlipidaemia	Cu-IUD CD	POP, DMPA, IMP, LNG-IUD	CHC	

(Continued)

(*Continued*)

Medical Condition	**Best Choice** *UK Category 1* No restriction for the use	**Alternative** *UK Category 2* Advantages generally outweigh the theoretical or proven risks	**Not Recommended** *UK Category 3* Theoretical or proven risks generally outweigh the advantages. Not recommended unless other more appropriate methods not available or acceptable *UK Category 4* Unacceptable risks	**Additional Information**
Valvular and congenital heart disease				• Among women with valvular heart disease, CHC use may further increase the risk for arterial thrombosis; women with complicated valvular heart disease are at the greatest risk • Prophylactic antibiotics solely to prevent endocarditis is *not* recommended for insertion or removal of IUDs
• Uncomplicated	POP, DMPA, IMP, Cu-IUD, LNG-IUD, CD	CHC		
• Complicated (pulmonary hypertension, atrial fibrillation, history of subacute bacterial endocarditis)	POP, DMPA, IMP, CD	Cu-IUD, LNG-IUD	CHC	

(*Continued*)

(*Continued*)

Medical Condition	**Best Choice** *UK Category 1* No restriction for the use	**Alternative** *UK Category 2* Advantages generally outweigh the theoretical or proven risks	**Not Recommended** *UK Category 3* Theoretical or proven risks generally outweigh the advantages. Not recommended unless other more appropriate methods not available or acceptable *UK Category 4* Unacceptable risks	Additional Information
Headaches				
• Non-migrainous	All methods			Women with migraine with aura had a higher risk for stroke than those without aura Women with a history of migraine who use CHC are about 2–4 times as likely to have an ischaemic stroke as nonusers
• Migraine without aura	Cu-IUD, CD	POP, DMPA, IMP, LNG-IUD. CHC may be initiated in a never user but should be advised to stop if migraine develops while patient is on CHC		
• Migraine with aura	Cu-IUD, CD	POP, DMPA, IMP,LNG-IUD	CHC	

(*Continued*)

(Continued)

Medical Condition	**Best Choice** *UK Category 1* No restriction for the use	**Alternative** *UK Category 2* Advantages generally outweigh the theoretical or proven risks	**Not Recommended** *UK Category 3* Theoretical or proven risks generally outweigh the advantages. Not recommended unless other more appropriate methods not available or acceptable *UK Category 4* Unacceptable risks	Additional Information
Epilepsy Anti-epileptic medications are associated with an increased risk of congenital malformations (foetal hydantoin syndrome, congenital cardiac and limb defects, cleft lip/ palate and neural tube defects) Hence effective contraception is important to prevent unplanned pregnancies	All contraceptive methods can be used in epileptic patients with no restrictions *First line choice*: • Cu-IUCD (metabolic neutrality, lack of drug interaction and high efficacy)			• The anti-epileptic medications (phenytoin, primidone, carbamazepine and phenobarbitone) act to induce the hepatic microsomal oxidase system which accelerates the metabolism of drugs including CHC and progesterone only pill • DMPA is not affected by enzyme inducers and no change in dosage needed • Does not seem to interfere with the contraceptive effectiveness of the LNG-IUD

(Continued)

(*Continued*)

Medical Condition	**Best Choice** *UK Category 1* No restriction for the use	**Alternative** *UK Category 2* Advantages generally outweigh the theoretical or proven risks	**Not Recommended** *UK Category 3* Theoretical or proven risks generally outweigh the advantages. Not recommended unless other more appropriate methods not available or acceptable *UK Category 4* Unacceptable risks	**Additional Information**
Epilepsy (continued)	• An increased risk of failure for CHC and POP users if an enzyme inducing epileptic is taken • Advise to use a CHC with higher oestrogen dosage (50 mcg) or double dosage of CHC with a lower oestrogen content (30 mcg) Double the normal dose of POP			

(*Continued*)

(Continued)

Medical Condition	**Best Choice** *UK Category 1* No restriction for the use	**Alternative** *UK Category 2* Advantages generally outweigh the theoretical or proven risks	**Not Recommended** *UK Category 3* Theoretical or proven risks generally outweigh the advantages. Not recommended unless other more appropriate methods not available or acceptable *UK Category 4* Unacceptable risks	**Additional Information**
Gall bladder disease	Cu-IUD, CD	POP, DMPA, IMP, LNG-IUD. CHC may be used in asymptomatic or previously treated by cholecystectomy	CHC not recommended in current symptomatic or medically treated gall bladder disease	CHC might cause a small increased risk for gallbladder disease and might worsen existing gallbladder disease
History of cholestasis • Pregnancy related	POP, DMPA,IMP, CU-IUD, LNG-IUD, CD	CHC		History of pregnancy-related cholestasis might predict an increased risk for COC-related cholestasis
• Past CHC related	CU-IUD, CD	POP, DMPA, IMP, LNG-IUD	CHC	

(Continued)

(Continued)

Medical Condition	Best Choice *UK Category 1* No restriction for the use	Alternative *UK Category 2* Advantages generally outweigh the theoretical or proven risks	Not Recommended *UK Category 3* Theoretical or proven risks generally outweigh the advantages. Not recommended unless other more appropriate methods not available or acceptable *UK Category 4* Unacceptable risks	Additional Information
Viral hepatitis	POP, DMPA, IMP, Cu-IUD, LNG-IUD, CD		Initiation of CHC is contraindicated in acute hepatitis/flares. However, may be safely used in carrier/chronic hepatitis	• COC use does not increase the rate or severity of cirrhotic fibrosis, nor does it increase the risk for hepatocellular carcinoma in chronic hepatitis • For women who are carriers, COC use does not appear to trigger liver failure or severe dysfunction
Cirrhosis • Mild (compensated without complications)	All methods can be used			
• Severe (decompensated)	Cu-IUD, CD		CHC, POP, DMPA, IMP, Cu-IUD, LNG-IUD	

(Continued)

(*Continued*)

Medical Condition	**Best Choice** *UK Category 1* No restriction for the use	**Alternative** *UK Category 2* Advantages generally outweigh the theoretical or proven risks	**Not Recommended** *UK Category 3* Theoretical or proven risks generally outweigh the advantages. Not recommended unless other more appropriate methods not available or acceptable *UK Category 4* Unacceptable risks	**Additional Information**
Liver tumours	• CU-IUD is the method of choice • CD	CHC, POP, DMPA, IMP, LNG-IUD may be used in focal nodular hyperplasia (no influence on either progression or regression)	CHC, POP, DMPA, IMP, LNG-IUD not advised in hepatocellular adenoma or malignant liver tumours	COC use in healthy women is associated with development and growth of hepatocellular adenoma; whether other hormonal contraceptives have similar effects is not known
Inflammatory bowel disease (IBD)	DMPA, IMP, Cu-IUD, LNG-IUD, CD	CHC, POP		Absorption among women with IBD may be reduced if the woman has substantial malabsorption caused by severe disease or small bowel surgery

(*Continued*)

(*Continued*)

Medical Condition	**Best Choice** *UK Category 1* No restriction for the use	**Alternative** *UK Category 2* Advantages generally outweigh the theoretical or proven risks	**Not Recommended** *UK Category 3* Theoretical or proven risks generally outweigh the advantages. Not recommended unless other more appropriate methods not available or acceptable *UK Category 4* Unacceptable risks	**Additional Information**
Systemic lupus erythromatosus (SLE) Patients with SLE are at an increased risk for IHD, stroke, VTE	Cu-IUD, CD are the only methods in patients *with* positive anti-phospholipid antibodies	CHC, POP, DMPA, IMP, LNG-IUD may be used in other patients *without* anti-phospholipid antibodies		Antiphospholipid antibodies are associated with a higher risk for both arterial and venous thrombosis
Thyroid disease	All methods may be used			

(*Continued*)

(Continued)

Medical Condition	**Best Choice** *UK Category 1* No restriction for the use	**Alternative** *UK Category 2* Advantages generally outweigh the theoretical or proven risks	**Not Recommended** *UK Category 3* Theoretical or proven risks generally outweigh the advantages. Not recommended unless other more appropriate methods not available or acceptable *UK Category 4* Unacceptable risks	**Additional Information**
HIV /AIDS				
Condom use has been shown to be highly effective in prevention of HIV infection in heterosexual couples in which one partner is infected. It also reduces transmission of other sexually transmitted infections which increase the risk for HIV seroconversion	CD + CHC, POP, DMPA, IMP	Cu-IUD and LNG-IUD	Repeated and high-dose use of the spermicide nonoxynol-9 was associated with increased risk for genital lesions, which might increase the risk of HIV infection	Hormonal contraception does not interfere with antiviral drug effectiveness The efficacy of oral contraceptives is not affected by administration of non-ritonavir boosted atazanavir or indinavir Depot medroxyprogestereone acetate may be safe to administer with efavirenz, nevirapine and nelfinavir

(Continued)

(Continued)

Medical Condition	**Best Choice** *UK Category 1* No restriction for the use	**Alternative** *UK Category 2* Advantages generally outweigh the theoretical or proven risks	**Not Recommended** *UK Category 3* Theoretical or proven risks generally outweigh the advantages. Not recommended unless other more appropriate methods not available or acceptable *UK Category 4* Unacceptable risks	**Additional Information**
Gestational trophoblastic disease	• All methods may be used with decreasing or undetectable levels of β-HCG. • CD are advised in patients with persistently elevated β -HCG levels but CHC, POP,DMPA, IMP may also be used		Cu-IUD and LNG-IUD are *contraindicated* in persistently elevated β-HCG levels or malignant disease	• After molar pregnancy evacuation, the balance of evidence found COC use *did not increase* the risk for postmolar trophoblastic disease. • Use of COCs during chemotherapy *does not* significantly affect the regression or treatment of postmolar trophoblastic disease compared with women who used a nonhormonal contraceptive method or DMPA

(Continued)

(*Continued*)

Medical Condition	**Best Choice** *UK Category 1* No restriction for the use	**Alternative** *UK Category 2* Advantages generally outweigh the theoretical or proven risks	**Not Recommended** *UK Category 3* Theoretical or proven risks generally outweigh the advantages. Not recommended unless other more appropriate methods not available or acceptable *UK Category 4* Unacceptable risks	**Additional Information**
Anatomical abnormalities/ uterine fibroids that distort the endometrial cavity	CHC, POP, DMPA, IMP, CD		Cu-IUD and LNG-IUD are contraindicated in patients with distorted uterine cavity incompatible with IUD insertion	
Breast disease	• All methods can be used in patients with benign breast disease or family history of cancer • Cu-IUD, CD are the only methods for patients with a current or past history of breast cancer	POP, DMPA, IMP, LNG-IUD are category 2 for an undiagnosed breast lump and carriers of known gene mutations, e.g. BRCA 1	CHC is contraindicated in patients who have breast cancer, are gene mutation carriers or have an undiagnosed lump	Breast cancer is a hormonally sensitive tumour, and the prognosis for women with current or recent breast cancer may worsen with hormonal contraceptive use

Combined Hormonal Contraception (CHC) is *not* recommended in:

1. Smokers aged ≥35 years
2. BMI ≥35 kg/m^2
3. Breast feeding patients <6 months postnatal
4. Non breastfeeding <21 days postpartum
5. Pregnancy not excluded
6. Patients with current or previous history of IHD or stroke
7. Hypertension
8. Hyperlipidaemia
9. Diabetic patients with underlying renal or vascular disease
10. Known thrombogenic mutations, personal or family history of VTE
11. Undergoing major surgery or having prolonged immobilisation
12. Complicated valvular and congenital heart disease
13. Migraine with aura
14. Current symptomatic or medically treated gall bladder disease
15. Past history of CHC related cholestasis
16. Active viral hepatitis or severe/decompensated cirrhosis, hepatocellular adenoma or liver cancer
17. Current or previous history of breast cancer, gene mutation carriers or have an undiagnosed breast lump
18. Women trekking to altitudes of >4500 m for >1 week may be advised to consider switching to an alternative method

Contraceptive Advice for Women Using Enzyme-inducing Drugs

Contraceptive Method	Short-term Use of Enzyme-inducing Drugs (<2 months)	Long-term Use of Enzyme-inducing Drugs (>2 months) or Difficulty Using Additional Contraceptive Precautions
Combined hormonal contraception (CHC) (a) Combined oral contraception (COC) (b) Combined transdermal patch (c) Combined vaginal ring	**Recommended option** Change to an alternative method unaffected by enzyme-inducing drugs. This could include temporarily stopping COC and having a one-off DMPA injection to cover the short-term treatment and 28 days after	Change to an alternative method unaffected by enzyme-inducing drugs
	Alternative options Use one COC pill daily (at least 30 µg EE), one patch weekly or one ring 3-weekly and use an extended or tricycling regimen with a hormone free interval of 4 days **Plus** Additional contraceptive precautions (e.g. condoms) while taking and for 28 days after stopping the enzyme-inducing drug **Or** Use two COC pills as per long-term treatment (see opposite). Not recommended if using the potent enzyme-inducers rifampicin or rifabutin	Use two COC pills containing at least 50 µg ethinyloestradiol (e.g. 20 and 30 µg COCs). Use an extended or tricycling regimen with a pill-free interval of 4 days **Note:** Not recommended if using the potent enzyme-inducers rifampicin or rifabutin

(Continued)

(*Continued*)

Contraceptive Method	Short-term Use of Enzyme-inducing Drugs (<2 months)	Long-term Use of Enzyme-inducing Drugs (>2 months) or Difficulty Using Additional Contraceptive Precautions
Progestogen-only contraception Progestogen-only pills (POPs) and progestogen-only implant	**Recommended option** Change to an alternative method unaffected by enzyme-inducing drugs (including one dose of progestogen-only injectable to cover the period of risk)	Change to an alternative method unaffected by enzyme-inducing drugs
	Alternative option Continue use of POP or implant Plus Additional contraceptive precautions (e.g. condoms) while taking and for 28 days after stopping the enzyme-inducing drug	No alternative—change advised
Progestogen-only injectable Levonorgestrel-releasing intrauterine system (LNG-IUS)	**No change required** Efficacy of DMPA and LNG-IUS unaffected by enzyme-inducing drugs and women can continue with the usual dose and dosing/replacement interval of 12 weeks or 5 years, respectively	

(*Continued*)

(Continued)

Contraceptive Method	Short-term Use of Enzyme-inducing Drugs (<2 months)	Long-term Use of Enzyme-inducing Drugs (>2 months) or Difficulty Using Additional Contraceptive Precautions
Non-hormonal methods Cu-IUD, barrier methods	**No change required** Efficacy unaffected	
Emergency contraception Cu-IUD Progestogen only emergency contraception (POEC)	Efficacy unaffected. Unless contraindicated, offer to all women (between 0–120 hours of unprotected sexual intercourse (UPSI) or within 5 days of expected ovulation) taking or within 28 days of stopping enzyme-inducing drugs	

Drugs that increase Contraceptive Hormone Levels

Drug Type	Drug	Interaction	Clinical Significance
Antibacterial	Erythromycin	Enzyme inhibitor	Modest to marked increases in oestradiol and dienogest levels. The clinical significance is not known but increased adverse events may be anticipated
Antifungal	Fluconazole Itraconazole Ketoconazole	Enzyme inhibitor	Modest increases in EE and progestogen. Breakthrough bleeding noted in studies. Evidence in relation to fluconazole has been broadly reassuring in relation to contraceptive efficacy
Antiretroviral	Atazanavir (unboosted)	Enzyme inhibitor	Modest to marked increases in EE when atazanavir is used unboosted. Concomitant use of combined methods not advised. Note when atazanavir is boosted with ritonavir the net effect is a reduction in EE levels

(*Continued*)

(*Continued*)

Drug Type	Drug	Interaction	Clinical Significance
Immuno-suppressant	Tacrolimus	Enzyme inhibitor	Theoretically inhibits the metabolism of oestrogens and progestogens leading to increased levels. The clinical significance is not known but the increase is likely to be small
Non-steroidal anti-inflammatory	Etoricoxib	Enzyme inhibitor	Doses of etoricoxib >60 mg raise ethinyloestradiol levels by approximately 40% or more. Potential risk of oestrogen-related adverse events
Statins	Atorvastatin Rosuvastatin	Enzyme inhibitor	Minor to modest increase in ethinyloestradiol and progestogens leading to increased levels. The clinical significance is not known but likely to be small

Drugs that are affected by Contraceptive Hormones

Drug Type	Clinical Effect
Antiepileptics	Ethinyloestradiol reduces plasma concentrations of lamotrigine. Possible increased risk of seizures. Consider increasing dose of lamotrigine monotherapy. To avoid toxicity in pill-free week, consider extended regimen. Ethinyloestradiol may also modestly reduce valproate levels
Antihypertensives	Hypotensive effect may be antagonised by combined hormonal contraception. Monitor effect
Antidiabetics	Oestrogens and progestogens antagonise the hypoglycaemic effect of antidiabetics. Monitor effect
Diuretics	Oestrogens may antagonise diuretic effect.
Thyroid hormones	Oestrogens may increase the requirements for thyroid hormones in hypothyroidism. Monitor thyroid function
Bronchodilators	Oestrogens reduce the excretion of theophylline resulting in increased plasma concentrations. A reduction of the theophylline dosage is recommended

(Continued)

(Continued)

Drug Type	Clinical Effect
Dopaminergics	Oestrogens increase plasma concentrations of ropinirole. Defined by the British National Formulary (BNF) as non-hazardous (i.e. does not usually have serious complications) Oestrogens and progestogens increase plasma concentrations of selegiline. Increased risk of toxicity. Concomitant use should be avoided
Immuno-suppressants	Plasma levels of tacrolimus possibly increased by ethinyloestradiol and gestodene. Monitor tacrolimus levels Cyclosporin levels possibly increased by oestrogens and progestogens (interaction unconfirmed and of uncertain clinical significance)
Muscle relaxants	Oestrogens and progestogens possibly increase plasma concentration of tizanidine potentially leading to toxicity
Potassium-sparing diuretics and aldosterone antagonists	Theoretical risk of hyperkalaemia when administered with drospirenone but COCs containing drospirenone not usually used in hypertensive patients
Retinoids	The adverse effects of oral contraceptives on lipids may be additive with those of isotretinoin. As retinoids are teratogenic, the benefits of COC use may outweigh risk and lipids should be monitored routinely during retinoid treatment

(Continued)

(*Continued*)

Drug Type	Clinical Effect
Triptans	COCs appear to modestly raise the level of frovatriptan, naratriptan, zolmitriptan and slightly increase the levels of sumatriptan. Before prescribing triptans in CHC users with migraine, health professionals should refer to UKMEC as CHC may be contraindicated in some women with a history of migraine

Chapter 60

INTRAUTERINE CONTRACEPTIVE DEVICE (IUCD) AND ASSOCIATED DILEMMAS

Missing IUCD Threads

Threads/Strings not visible — if the IUCD strings are not visible on speculum examination, the possibilities from most to least common are:

- The IUCD is *in situ*, but the strings are curled and retracted into the endocervical canal or uterine cavity, or they are broken. Uterine enlargement secondary to fibroids or pregnancy, or rotation of the IUCD can also cause retraction of strings;

- The IUCD has been expelled;
- The IUCD has perforated the uterus and is in the myometrium or abdomen.

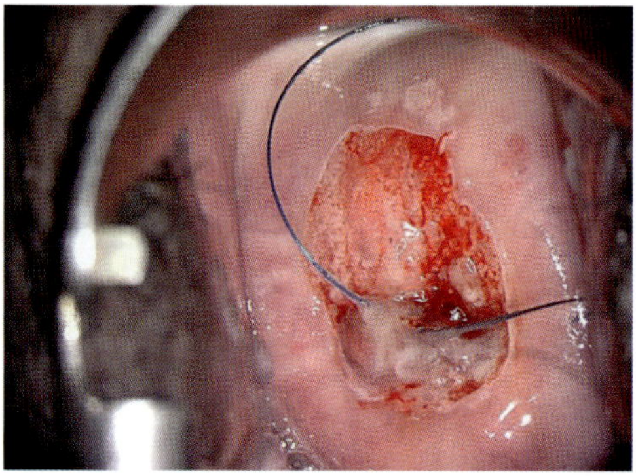

Figure 1. Ectropion with IUCD thread in situ.

Management of Missing IUCD (Intrauterine Contraceptive Device)

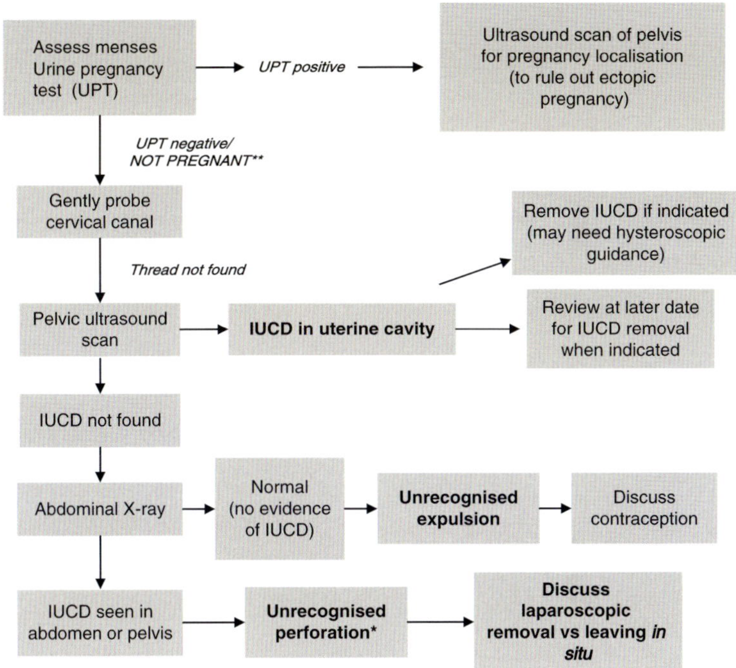

* Perforation

Although serious complications following perforation are rare, any perforated IUCD should be removed unless the surgical risk is excessive. The major concerns of nonintervention are adhesion formation and perforation into bowel, bladder or blood vessels.

If the IUCD is in the abdomen or perforating through the myometrium, operative laparoscopy is the preferred method of removal. It can be performed electively in asymptomatic patients, and is usually successful. If laparoscopy is unsuccessful due to extensive adhesions, the procedure should be converted to a laparotomy.

If the IUCD is embedded in the myometrium, operative hysteroscopy may be required for removal. An intraoperative X-ray can help localise the IUCD.

For patients whose IUCDs have perforated and recovered, another IUCD may be offered in future.

Pregnancy with IUCD

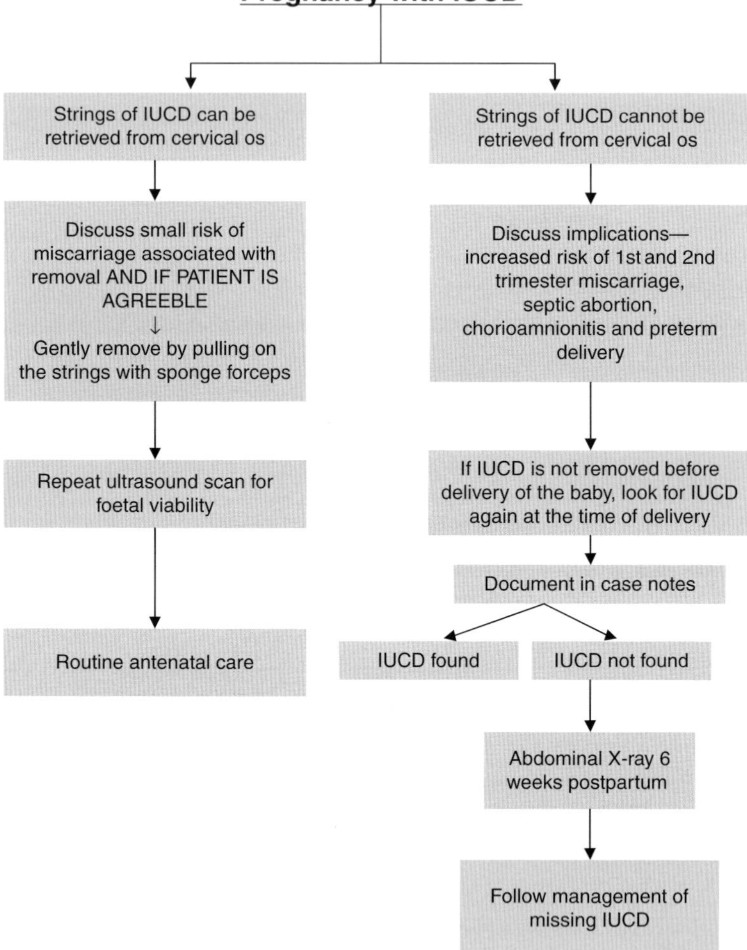

Other IUCD dilemmas

1. *Malpositioned IUCD*

An IUCD that is >20 mm from the fundus in a normal uterus. IUCDs in *symptomatic* women should be removed. In *asymptomatic* women who wish to continue IUCD use, the IUCD may be left in place if it is located *above the internal os* and if the woman would not replace it or choose another highly effective method of contraception. Suggest removal of malpositioned *IUCDs located below the level of the internal os*. In women with a history of expulsion, perforation or malposition of a previous IUCD, the next IUCD should be placed under ultrasound guidance.

2. *Pain with IUCD*

If a woman with a longstanding IUCD develops new severe cramping pain or abdominal tenderness, she should be evaluated for pelvic inflammatory disease (PID), ectopic pregnancy, miscarriage, IUCD expulsion or perforation.

Mild and moderate dysmenorrhoea can often be controlled with nonsteroidal anti-inflammatory drugs (NSAIDs).

3. *Abnormal uterine bleeding (AUB) and IUCD*

Possible causes of new onset abnormal bleeding in women after prolonged use of IUCDs include displacement of the device, pregnancy (intrauterine or ectopic), infection as well as gynaecological disorders of the cervix or uterus (e.g. leiomyomas, polyps, endometrial cancer). In women over age 40 or with risk factors for endometrial cancer who develop abnormal bleeding, the endometrium should be evaluated. Any LNG IUD user presenting with new onset of amenorrhoea should have a pregnancy test.

4. *Pelvic inflammatory disease (PID) and IUCD*

a) Symptomatic PID — administer appropriate antibiotics followed by removal of IUCD and prescribe alternative contraception.
b) Asymptomatic PID (laboratory evidence of Gonorrhoea or Chlamydia) — administer standard antibiotic treatment without IUCD removal. Assess appropriateness for continued IUCD use.
c) Asymptomatic + Actinomyces — No treatment is required.

Chapter 61

EMERGENCY CONTRACEPTION

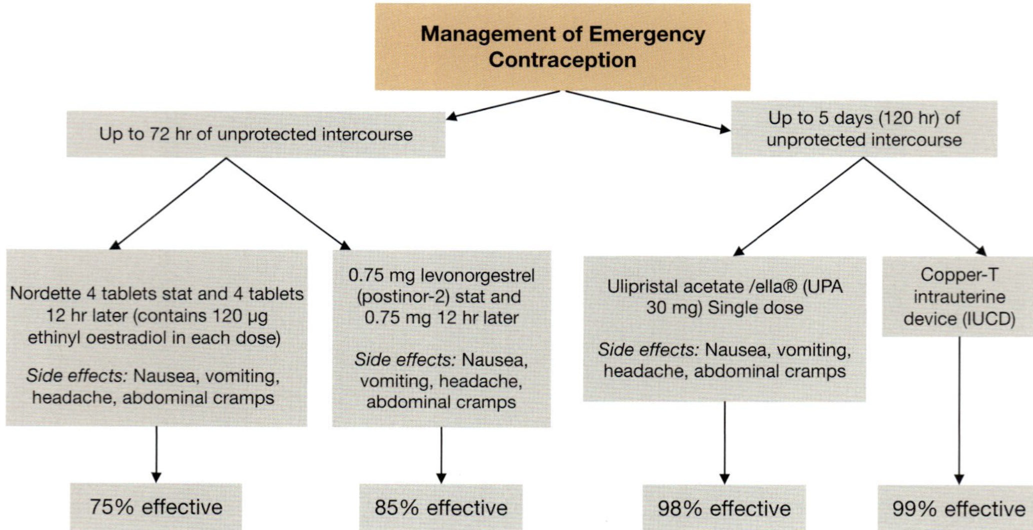

Note
- Compared to levonorgestrel, ulipristal acetate (ella®) almost halves the risk of pregnancy among women using it within 120 hours of sexual intercourse

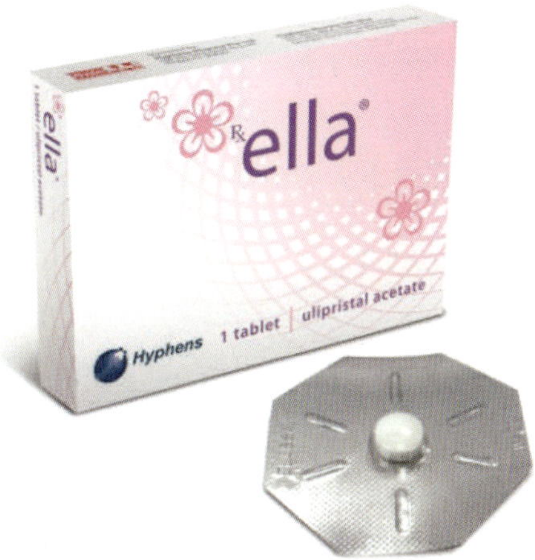

Figure 1. Ulipristal acetate (UPA).

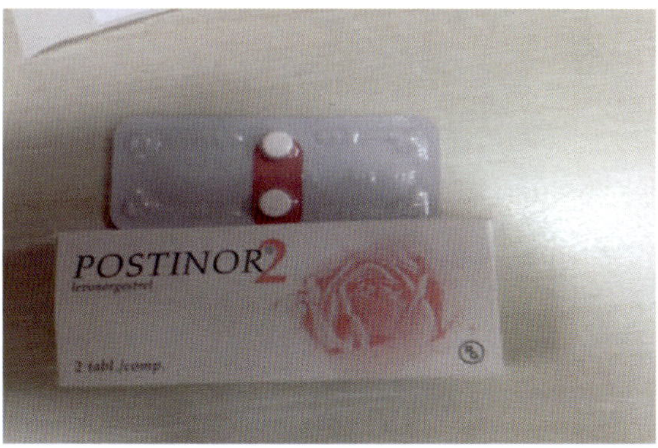

Figure 2. Postinor 2.

Chapter 62

MENOPAUSE

Definition

- Clinical retrospective diagnosis: 12 months of amenorrhoea after the final menstrual period

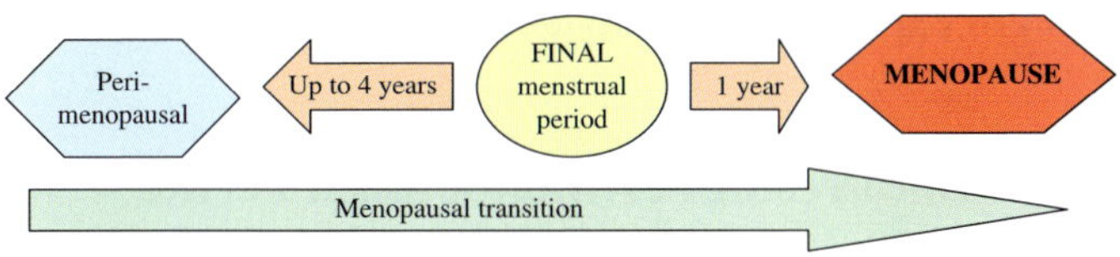

- Women have a finite number of ovarian oocytes, which undergo atresia with time with ovarian function decline
- Average age of menopause: 51 years
- Menopause before age 40: premature ovarian failure (POF)
- Menopause transition (perimenopausal period) may last for up to four years
- Surgical menopause may be induced if bilateral oophorectomy is performed before natural menopause sets in

Factors Affecting Age of Menopause

- Familial: family history of early menopause increases risk for earlier menopause
- Smoking: reduces age of menopause by average of 2 years
- Iatrogenic:
  - History of chemotherapy or radiotherapy
    - Surgery: bilateral salpingo-oophorectomy
- Autoimmune: history of type 1 diabetes mellitus, thyroid disease
- Genetics: history of chromosomal abnormalities, e.g. Turner syndrome
- *In utero* exposure to diethylstilbestrol (DES)

Clinical Features in Perimenopausal Period

- Irregular periods

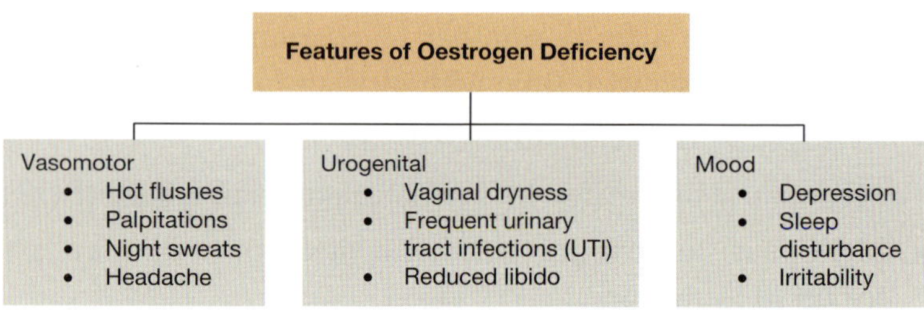

Menopausal Transition

- Stages of menopausal transition can be defined using the STRAW staging system (**ST**ages of **R**eproductive **A**geing **W**orkshop, 2001)

The Stages of Reproductive Ageing Workshop +10 staging system for reproductive ageing in women

Menarche (stage -5) FMP (0) (stage +1a)

Stage	-5	-4	-3b	-3a	-2	-1	+1a	+1b	+1c	+2
Terminology	**REPRODUCTIVE**				**MENOPAUSAL TRANSITION**		**POSTMENOPAUSE**			
	Early	Peak	Late		Early	Late	Early			Late
					Perimenopause					
Duration	*Variable*				*Variable*	1-3 years	2 years (1+1)		3-6 years	*Remaining lifespan*
PRINCIPAL CRITERIA										
Menstrual cycle	Variable to regular	Regular	Regular	Subtle changes in flow/ strength	*Variable length:* Persistent ≥7-day difference in length of consecutive cycles	Interval of amenorrhea of >=60 days				
SUPPORTIVE CRITERIA										
Endocrine FSH AMH Inhibin B			Low Low	Variable* Low Low	$\uparrow$ Variable* Low Low	$\uparrow$ >25 IU/L• Low Low	$\uparrow$ Variable Low Low		Stabilizes Very low Very low	
Antral follicle count			Low	Low	Low	**Low**	Very low		Very low	
DESCRIPTIVE CHARACTERISTICS										
Symptoms						Vasomotor symptoms *Likely*	Vasomotor symptoms *Most likely*			*Increasing* symptoms of urogenital atrophy

Arrow: elevated.
* Blood draw on cycle days 2-5.
• Approximate expected level based on assays using current international pituitary standard.
Reproduced with permission from: Harlow SD, Gass M, Hall JE, et al. Executive Summary of the Stages of Reproductive Aging Workshop + 10: Addressing the Unfinished Agenda of Staging Reproductive Aging. J Clin Endocrinol Metab 2012. Copyright © 2012 The Endocrine Society.

Long-term Implications

- Osteoporosis
- Cardiovascular disease
- Dementia

Assessment of Menopause

- **History**
    - **Clinical diagnosis: 12 months of amenorrhoea**
    - Perimenopausal symptoms (as described above)
- **Examination**
    - Vaginal and labial atrophy
- **Investigations**
    - Not diagnostic
        - Elevated FSH > 30 IU/L suggests menopause

Management of Menopause

- Dependent on patient's preference and severity of symptoms
- **Non-hormonal:**
    - Evening primrose oil
    - Cimicifugae extract (black cohosh), e.g. Remifemin — also found in Dang Quai (traditional Chinese Medicine)
    - Isoflavone: phytoestrogens

- **Hormone replacement therapy**
  - Effective for symptomatic relief, especially when symptoms adversely affect quality of life
  - The lowest effective dose should be used for the shortest period necessary
  - Review at 3–6 months

Chapter 63

OSTEOPOROSIS

Definition

- Progressive systemic skeletal disease characterised by:
  - Low bone mass
  - Micro-architectural deterioration of bone tissue
  - With consequent increase in bone fragility and susceptibility to fractures

WHO Classification of Bone Mineral Density (BMD)	
Normal	T score ≥−1.0
Osteopenia	T score between −1.0 and −2.5
Osteoporosis	T score ≤−2.5

Risk Factors for Fractures

- Age
- BMI ≤20
- Genetics: history of osteoporotic fracture in a first degree relative
- Personal history of fragility fractures after age of 40
- Immobility
- Smoker
- Alcohol use of >2 units a day
- Excessive caffeine intake >4 cups of coffee a day
- Premature menopause before age of 40
- Malnutrition with poor calcium intake of <500 mg of elemental calcium a day

- Chronic disease
  - Primary hyperparathyroidism
  - Malabsorption syndromes, e.g. Coeliac disease
  - Rheumatoid arthritis

- Long-term medications causing osteoporosis
  - Systemic steroids, e.g. prednisolone >5 mg for >3 months
  - GnRH analogues
  - Anticonvulsant therapy

  - Aromatase inhibitors
  - Omeprazole
  - Long-term heparin use

Screening Assessment Tools

- FRAX WHO Fracture Risk Assessment Tool
  - Computes the 10-year probability of hip fracture or a major osteoporotic fracture
  - A *major* osteoporotic fracture is a clinical spine, hip, forearm or humerus fracture

- OSTA (Osteoporosis Self-Assessment Tool for Asians)
  - Calculated by using age — weight
  - If low risk, no need BMD
  - If medium risk, measure BMD if risk factors present
  - If high risk, measure BMD

OSTA CHART

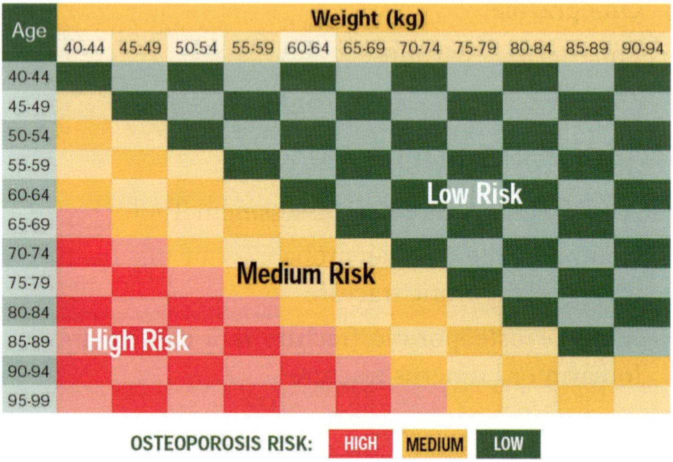

*Koh LKH *et al*. A simple Tool to Identify Asian Women at Increased Risk of *Osteoporosis Int* (2001) **12**: 699–705.

OSTA CHART

When to do BMD for a Woman?

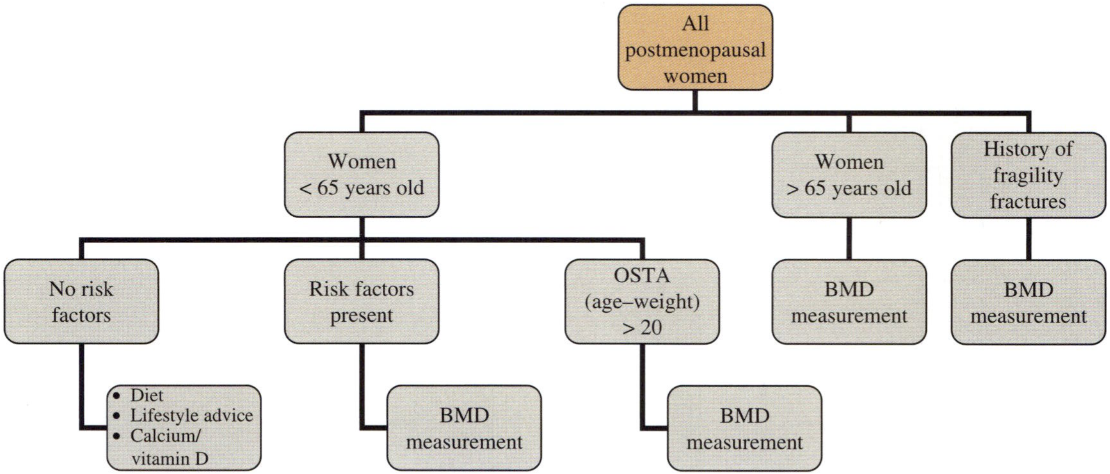

BMD Measurement

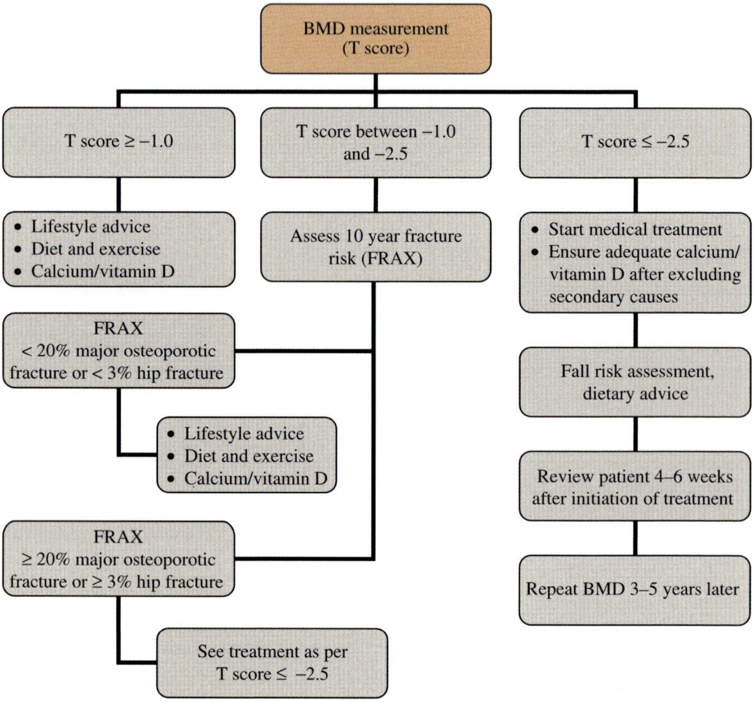

When to Repeat BMD

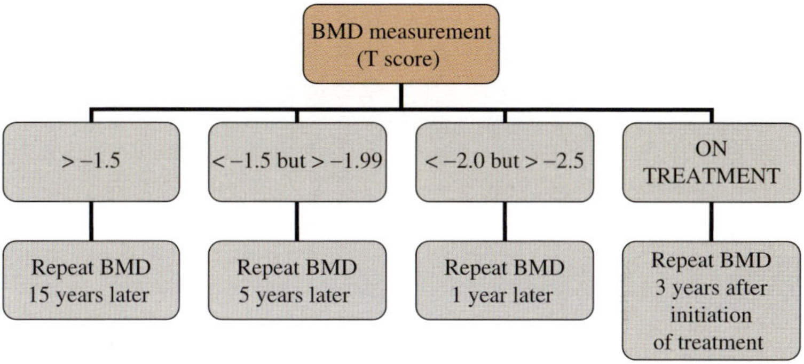

Management of Osteoporosis

- Lifestyle modifications
  - Stop smoking, alcohol and caffeine use
  - Fall prevention and home assessment
  - Adequate nutrition
  - Encourage weight-bearing exercises such as walking, dancing, low impact aerobics, stair climbing, free weights resistance bands push-ups
- Pharmacotherapy (see table below)
  - Calcium and vitamin D: recommended daily intake of Vit D_3 is 800–1200 IU per day
  - Bisphosphonates
  - Strontium ranelate
  - Raloxifene (SERM)
  - Tibolone
  - Denosumab

Medications used for Osteoporosis

Drug Type	Trade Name	Dosing	Vertebral	Hip	Caution
Bisphosphonates	Aledronate® (FOSOMAX)	Oral 70 mg weekly with Vit D3 5600 IU	Yes	Yes	*Osteonecrosis of the jaw* — most commonly with zoledronate (incidence 1.3–7%) — rare with oral preparations (1 in 100 000 patient years)
	Risedronate® (ACTONEL)	Oral 35 mg weekly or 150 mg monthly	Yes	Yes	
	Zolendronate (ACLASTA®)	IV infusion 5 mg over 15 minutes once a year	Yes	Yes	Infusion related reactions — include fever, myalgia, flu like symptoms Check for renal impairment before initiation
Strontium Ranelate	Protos®* (STRONTIUM)	Oral 2 mg daily	Yes	Yes	Risk of *DRESS (Drug Rash, Eosinophilia and Systemic Symptoms), SJS (Steven Johnson syndrome) and TENS (Toxic Epidermal Necrolysis)* — highest risk of occurrence is within the first 8 weeks of treatment with poorer prognosis in the elderly — increased risk reported in local population

*European Medicine Agency contraindicates its use in osteoporosis due to recent association of Protos® with an increased risk of non-fatal myocardial infarction.

(*Continued*)

Medications used for Osteoporosis *(Continued)*

Drug Type	Trade Name	Dosing	Vertebral	Hip	Caution
Selective oestrogen Receptor Modulator (SERM)	Raloxifene® (EVISTA)	Oral 60 mg daily	Yes	No	Vasomotor symptoms and leg cramps are common Risk of VTE Rare risk of fatal stroke in RUTH trial
Hormone use	Tibolone® (LIVIAL)	Oral 2.5 mg ON	Yes	No	Risk of cardiovascular events Risk of stroke
Human Monoclonal Antibody	Denosumab (PROLIA®)	Subcutaneous injection 60 mg twice a year	Yes	Yes	Better compliance for patients with creatinine clearance < 35 mL/min (renal impairment) Requires calcium 1000 mg daily and at least 400 IU vitamin D Correct for hypocalcaemia before initiation

Chapter 64

HORMONE REPLACEMENT THERAPY (HRT)

> "Short term hormone replacement therapy is acceptable and relatively safe for healthy, symptomatic, recently postmenopausal women."
>
> Women's Health Initiative (WHI)
> July 2012

WHO to Give?

- Symptomatic relief of menopausal symptoms which adversely affect the quality of life
- Women with premature menopause for treating menopausal symptoms and preventing osteoporosis till 50 years old
- Addback therapy when gonadotrophin-releasing hormone agonists are used
- Women who had early surgical menopause (bilateral oophorectomy)

How to Give?

- The **lowest effective dose** should be used for the **shortest period necessary**
- **Individualised treatment tailored to needs**
- Reappraise annually
- Short duration of up to 5 years usually

— If **absent** uterus, use oestrogen only
  - Except in patients with history of endometriosis as oestrogens alone may induce a recurrence of the disease

— If **intact** uterus, use oestrogen and progesterone
  - Progesterone is needed to prevent endometrial hyperplasia and malignancy

Benefits of HRT?

- Symptomatic relief
- Prevention of osteoporosis

Risks of HRT?

- Venous thromboembolism (VTE)
- Breast cancer
- Stroke
- Myocardial infarction
- Gall bladder disease

Contraindications of HRT:

- History of breast cancer
- History of coronary heart disease
- Previous venous thromboembolic event
- Previous stroke
- Active liver disease

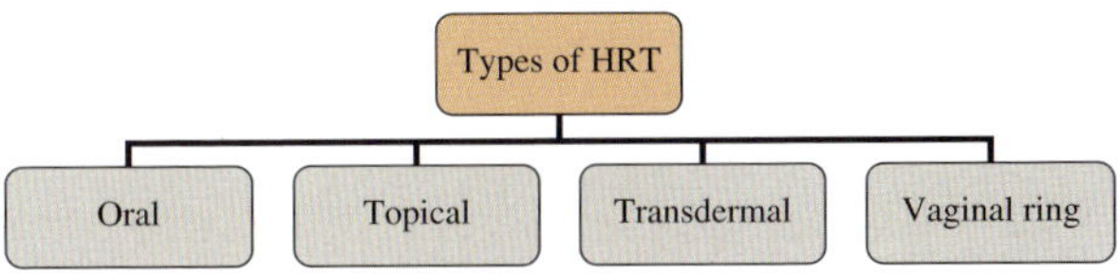

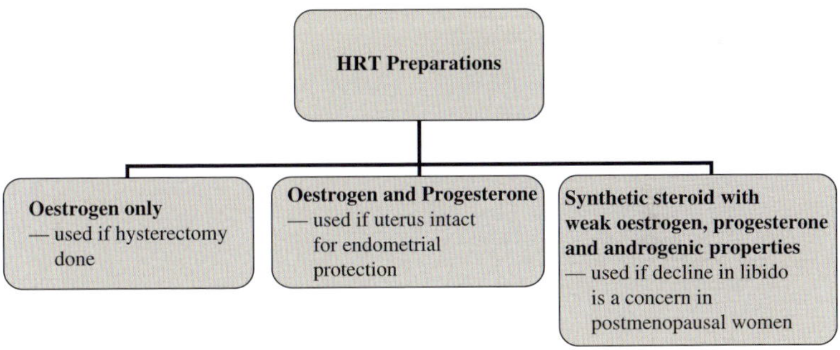

Selective Oestrogen Receptor Modulators (SERMs)

- Competitive inhibitors of oestrogen binding receptors
  - E.g. tamoxifen, raloxifene (Evista®)
- SERMs protects against:
  - Menopausal related bone loss

    - Breast cancer (especially tamoxifen)
    - High total cholesterol concentrations
- Uses: prevention and treatment of osteoporosis
- Side effects: can worsen hot flushes

Oral preparation of HRT

Drug Type	Trade Name	Active Ingredient	Dose	Comments
Oestrogen only — no uterus	Estrofem®	17β-oestradiol	1 mg or 2 mg daily (28 days)	To be taken daily. In women with intact uterus, add progestogen 12–14 days each cycle
Oestrogen only	Premarin®	0.625 mg conjugated oestrogen	Continuous	Hormone replacement therapy for oestrogen deficiency symptoms in postmenopausal women
Oestrogen only	Progynova®	Oestradiol valerate	2 mg daily May be reduced to 2 mg every other day or 1 mg daily	Should be taken daily. In women with intact uterus, add progestogen 12–14 days each cycle
Oestrogen and Progesterone — intact uterus	Activelle®	Oestradiol Norethisterone acetate	Oestradiol 1mg Norethisterone 0.5 mg	Used only in postmenopausal women. Useful for prevention of osteoporosis if high risk of future fractures and intolerant of other medicinal products. (Approved for prevention of osteoporosis)

(*Continued*)

Oral preparation of HRT *(Continued)*

Drug Type	Trade Name	Active Ingredient	Dose	Comments
Oestrogen and Progesterone	Femoston®	17β-oestradiol Dydrogesterone	1 tablet daily orally Femoston 1/10 tablets —14 tablets oestradiol 1 mg —14 tablets oestradiol 1 mg and dydrogesterone 10 mg	If patient is still menstruating; begin on 1st day of cycle
Oestrogen	Premarin®	0.625 mg conjugated oestrogen	May be continuous or cyclical One tablet daily; in women with intact uterus, add progestogen 12–14 days each cycle.	Hormone replacement therapy for oestrogen deficiency symptoms in postmenopausal women
Oestrogen and Progesterone	Progyluton®	Oestradiol valerate Norgestrel	Dose : 11 tablets of oestradiol 2 mg (white) and 10 tablets of oestradiol 2 mg and norgestrel 0.5 mg (brown)	Start on 5th day of cycle, 1 white tablet daily for the first 11 days, followed by 1 light brown tablet for 10 days (total 21 days), then stop for 7 days

(Continued)

Oral preparation of HRT (*Continued*)

Drug Type	Trade Name	Active Ingredient	Dose	Comments
Oestrogen and Progesterone	Trisequens®	Oestradiol Norethisterone acetate	• 12 blue tablets of oestradiol 2 mg • 10 white tablets of oestradiol 2 mg and norethisterone acetate 1mg and • 6 red tablets of oestradiol 1mg	Start with blue tablets. Take continuously for 28 days
Synthetic steroid	Livial®	Tibolone	One tablet daily (2.5 mg)	Can experience amenorrhoea or breakthrough bleeding and spotting
Local preparation of HRT				
Oestrogen	Divigel®	Oestradiol hemihydrate	One sachet daily (0.25 mg oestradiol)	Useful for climacteric symptoms, e.g. hot flushes and night sweats
Oestrogen	Estring® (Oestradiol vaginal ring)	Oestradiol	2 mg in one ring (lasts for 90 days)	Inserted to upper third of vaginal vault *Caution* : toxic shock syndrome cases have been reported

(*Continued*)

Local preparation of HRT *(Continued)*

Drug Type	Trade Name	Active Ingredient	Dose	Comments
Oestrogen	Oestrogel® (oestradiol 0.06% gel)	17β oestradiol	For cutaneous application only. Start with ½ ruler (1.25 g) and slowly increase to 1 ruler (2.5 g) daily Average dose is 1 ruler/day, for 24-28 days every month	Vaginal bleeding reminiscent of menstrual flow may occur during the period of treatment interruption
Oestrogen	Premarin® vaginal cream	Conjugated oestrogens	0.5–2 g daily, intravaginally or topically, depending on the severity of the condition. Administration should be cyclic (e.g, three weeks on and one week off)	Treatment of atrophic vaginitis

(Continued)

Local preparation of HRT *(Continued)*

Drug Type	Trade Name	Active Ingredient	Dose	Comments
Oestrogen	Vagifem® vaginal tablets	Oestradiol	*Initial*: 1 vaginal tablet (25 mcg) daily for 2 weeks *Maintenance*: 1 vaginal tablet twice a week	Treatment of atrophic vaginitis due to oestrogen deficiency
Transdermal Preparations of HRT				
Oestrogen	Estraderm® patch	Oestradiol	25 µg/day (One patch twice a week)	In women with an intact uterus, supplemented by sequential administration of a progestogen to be taken on the last 12 days of each 4-week treatment cycle

Chapter 65

SUBFERTILITY, SEMEN ANALYSIS AND MANAGEMENT OF AZOOSPERMIA

Definition

Subfertility is defined as the failure to conceive after one year of regular unprotected sexual intercourse in the absence of known reproductive pathology. It affects 10–15% of couples trying to conceive.

In all cases of infertility, the prognosis of a pregnancy is greatly influenced by:

1. Age of woman
2. Duration of infertility
3. Occurrence of a previous pregnancy

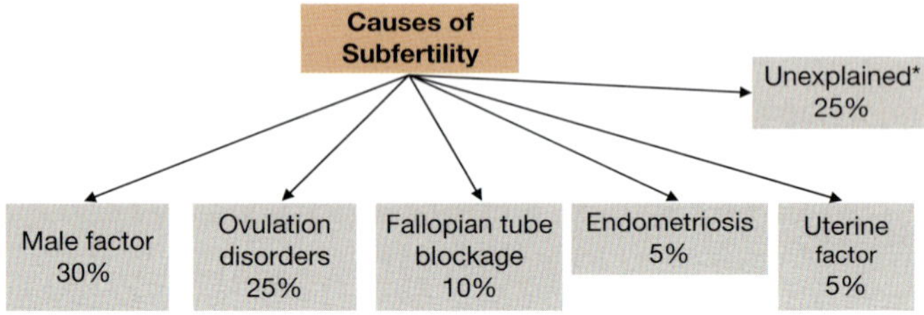

* Not identifying a cause for infertility does not necessarily mean that the couple is normal or has no cause.

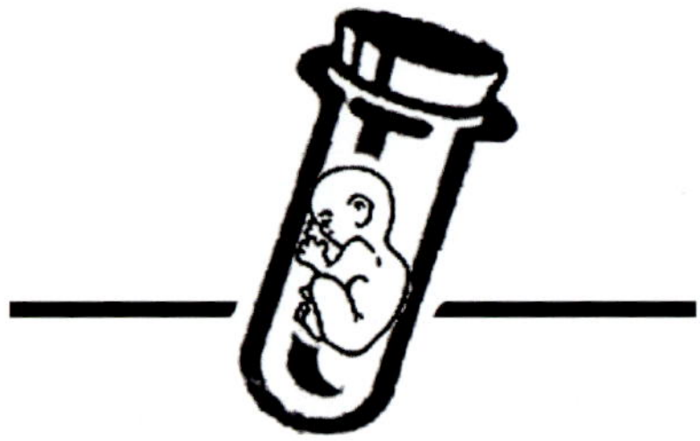

Management of Subfertility

General Advice

- Stop smoking or alcoholic binging
- Reduce weight if body mass index >30 kg/m^2
- Timed coitus (3 times/week)
- Pre-conceptional folic acid supplementation
- Screening for rubella +/– varicella immunity. Vaccinate if non-immune
- Pap smear
- Thalassaemia screen (MCV)

INVESTIGATIONS OF SUBFERTILITY

Male partner

- Look for hypospadias scrotal varices, genetic syndrome in male partner
- Seminal analysis for male partner

Female partner

If irregular menses (oligoamenorrhoea)

1. *Ultrasound of pelvis* looking for polycystic ovaries
2. *FSH/LH*
3. *Prolactin*
4. *Thyroid function test*
5. *Testosterone 17-hydroxyprogesterone* (only in the presence of clinical or biochemical evidence of hyperandrogenism)

Assess ovulation

- *Mid-luteal Progesterone* level: (taken 7 days before next expected period). Low level (<30 nmol/l) suggest ovulatory dysfunction

Pelvic assessment

- *Transvaginal ultrasound scan* (TVUS) to exclude pelvic pathology like fibroids or endometriotic cysts
- *Saline infusion sonohysterography* (SIS) may be used if history suggests presence of polyps, submucosal fibroid and synechiae

Tubal assessment:

- *Chlamydia antibody titre*
- *Hysterosalpingogram (HSG)* in the absence of co-morbidities such as pelvic inflammatory disease (PID), previous ectopic and endometriosis
- Laparoscopy and hydrotubation of fallopian tubes

Ovarian reserve

- *Day 2–3 FSH* (follicular stimulating hormone) level: if raised >10 IU/L suggests poor ovarian reserve
- *Antral follicle count* on pelvic ultrasound: < 6 follicles per ovary suggests lower ovarian reserve
- *Anti Mullerian hormone* (AMH): < 1 ng/mL suggests poor ovarian reserve

Preconception investigation:

1. PAP smear
2. Rubella immunity
3. Thalassaemia screen (MCV)
4. +/− Varicella immunity

Refer if

- Woman's age >35 years old
- Woman's age >30 and after trying for >1 year
- Woman's age <30 and after trying for >2 years
- Duration of subfertility >3 years
- Known history of reproductive pathology, eg. amenorrhoea, pelvic inflammatory disease (PID), endometriosis
- Known history or reason for infertility, e.g. tubal ligation/vasectomy, premature ovarian failure (POF)
- Follicle stimulating hormone >10 IU/L
- Sexual dysfunction
- Pelvic abnormalities on ultrasound scan like large fibroids or endometriotic cysts
- Blocked fallopian tubes or abnormal uterine cavity on HSG
- The presence of male problems, e.g. history of urogenital surgery, varicocoele, significant systemic illness
- Abnormal seminal fluid analysis

  Sperm count $<15 \times 10^6$/mL

  Sperm motility <40%

Principles of Subfertility Treatment

- Start with clomiphene citrate 50 mg OM on day 2–6 of menses if the patient is anovulatory (after a course of dydrogesterone 10 mg om × 5 days to induce withdrawal bleeding). Check serum progesterone on day 21/22 of menses for evidence of ovulation (or 7 days before expected menses for women with longer menstrual cycles)
- *Side-effects of clomiphene*: nausea, giddiness, headaches, hot flushes, mood swings, blurred vision and multiple pregnancies (10%). Although there is no known risk of ovarian cancer, it is recommended not to prescribe more than 6 ovulatory cycles of clomiphene
- Consider adding metformin 500 mg tds or 850 mg bd to clomiphene if patient has polycystic ovarian syndrome (PCOS) and high BMI (>35 kg/m^2) with clomiphene resistance. Metformin may be started at 500 mg om and slowly increased till the optimal dose is reached to reduce the gastrointestinal side effects
- Consider induction of ovulation with gonadotrophins or laparoscopic ovarian drilling for clomid-resistant polycystic ovarian syndrome (PCOS)
- Intrauterine insemination, especially for coital dysfunction

(*Continued*)

Principles of Subfertility Treatment (*Continued*)

- Laparoscopic treatment of endometriosis
- Super-ovulation intrauterine insemination (SO-IUI) for mild male factor, minimal or mild endometriosis, unexplained infertility with bilateral patent fallopian tubes
- *In vitro* fertilisation (IVF)/intracytoplasmic sperm injection (ICSI) for tubal infertility, moderate or severe endometriosis, failed SO-IUI, severe male factor
- Laparoscopic/ microsurgical surgery for tubal blockage or peritubal adhesions

Ovarian Hyperstimulation Syndrome (OHSS)

OHSS is an iatrogenic complication of the luteal phase and early pregnancy after ovulation induction or ovarian stimulation. It is a systemic disease resulting from vasoactive products released by hyperstimulated ovaries. The pathophysiology is characterised by increased capillary permeability, leading to leakage of fluid from the vascular compartment, with third space fluid accumulation and intravascular dehydration. Its occurrence is dependent on the administration of human chorionic gonadotrophin (HCG).

Early and late form of OHSS

The early form of OHSS (<10 days after the ovulation triggering injection of HCG) is related to an exaggerated ovarian response to gonadotrophin stimulation, whereas the late form (≥10 days after HCG) is mainly related to the secretion of placental HCG. Those cases which constitute both early OHSS and followed by pregnancy are serious and long-lasting.

Mild ovarian hyperstimulation probably occurs in up to 33% of stimulated cycles, while 3–8% of IVF cycles are complicated by moderate to severe forms.

Symptoms of OHSS

Most frequent symptoms and signs

- Lower abdominal distension
- Progressive increase in abdominal circumference measured at the level of the umbilicus
- Ovaries enlarged up to >12 cm.
- Nausea and vomiting, preventing intake of food and fluids
- Dyspnoea and respiratory distress due to an elevated diaphragm and hydrothorax
- Diarrhoea
- Quick weight gain

More severe signs and symptoms of OHSS

- Ascites
- Hypotension
- Pleural effusion (more frequently on the right side)
- Pericardial effusion
- Adult form of respiratory distress syndrome
- Oliguria and anuria
- Multiple organ failure
- Death (1/500 000 cycles)

Laboratory Investigations:

- Electrolyte disorders (hyponatraemia or hyperkalaemia)
- Hypovolaemia
- Haemoconcentration (haematocrit >45%)
- Leucocytosis >15 000/mm^3
- Creatinine clearance <50 mL/min; serum creatinine >1.2 mg/dL
- Elevated liver enzymes
- Hypercoagulability

Additional complications of OHSS

- Ovarian torsion

Causes sudden, extreme abdominal pain and nausea. Incidence of 1/5000 stimulation cycles but more frequent if OHSS and pregnancy are present.

- Ovarian bleeding

Caused by ovarian rupture or intraovarian bleeding; may be caused by pressure or bimanual examination. Signs of acute haemorrhage include hypotension, nausea, sudden drop in haematocrit count.

- Thromboembolic symptoms

The incidence of thrombosis with OHSS is 0.7–10% and that there is an apparent preponderance of upper body sites and frequent involvement of arterial system.

Refer to Chapter 8 on "Management of OHSS."

Semen Analysis and Management of Azoospermia

Basal Seminal Analysis

	Normal Range (WHO Criteria 2009)	Pathological term
Abstinence (days)	2–7	
pH	≥ 7.2	
Volume (mL)	> 1.5	Aspermia (no semen)
Density ($\times 10^6$/mL)	≥ 15	Azoospermia (no sperm) Oligozoospermia ($< 15 \times 10^6$/mL)
Motility	$\geq 40\%$ forward progression	Asthenozoospermia
Morphology	$\geq 4\%$	Teratozoospermia (malformed)
WBC ($\times 10^6$/mL)	< 1	

- Semen analysis is not a test of fertility but a component of the investigation in infertility
- Semen specimens are obtained by masturbation after at least 3 days of abstinence
- 2–3 samples of semen analysis obtained over a 3-month period before a final diagnosis of male factor can be made
- If the first semen analysis is normal, there is no need for a repeat test

Abnormal semen analysis: What to do?

- Check for collection problems or any recent illness. Review use of medications, occupational and environmental exposures of teratogens
- Repeat test 12 weeks later to exclude a spurious result

Likely Causes

1. *Azoospermia* — obstructive and non-obstructive (hypogonadotrophic hypogonadism, conditions affecting spermatogenesis such as radiotherapy)
2. *Asthenospermia* — endocrine disorders, infection of accessory glands, varicocoeles and epididymal dysfunction. Many are idiopathic
3. *Teratozoospermia* — temporary insults to spermatogenesis (recent febrile illness, medication), varicocoeles

Semen Analysis

Several factors can affect the sperm count and other semen analysis values.

- physical damage to the testicles
- extremely high fever
- infection such as sexually transmitted infections (STIs), mumps
- varicocoele
- history of radiation treatment of testicles or environmental insult from toxins
- exposure to certain drugs (such as azathioprine or cimetidine)
- higher level of oestrogens may have lower sperm counts
- obstruction of vas deferens or ejaculatory ducts
- genetic conditions

Predictive value of sperm morphology in determining pregnancy rate is low. Most important parameters are *concentration of sperm in the semen* and *motility*

Enhancing male sperm quality

Prevention

- Avoid tight trousers and underwear or heat such as frequent sauna visits

- Avoid excessive ejaculation or prolonged abstinence
- Avoid drugs that affect sperms, i.e. anabolic steroid, testosterone
- Stop smoking, limit alcohol use
- Prevent STIs by adopting safer sexual practices
- Adopt healthy diet and exercise regularly to prevent obesity which is associated with higher oestrogen levels

Therapeutic — *potentially treatable*

- Varicocoele surgery
- Antibiotics for infection
- Surgery for genital tract obstructions
- Hormonal therapy for gonadotrophin deficiency
- Reversible drug or toxin effects

Untreatable subfertility *(idiopathic oligozoospermia, asthenozoospermia and teratozoospermia)*

Various therapies have been proposed but few have clear evidence of benefit

- Centrum®/vitamins A, C, E/multivitamin with zinc
- Selenium (200 μg daily)
- L-carnitine and acetylcarnitine (Proxeed)
- Arginine, L-arginine

- Vitamin B12 (1000 μg daily)
- Zinc (150–30 mg daily)
- Antioxidant: vitamin C (1000 mg daily), vitamin E (400 IU bd)
- Coenzyme Q10 (10 mg daily)
- Tribestan (non-hormonal herbal product that stimulates the function of the reproductive system)

Drugs that can affect sperm production or function

- alcohol
- alkylating agents
- allopurinol
- anabolic steroids
- cimetidine
- colchicine
- cyclosporin
- erythromycin
- gentamicin
- neomycin
- nitrofurantoin
- spironolactone
- sulfasalazine
- tetracyclines

Azoospermia

The diagnosis of azoospermia requires two or more centrifuged semen samples, 3 months apart, to confirm that sperms are totally absent. Baseline investigations with FSH, LH, testosterone may be requested while waiting for second sample.

Table 1. Evaluation of the Azoospermic Patient

History	Examination	Investigations
Prior fertility	Testis size (N* = 4 – 5.5 cm long/25 mL) and consistency	FSH, LH, prolactin
Childhood illnesses	Presence of varicocoeles	Total testosterone
Genital trauma/ pelvic or inguinal surgery	Presence of inguinal or scrotal scars	Ultrasound imaging of the urogenital tract and testes
Exposure to gonadotoxins	Secondary sexual characteristics (body habitus, hair distribution, and gynaecomastia)	Karyotype analysis and Yq microdeletion analysis
Medications	Presence of vas deferens (absent in patients with cystic fibrosis)	MRI pituitary gland
Family history of birth defects, mental retardation, reproductive failure or cystic fibrosis	Consistency of the epididymis (which may be thickened from fibrosis due to infections)	

*N = normal

Management of azoospermia

1. *Testicular failure — elevated FSH level*

   There is no known upper limit of FSH level that implies testicular failure. Usually, we use the cutoff of 2x above normal limit. However, there may still be sperms present in the testis which could be retrieved surgically. Referral to urology/reproductive andrologist for assessment and counselling is warranted.

2. *Hypogonadotrophic hypogonadism — low FSH, LH and testosterone levels*

   Pituitary MRI to exclude a pathological lesion. If negative, HCG may be given to initiate spermatogenesis. It may take up to one year to induce sufficient spermatogenesis resulting in acceptable semen parameters.

3. *Obstructive Causes*

   Treatment options are surgical correction to by-pass the obstruction, allowing for natural conception or surgical sperm retrieval followed by ICSI.

Approach to Azoospermia

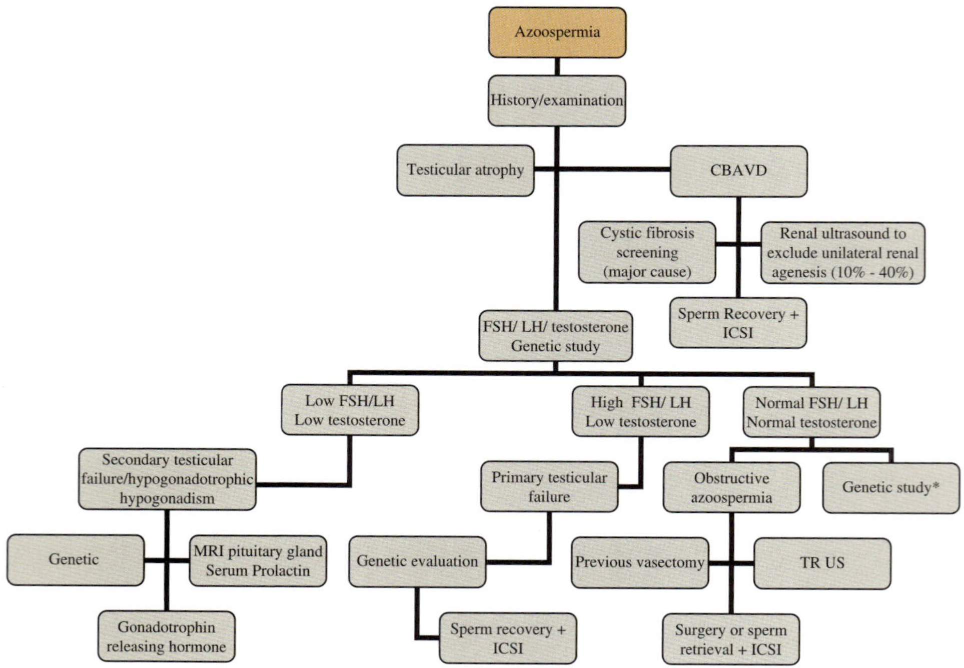

* *Genetic study* should be offered as obstructive azoospermia and impaired spermatogenesis secondary to genetic causes are not mutually exclusive.

CBAVD – Congenital bilateral absence of vas deferens.
ICSI – Intracytoplasmic sperm insemination.
TRUS – Transrectal ultrasound scan.

Chapter 66

APPROACH TO HYPERPROLACTINAEMIA

Physiological	Pharmacological	Pathological

• Lactation
• Pregnancy
• Stress
• Coitus
	(Due to dopamine–antagonist mechanism of action)
	• Antipsychotics
	  • Typical
	    — phenothiazine
	    — butyrophenone
	  • Atypical
	    — Risperidone
	    — Olanzapine
	• Antidepressants
	• Anticonvulsants
	• Antiemetics
	  — Metoclopramide
	• Antihypertensives
	  — Methyldopa
		• *Hypothalamic-Pituitary Disorders*
		  • Pituitary Stalk Section
		  • Infiltrative
		    ▪ Sarcoidosis
		    ▪ Granulomas
		    ▪ Tuberculosis
		    ▪ Histiocytosis
		  • Trauma
		  • Cranial irradiation
		  • Previous surgery
		  • Tumours
		    ▪ Craniopharyngioma
		    ▪ Meningioma
		    ▪ Germinoma

(Continued)

(*Continued*)

Physiological	Pharmacological	Pathological

	• Oestrogens
	• Opioids
	• MAO inhibitors (monoamine oxidase)
	• Cimetidine
		• Pituitary Diseases
		  • Empty Sella Turcica syndrome
		  • Tumours
		    ▪ Pituitary adenoma
		      — Prolactinoma
		      — Non-functioning adenoma
		  • Acromegaly
		  • Cushing disease
		• Systemic diseases
		• Chronic renal disease
		• Liver cirrhosis
		• Hypothyroidism
		• Polycystic ovarian syndrome (PCOS)

Patient usually Presents with Symptoms of

- **Features of hyperprolactinaemia**
  - Galactorrhoea
  - Oligomenorrhoea
  - Subfertility
- **Take history to screen for underlying aetiology**
  - Drug history
  - Neurological symptoms, e.g. visual disturbances, headaches
  - Other medical diseases, e.g. hypothyroidism, chronic renal or hepatic disease
  - Previous neurological surgery/irradiation
  - Excessive exercise or stress

↓

On Examination

- **Breast examination**
  ** Refer to Chapter 67 on "Approach to Galactorrhoea"*
- **Gynaecological examination**
- **Neurological examination**
  — Bitemporal haemianopia
  — Signs of space occupying lesions
- **Systemic review**
  — Chronic renal failure
  — Liver cirrhosis
  — Hypothyroidism
  — Acromegaly

⬇

Investigations

- **Serum prolactin**
  — Normal < 25 μg/L
- **MRI hypothalamic-pituitary axis to exclude pituitary tumour**
- **Endocrine screen**
  — Thyroid panel
  — Growth Hormone, Adrenocorticotropic hormone (ACTH)

⬇

Management of Hyperprolactinaemia

- Drug-induced/pharmacological hyperprolactinaemia
  — Assess indication of medication
  — Discontinue medicine and reassess serum prolactin levels
  — Do not need to treat asymptomatic drug-induced hyperprolactinaemia
  — If possible — reduce dosage or switch to a drug with less dopamine-antagonist effect
  — If not possible — cautious administration with close surveillance
- Systemic or endocrine disorders
  — Treat any underlying chronic disease

Management of Micro- and Macroprolactinoma

Medical (1st line)
Dopamine Agonists (Bromocriptine/Cabergoline)

↓

Surveillance

- Serial prolactin level to assess resumption to normal level
- Repeat MRI* scan in one year

↓

Stop treatment

After one year of treatment, if serum prolactin returns to normal and with no evidence of remnant tumour on MRI* scan

Surgery

- Failure of medical therapy
- Expanding prolactinoma (patient with neurological and opthalmological deficits not responding to dopamine agonists
- Infarction/haemorrhage into prolactinoma with visual disturbances, severe headache, altered consciousness, vascular collapse
- Resistant/malignant prolactinoma

Radiotherapy

- Limited scope
- Resistant to medical and surgical therapy

*MRI = Magnetic resonance imaging.

Management of Pituitary Adenomas/Prolactinomas in Pregnancy

— Microadenoma < 10 mm diameter

— Macroadenoma > 10 mm diameter

Risk of enlargement of microprolactinomas in pregnancy

— Low risk of expansion

— Usually bromocriptine is discontinued.

Risk of enlargement of macroprolactinomas in pregnancy

— Higher risk (30%) of expansion

— Continue medical treatment

— Monitor visual fields in each trimester

— Look out for visual symptoms

10% of macroadenoma in pregnancy may require surgery.

Chapter 67

APPROACH TO GALACTORRHOEA

Galactorrhoea is defined as excessive lactation unrelated to breastfeeding and postpartum.

Physiological lactation usually occurs in the immediate postpartum, and is caused by a sudden drop in progesterone in the presence of high levels of prolactin.

Most patients present with nipple discharge.

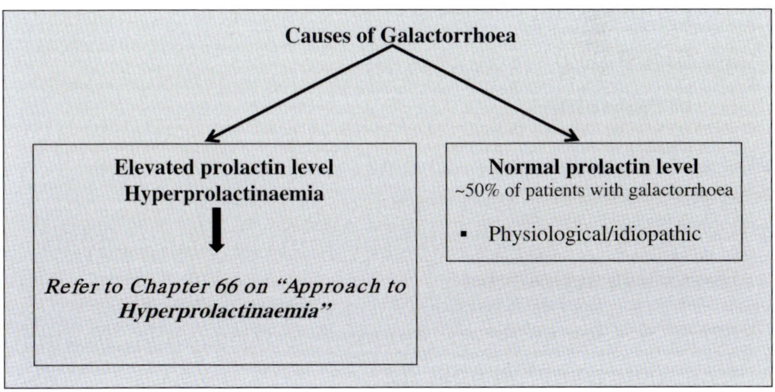

Normal prolactin level usually quoted as < 25 μg/L
Normal prolactin range used in KKH 6.98–32.94 μg/L

History

- **Details of discharge**
  - Unilateral or bilateral
  - Colour (clear, white, green, bloody)
  - Amount
  - Duration
  - Odour

- **Associated symptoms**
  - Nipple/skin changes
  - Breast pain
  - Breast lumps
  - Fever

- +/– **Details suggestive of hyperprolactinaemia and its respective aetiologies**

  (Refer to Chapter 66 on "Approach to Hyperprolactinaemia" for a more comprehensive list)

Examination

- **Vital parameters**
- **Bilateral breast examination**
  - — Unilateral or bilateral
  - — Uniductal or multiductal
  - — Discharge: colour, consistency, blood, amount, smell
  - — Associated signs: nipple/skin changes, tenderness, lumps
  - — Bilateral axillary examination: enlarged lymph nodes
- +/– **Signs suggestive of hyperprolactinaemia and its respective aetiologies**

  (refer to Chapter 66 on "Approach to Hyperprolactinaemia" for a more comprehensive list)

Pathological Nipple Discharge

— unilateral, uniductal, persistent, spontaneous

— may be blood-tinged

— important to identify and refer to breast surgeon expediently as malignancy may occur in 10% of pathological nipple discharge

Approach to Galactorrhoea

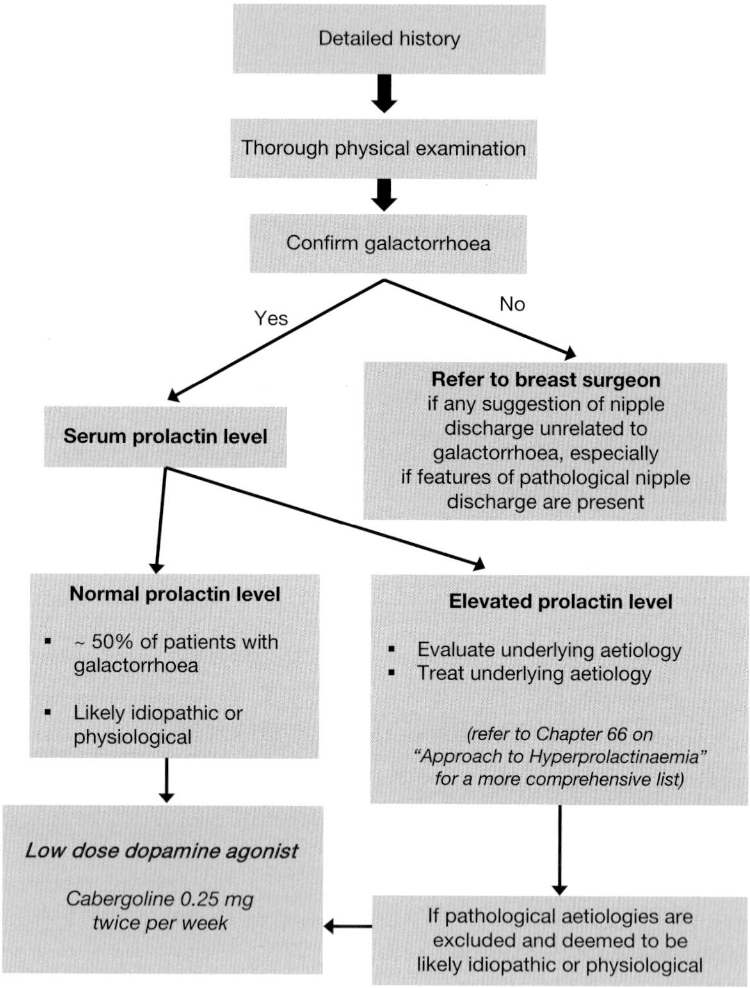

Chapter 68

SEXUAL DYSFUNCTIONAL PROBLEMS

Introduction

- About 50% of married couples have sexual problems or concerns
- The numbers seen in practice is much lower because
    - Patients seldom complain of sexual problems
    - Failure of doctors to take a sexual history
    - Doctors are too inhibited and talking of sexual matters is considered a taboo
    - Doctors are uncomfortable when discussing about sex

Uncovering sexual problems

Two ways:

1. Respond to patient's stated complaint about a sexual problem or other problems that may affect activity, e.g. chronic vaginismus

2. Ask questions routinely as part of psychosocial history-taking
   - If a problem or concern is identified, then taking a sexual problem history is applicable
   - Embarrassment will be prevented if this is done in a routine and comfortable way
   - Routinely asking question about sexual functioning helps to uncover the problems. Many problems will be missed by not enquiring about sexual difficulties

How to Help Dissatisfied Women with their Sexual Response?

- Be knowledgeable about current information on sexual behaviour
- Be objective about sexual behaviour
- Be approachable
- Be willing to listen and clarify problems
- As an educator, the doctor can use gynaecological examination to educate the patient on female genital and body functions
- Recommend reading materials
- As a therapist, the doctor can diagnose and treat sexual problems

- Facilitate improved communication between patient and partner
- **Refer to OBGYN** for sexual dysfunction problems when applicable

How to Ask Your Patient?

- Are you currently sexually active?
- What is your frequency of sexual intercourse?
- Does your partner encounter any difficulty with erection or ejaculation?
- Do you have difficulty with getting sexually aroused, lubricating or reaching orgasm?
- Do you experience pain during sexual intercourse?
- Are you satisfied with your sex life? If not, why?
- Do you have any questions or concerns related to sex that you wish to discuss?

History of sexual problem

- Description of current problem
- Onset and cause of the problem
- Patient's perception of cause and maintenance of the problem

- Past treatment and outcome:
  - Medical evaluation
  - Professional help
  - Self treatment
- Current expectations and goals of treatment

Types of problems encountered

Female problems

- Dyspareunia/painful intercourse
- Non-consummation
- Vaginismus
- Anorgasmia
- Low libido

Male problems

- Erectile dysfunction (ED)
- Premature ejaculation
- Retarded/anejaculation
- Low libido

The Psychosexual Dysfunction

- Inhibition in the sexual response cycle (arousal, excitement, orgasm and resolution phases) can occur at one or more of the phases. This causes disturbances in the subjective sense of pleasure and objective performance

- Dysfunction can be lifelong or acquired, generalised or situational, total or partial

Associated features

- Usually no obvious sign of disturbance is seen
- There could be a sense of not living up to ill-defined concept of normality or complaints, e.g. dyspareunia, anxiety, guilt, shame, frustration and somatic symptoms
- There is a fear of failure and development of a "spectator" attitude (self-maintaining) and sensitivity to the sexual partner's reaction
- This impairs performance and satisfaction further and leads to secondary avoidance of sexual activity and impairs communication with the sexual partner
- The cause is variable — life-long or short-lived episodes. Episodes of sexual dysfunction can recur. The relationship with the partner suffers and marital relationship can be disrupted
- Main predisposing causes are anxiety and a negative attitude toward sexuality due to experiences, internal conflicts or rigid cultural values
- The milder forms are extremely common

The Psychosexual Dysfunction

Phase	*Dysfunction*
Desire	Hypoactive sexual desire Inhibited sexual desire
Excitement	Erectile dysfunction (male) Difficulty in arousal/lubrication (female)
Orgasm	Premature ejaculation (male) Retarded ejaculation (male) Anorgasmia (female)
Others	Vaginismus/pain on sex Ejaculating pain Sexual phobia/avoidance

Assessing Categories of Aetiology

- History details provide the best important diagnostic clues
- Organically induced sexual problems are persistent and progressively worsening
- Psychosexual problems are episodic or situational

Physical Examination

- Only second in importance to history-taking
- Vaginismus is unique. It is the only condition that can be diagnosed at physical examination

Investigations

- When an organic aetiology is suspected (e.g. premature menopause causing vaginal dryness and loss of libido), the biochemical and endocrine parameters need to be assessed
- Vaginal swab and culture to exclude infective causes
- Diagnostic laparoscopy to exclude dyspareunia due to endometriosis if indicated
- Other special tests, e.g. arteriography and penile blood flow studies may be warranted

Management of Sexual Dysfunction Problems

- This may include counselling or medications or both
- The approach depends on:
  - Knowledge and skill (of therapist)
  - Time available
  - Professional interest
- An informed, interested and sensitive physician can contribute significantly to solving the sexual problems of the patient
- The informed non-specialist will frequently be successful in treating patients with dyspareunia, premature ejaculation, secondary erectile failure and sexual problems resulting from illness, drugs or surgery

To Treat or to Refer?

- Long-standing sexual dysfunction, marital discord, psychiatric illness and problems with self-image, self-esteem and denial are best referred to an expert

Intervention

- Medical specialist should be able to provide effective treatment for patients with sexual problems in 80% or more of the cases encountered in practice
- Four levels of intervention are possible. Each descending level of approach requires increasing degree of knowledge, training and skill

Level 1: Permission

- People want to know or hear that they are normal and they need a professional to tell them this
- Permission involves saying it is okay to be sexual, have sexual thoughts, dreams or fantasies and to talk and discuss about sex
- It is okay to carry on with any sexual activity they are involved in, for example, masturbation, oral sex

Level 2: Limited information

- Involves patient education by discussion, seminars, books, pamphlets, videos, etc.

- Education means talking about normality of this feeling, e.g. sex after hysterectomy or during pregnancy
- Education helps to dispel myths

Level 3: Specific suggestions

- There are attempts to help patient change his or her behaviour and reach stated goals
- The approach is time- and problem-oriented
- This approach is helpful in problem of arousal, erection, ejaculation, orgasm or painful intercourse

Level 4: Intensive therapy

- Cases that may require appropriate treatment if he or she is interested to undertake therapy
- The main objective of treatment is to modify the immediate antecedents or cause of sexual symptoms
- Suggested exercises are conducted within a flexible time frame
- The patient proceeds to the next level when he or she is comfortable with the preceding ones
- Progress is at his or her own pace and is dictated by patient's and partner's anxiety level

Vaginismus

Introduction

- Vaginismus is an involuntary contraction of the muscles surrounding the entrance to the vagina, making penetration impossible or painful
- The primary muscle group involved is the pubococcygeus (PC)
- There could be deep-seated subconscious negative feelings such as anxiety or fear associated with vaginal penetration. The vaginal PC muscles, as they contract, are in effect often acting as a protective mechanism against penetration
- *Primary vaginismus* occurs when a woman has never, at any time, been able to have pain-free sexual intercourse due to the PC muscle spasm. The vaginismus condition becomes evident during initial attempts at sexual penetration or gynaecological examination and continues to persist
- *Secondary vaginismus* occurs when a woman who had previously enjoyed sexual intercourse without pain, develops the vaginismus condition later, possibly following some trauma or surgery. She is no longer able to have intercourse, even though the physical concerns have been resolved
- Women with vaginismus are sexually responsive and have deep desire to make love. It is extremely frustrating to not be able to engage in pleasurable sexual intercourse

Factors associated with vaginismus

- Past sexual abuse
- Exposure as a child to shocking sexual imagery
- Domestic violence
- Rigid parenting
- Inadequate sex education
- No known experience

Management of vaginismus

- Obtain proper diagnosis
- Educating the patient about the condition and anatomy is important
- Identify the negative events and consciously over-ride them through written and verbal reassurances
- **REFER to sex therapy doctor**
- Retraining of the PC muscles through the use of vaginal dilator exercises
- Complete a series of exercises with the partner to educate each other, build sexual trust and progress to full sexual intercourse

Sexual Position for Conception

- Many experts believe that the missionary position (man on top) affords the best opportunity for baby-making. This position allows for the deepest penetration and as a result, places the sperms closer to the cervix

- For additional effectiveness, the woman can try elevating her hips with a pillow so that her cervix is exposed to the maximum amount of semen
- Other effective positions include:
  - Rear-entry, when the man enters the woman from behind, either lying down or kneeling, can also deposit the sperms close to the cervix and aid conception
  - Lying side-by-side — this can be a relaxing position and easier on a partner who is overweight or has chronic back problem
- A woman can further increase the likelihood of conception by remaining in bed for up to half an hour following intercourse, preferably on her back and with a pillow under her pelvic region. In theory, this provides the sperms with additional travel time up to the fallopian tube along with help from the forces of gravity
- Avoid having sex while sitting, standing or with female partner on top. These positions defy gravity and may discourage the upward mobility of the sperms
- The contractions that accompany the female orgasm may help carry the sperms further into the cervix

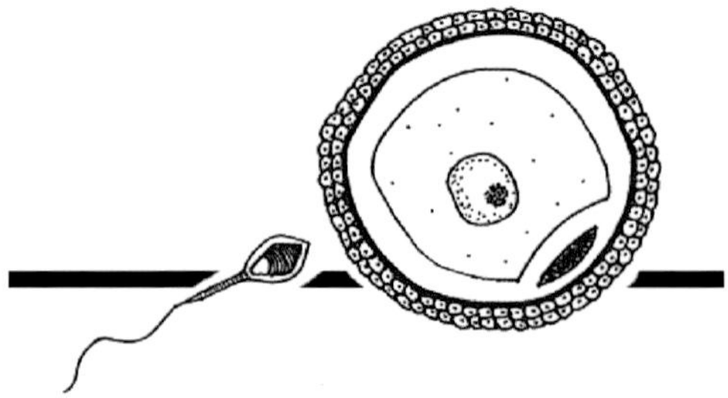

Chapter 69

MAMMOGRAM, BREAST ULTRASOUND SCAN AND BREAST BIOPSY

Introduction

- *Common benign conditions* seen in the breast include fibrocystic change and benign tumours such as fibroadenomas, papillomas and phyllodes tumours
- *Common malignant lesions* are *in situ* cancers such as ductal carcinoma *in situ* (DCIS) and infiltrative cancers

Mammogram

Mammographic features suspicious for cancer include:

1. Spiculated or ill-defined masses
2. Clusters of heterogeneous or pleomorphic microcalcifications with linear, branching or casting configuration
3. Architectural distortion

4. Others — lymph node enlargement, skin thickening, nipple retraction
    - Using standard nomenclature and terminology, mammograms are reported using the **BIRADS** scoring system (**Breast Imaging Reporting and Data System**)
    - The risk of malignancy can be estimated based on the BIRADS score

Table 1. BIRADS Classification

BIRADS Category	Assessment	Cancer Risk*	Recommendations
0	Needs further imaging evaluation	—	Complete radiological evaluation, e.g. spot views, ultrasound
1	Negative	Nil	Routine screening
2	Benign	Nil	Routine screening
3	Probably benign	<2%	Short term e.g. 4–6 months mammographic follow up for interval change
4	Suspicious	30–40%	Biopsy urged
5	Highly suggestive of malignancy	98–99%	Biopsy required

*False negative rates of screening mammography vary with age group screened and can be up to 20%.

Breast Ultrasound Scan

- An ultrasound scan of the breast is a useful adjunct to distinguish between cystic and solid masses seen on mammograms

- Lesions that are solid, hypoechoic, irregular, taller-than-wide, and have shadowing or increased vascularity, have an increased risk of malignancy
- If a biopsy is not performed, the lesions should be followed up closely for interval change

Breast Biopsy

- When assessing for biopsy, in addition to radiological features, consider other factors such as the age of the patient, duration of the lesion, family and personal history of breast cancer
- In the presence of a palpable mass, normal radiological imaging should not deter the clinician from performing a biopsy
- For lesions that are seen on mammography and/or ultrasound but not palpable, image guidance (using X-rays or ultrasound scan) may be necessary to guide the clinician during the biopsy procedure

Chapter 70

BREAST CANCER SCREENING

Screening Mammogram Schedule

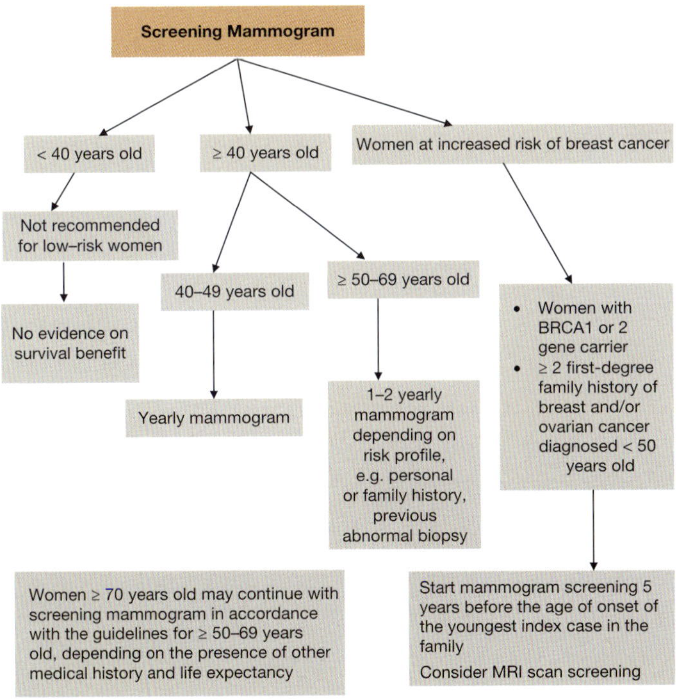

Part 4

INVESTIGATIONS IN GYNAECOLOGY

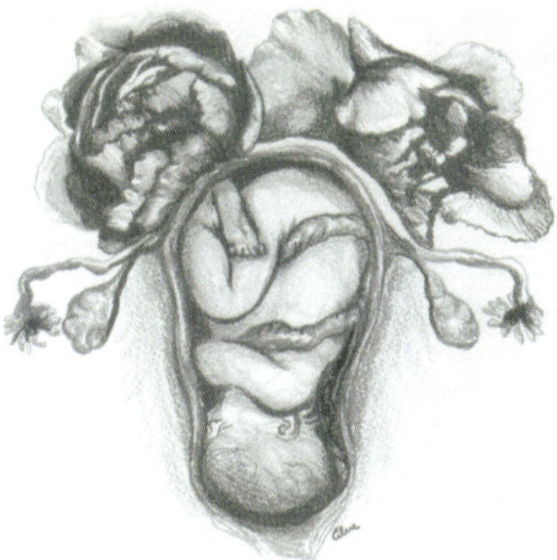

"The Dream" 2013

Description: "For the womb has dreams" — Anais Nin

Chapter 71

OVARIAN TUMOUR MARKERS

Ovarian Tumour Markers

Test	Purpose	Normal Range	Interpretation and Management Guidelines
Cancer antigen 125 (CA125)	• To exclude epithelial ovarian cancer • Can be used for monitoring of women with known ovarian cancer (monitor response to treatment/to detect recurrence)	• 0–35 U/mL	• Can be raised in cancers like ovary, fallopian tube and endometrium • Increased in benign conditions like pelvic inflammatory disease, uterine fibroids, endometriosis, adenomyosis, pregnancy and during menstruation • Derived from pericardium, pleura and peritoneum and can be increased in conditions relating to these • Perform pelvic ultrasound scan to exclude pelvic pathology
Carcinoembryonic antigen (CEA)	• To exclude primary colorectal cancer • As a tumour marker, to identify recurrences after surgical resection, to localise cancer spread • Not so useful as a screening tool	• <2.5 ng/mL (non smoker) • <5 ng/mL (smoker)	• Expressed in adenocarcinomas • Elevated levels are found in cancers like ovary, breast, colorectum, gastric, pancreatic, lung and medullary thyroid carcinoma • Also increased in benign conditions like cirrhosis of liver, ulcerative colitis, Crohn's disease, chronic obstructive lung disease and pancreatitis

(*Continued*)

Ovarian Tumour Markers *(Continued)*

Test	Purpose	Normal Range	Interpretation and Management Guidelines
Alpha foetoprotein (αFP)	• To exclude liver cancer or yolk sac ovarian tumour	• 0–40 ng/mL (non pregnant) • 10–150 ng/mL (between 15–18 weeks of pregnancy)	1. *Non pregnant + elevated αFP* • Hepatocellular cancer • Ovarian cancer (yolk sac tumours) • Non-neoplastic conditions like cirrhosis or hepatitis 2. *Pregnant + elevated αFP* • Wrong dates • Multiple gestation • Neural tube defect in foetus • Omphalocoele • Intrauterine death (IUD) 3. *Pregnant + low levels of αFP* • Wrong dates • Trisomy 21/18

(Continued)

Ovarian Tumour Markers *(Continued)*

Test	Purpose	Normal Range	Interpretation and Management Guidelines
Carbohydrate antigen 19–9/ cancer antigen 19–9 (CA 19–9)	• Not useful as a screening tool (high false negative and false positive). • Can have prognostic significance to evaluate effectiveness of treatment of cancer of exocrine pancreas	• 0–37 μg/mL (<40 μg /mL)	• Elevated levels are associated with pancreatic, oesophageal, colorectal, hepatocellular, gall bladder cancers • Also increased with benign conditions like pancreatitis, cirrhosis of liver, disease of biliary tract
Note: Ovarian tumour markers are *not* useful in pregnant women as they would be raised in normal pregnancies.			

Chapter 72

FEMALE HORMONAL PROFILE

Female Hormonal Profile

Test	Purpose	Normal Range	Interpretation and Management Guidelines
Follicular stimulating hormone (FSH) (Day 2–3)	Young women for ovarian reserve Perimenopausal	3–10 IU/L	• Poor ovarian function if FSH >10 IU/L • Impending menopause if FSH >30 IU/L • Clinical diagnosis of menopause if amenorrhoea for *ONE* year
Luteinising hormone (LH) (Day 2–3)	Polycystic ovarian syndrome (PCOS)		• LH : FSH > 3 : 1 suggests PCOS
Prolactin	Hyperprolactinaemia	0–32.9 μg/L	• Refer to endocrinologist if persistently high *Common causes* Prolactinomas, hypothyroidism, medications (tricyclic antidepressants, metoclopramide, phenothiazines, methyldopa, H2 blockers), polycystic ovarian syndrome • Refer to Chapter 66 on "Approach to Hyper-prolactinaemia"

(*Continued*)

Female Hormonal Profile *(Continued)*

Test	Purpose	Normal Range	Interpretation and Management Guidelines
Dehydroepiandrosterone acetate (DHEA)	Hirsutism/virilisation	<2500 nm/L	• Consider MRI scan to exclude adrenal tumours if DHEA >2500 nm/L
Testosterone	Hirsutism/virilisation	0–2.5 nmol/L	• If testosterone >5 nmol/L, exclude testosterone-secreting tumour
Oestradiol (E2)	Fertility investigation	• Follicular phase 30–90 pg/mL • Luteal phase 70–300 pg/mL • Post-menopausal 0–30 pg/mL	• Wide range for normality • If FSH high/E2 normal, denotes poor ovarian reserve, i.e. poor prognosis for fertility • Day 3 FSH is normal, E2 high, ovarian reserve may still be affected • Not useful in perimenopausal women. • High levels may be associated with oestrogen-secreting ovarian tumours • Low levels may be associated with ovarian failure, decreased ovarian reserve and Turner syndrome

(Continued)

Female Hormonal Profile *(Continued)*

Test	Purpose	Normal Range	Interpretation and Management Guidelines
Progesterone	Ovulatory function	Day 21 progesterone >30 ng/mL	Ovulatory cycle if day 21/22 progesterone >30 ng/mL. Irregular menses — to do blood test 7 days before next expected menses
Anti-Mullerian hormone (AMH) — produced by granulosa cells of pre-antral and small antral follicles of ovary	• Useful in artificial reproductive technique cycles (ART) to customise treatment protocol • Can predict ovarian responsiveness but not embryo quality/pregnancy/live birth after IVF or ICSI	• *13–45 years*: 1–10 ng/mL • *>45 years*: <1 ng/mL	• As the number of ovarian follicles diminishes with age, AMH can be a marker for ovarian ageing • Useful adjunct to serum FSH/oestradiol levels and antral follicle count when estimating ovarian reserve • Poor response to IVF indicative of diminished ovarian reserve is associated with low AMH

Chapter 73

IMAGING MODALITIES IN GYNAECOLOGY

Indications for Ultrasound in Gynaecology

Evaluation of uterus, cervix, cul de sac, adnexae for various pathologies.

(i) Congenital abnormalities of uterus (didelphys/bicornuate/septate uterus)
(ii) Uterine/cervical fibroids
(iii) Adenomyosis
(iv) Endometrial/cervical polyps
(v) Ovarian cyst (endometriotic/follicular/dermoid/polycystic ovaries)
(vi) Hydrosalpinx
(vii) Tuboovarian mass/abscess
(viii) To differentiate between simple and complex ovarian cysts
(ix) Hydrometra/pyometra/haematometra
(x) Localisation of intrauterine contraceptive device (IUCD)

Indications for Transabdominal Ultrasound Scan

(i) Patient is unable to tolerate transvaginal probe
(ii) Patient is a virgin
(iii) For evaluation of abdomen and upper pelvis (e.g. large fibroids/ovarian masses that extend into the upper pelvis or abdomen)

1. Transvaginal Ultrasound Scan (TVUS)

- Evaluates pelvic structures better (uterine size, endometrial thickness, endometrial polyps)
- Useful tool for obese patients
- Evaluates early pregnancy location

2. Hysterosalpingography (HSG)

Radiographic evaluation of uterine cavity and fallopian tubes after injection of radio-opaque medium through the cervical canal.

Indications

(i) Evaluation of tubal patency (for subfertility)
(ii) Evaluation of endometrial pathology (polyps/myoma/synechiae)

(iii) Evaluation of tubal pathology (cornual block, hydrosalpinx, salpingitis isthmica nodosa)

Advantage

- Provides better delineation of contour of uterine cavity
- Outlines lumen of fallopian tubes and cornua
- Outlines width of cervical canal
- Spill of contrast from fimbrial ends of fallopian tubes to evaluate tubal patency

Disadvantage

- Pain/radiation/contrast allergy/perforation/syncope

Contraindication

(i) Recent or acute pelvic infection
(ii) Pregnancy

3. Saline Infusion Sonohysterography (SIS)

Fluid enhanced endovaginal scanning to aid evaluation of uterine cavity. Fluid is instilled into uterine cavity transcervically and visualisation of endometrial cavity carried out simultaneously by transvaginal scan.

Indications

(i) Evaluation of tubal patency (subfertility)
(ii) Evaluation of endometrial pathology (investigating for postmenopausal bleeding, abnormal uterine bleeding, secondary amenorrhoea, recurrent pregnancy loss)
(iii) Evaluation of congenital abnormalities of uterus.

Advantage

- Better delineation of focal endometrial abnormalities such as polyps, hyperplasia, cancer, leiomyomas and adhesions

Disadvantage

- Infection, false positive due to blood clots, mucous plugs and possible dissemination of cancer

Contraindication

(i) Recent or acute pelvic infection
(ii) Pregnancy

4. CT Scan
5. MRI Scan
} Refer to Chapter 74 on "Role of Interventional Radiology in Obstetrics and Gynaecology"

Chapter 74

ROLE OF INTERVENTIONAL RADIOLOGY (IR) IN OBSTETRICS AND GYNAECOLOGY

Modalities

1. Ultrasound Scan (US)

a) Most frequently applied due to the following advantages:
   i. Real-time imaging enables tracking of needle trajectory at all times
   ii. Detailed characterisation of cystic collections
   iii. Colour and pulse Doppler to identify vessels and vascularity
   iv. Non ionising radiation
   v. Availability of different probes for different regions (transcutaneous, transvaginal, transrectal)
   vi. Quick start-up time
   vii. Equipment fairly inexpensive

b) Limited by penetration of ultrasound scan
   i. Deep-seated lesions
   ii. Overlying lung, gas-filled bowel, calcifications/calculi/bone
   iii. Obese patients
   iv. Not all lesions seen on CT or MRI are visible

c) Portability
   i. Flexibility of performing location, though would be best to be in a sterile environment
   ii. Possibility of intraoperative assessment and localisation of lesions that may be occult on palpation

2. Computed Tomography (CT Scan)

a) Frequently used for
   i. Deep-seated lesions/collections, structures such as retroperitoneal masses/nodes, pelvic masses beyond the reach of the transvaginal/transrectal approach
   ii. Pulmonary/thoracic applications
   iii. Bone biopsy/ablation

b) Easier and better appreciation of anatomy
   i. Easier to appreciate relationship of structures with complete view of section
   ii. Accurate needle placement in experienced hands

c) Limitations
   i. Ionising radiation to patient and staff
   ii. CT fluoroscopy when used intermittently has the potential for shift of needle position between imaging
   iii. Need time to warm up machine
   iv. Vessels may not be delineated from adjacent structures on unenhanced CT scan

3. Magnetic Resonance Imaging (MRI) Scan

a) Applications
   i. For biopsy of lesions that are occult on ultrasound and CT scan
   ii. Where use of ionising radiation is to be avoided (e.g. in children, young women)

b) Limitations
   i. High cost
   ii. Specialised MR compatible equipment required (monitoring devices, needles, etc.)

General Risks of Procedures

1. Anxiety/discomfort/pain
   a) Most procedures are performed with the patient being conscious

   b) Occasionally, patients who are sensitive may feel passage of needle or catheter in body
   c) Prolonged procedure or inability to adequately anaesthetise needle/catheter tract due to limitation of needle length or proximity of major vessel to site

2. Bleeding/haemorrhage
   a) Usually related to inadvertent puncture of artery and may not be immediately noticed as incisions are usually small
   b) Haematoma may take days to weeks to resolve
   c) May require transfusion with blood products

3. Infection
   a) Usually very remote risk as skin preparation follows surgical standards and incisions are usually tiny
   b) Related to inadvertent transgression of infected collections or hollow viscous
   c) Immunocompromised patient

4. Radiation exposure (fluoroscopy and CT guided procedures)
   a) Local skin discolouration/burn
   b) Long-term potential cancer risk

Common Procedures Performed at KK Hospital

1. Aspiration and drainage
2. Biopsy

3. Vascular access devices
4. Prophylactic placement of bilateral internal iliac artery balloons
5. Angioembolisation
6. Percutanceous nephrostomy
7. Antegrade ureteric stenting
8. Varicose vein ablation

1. Aspiration and drainage

a) Terminology

i. *Aspiration*

1. usually with a 18/19 G sheathed needle or 21/22 G Chiba needle
2. tract is usually not dilated
    a. may safely transgress structures with minimal to no significant damage
    b. may be considered as an alternative to drainage if bleeding risk is increased yet fluid sample or decompression of a collection is necessary
3. For small collections (<3 cm diameter) unsuitable for drain insertion
4. Reduced recovery time compared to drainage

ii. *Drainage*

1. a pigtail drainage catheter is usually inserted, either directly or after tract dilatation over a guidewire to allow further egress of fluid, when volume is large

2. complex/inspissated collections
    a. allow time for liquefaction
    b. allow daily flushing to thin out fluid for easier drainage

b) Indications
  i. Diagnostic
    1. microbiology
    2. cytology
  ii. Therapeutic
    1. abscess drainage
    2. decompress pressure symptoms

c) Modality
  i. Ultrasound — most commonly applied
  ii. CT scan — for deep-seated collections, collections complicated by presence of large amount of gas
  iii. Fluoroscopy — usually used in combination with ultrasound scan to delineate extent of collection

d) Preparation (similar to pre-surgical investigations as risks of bleeding or damage to adjacent structures may require surgery)
  i. Prior discussion of case with Interventional Radiologist
  ii. Clearly filled procedure forms with relevant history and details

iii. Informed consent
iv. Blood tests
    1. Haemoglobin
    2. Platelet count
    3. PT/PTT
    4. Type and screen if low bleeding risk. Group and match if blood parameters deranged or coagulopathic
v. Fasting:
    1. at least 3–6 hours to avoid risks associated with reflux/vomiting and aspiration
    2. commence IV fluids containing dextrose if diabetic or prolonged fasting
    3. IV sedation usually required for transvaginal/transrectal procedures
vi. Antibiotic cover
    1. Infected/likely infected collections
    2. Possibility of transgression of bowel
    3. Obstructed ductal systems
vii. Cessation of antiplatelet and anticoagulation therapy to reduce risk of prolonged/profuse bleeding
viii. Appropriately filled and labelled specimen forms and bottles

e) Post-procedure care
   i. Vital signs — surrogate marker for haemorrhage, peripheral pulse quality may hint at extrinsic compression on pelvic vessels by haematoma; first 4–6 hours is crucial to identify arterial bleed
   ii. Observe wound site (open dressing to inspect) — bleeding, infection
   iii. Observe patient for pain and other unexpected symptoms such as increasing swelling/girth around biopsy site
   iv. Maintain IV access or IV fluids to replace blood volume loss
   v. Low threshold for imaging if massive blood loss suspected, include arterial phase if CT scan is to be performed

2. Biopsy

a) Indication
   i. Histological confirmation of disease before proceeding with definitive treatment
   ii. Imaging features are atypical/inconclusive
   iii. To exclude secondary pathology

b) Modality
   i. Ultrasound guidance (90%)
   ii. CT guidance for lungs, bones and deep-seated soft tissue lesions or complex anatomy
   iii. MR guidance for lesions that are occult on ultrasound and CT scan

c) Routes
   i. Transabdominal route is less invasive, although some pelvic masses may be better accessed via transvaginal or transrectal routes
   ii. Transthoracic for pulmonary lesions

d) Preparation
   i. Prior discussion of case with Interventional Radiologist
   ii. Clearly filled procedure forms with relevant history and details
   iii. Informed consent
   iv. Blood tests
      1. Haemoglobin
      2. Platelet count
      3. PT/PTT
      4. Type and screen if low bleeding risk. Group and match if blood parameters deranged or coagulopathic

   v. Fasting
      1. at least 3–6 hours to avoid risks associated with reflux/vomiting and aspiration
      2. commence IV fluids containing dextrose if diabetic or prolonged fasting
      3. IV sedation usually required for transvaginal/transrectal procedures

vi. Antibiotic prophylaxis is not routinely required

vii. Cessation of antiplatelet and anticoagulation therapy to reduce risk of prolonged/profuse bleeding

viii. Appropriately filled and labelled specimen forms and bottles

e) Post-procedure care

i. Similar to aspiration and drainage

ii. Angiography and embolisation if arterial bleeding or large pseudoaneurysm identified on imaging subsequently

f) Specific risks

i. Collateral injury — bowel, bladder, vessels (depending on location of biopsy target)

ii. Pseudoaneurysm — apposition of artery to vein with subsequent healing

iii. Haemorrhage — especially if artery transgressed

iv. Spillage of bowel content

v. Urine leakage

3. Vascular Access Devices

a. Indication

i. Difficult venous access

ii. Parenteral nutrition

iii. Administration of medications — chemotherapeutic agents, blood clotting factors
iv. Frequent blood sampling

b. Types
  i. Peripherally inserted central venous catheter (PICC)
    1. Normal versus power injector compatible
      a. Power injectable PICC may withstand the high flow rates and injection pressures required for contrast administration for future CT scans
      b. Slightly costlier compared to regular PICCs
    2. Cuffed versus uncuffed
      a. Fibrous cuff buried under the skin at the catheter entry site; usually takes in 2–3 weeks, thereafter does not easily slip/dislodge
      b. Fibrous ingrowth around the cuff potentially excludes the catheter from ascending infection; secures catheter *in situ*, reduces chances of accidental pull-out of catheter
      c. Requires blunt dissection to loosen the cuff at removal
    3. Single, double or triple lumen options
      a. Normally external diameters of the catheters do not differ very much; as such, more lumens generally mean smaller lumen sizes, and potentially higher likelihood of blockage of each lumen

b. Catheters are usually cut to length and both lumens are flush (at same level)

ii. Central venous catheter

1. Tunnelled

a. Usually inserted via infraclavicular subcutaneous tunnel into the internal jugular vein with catheter tip positioned within the superior vena cava (SVC). External jugular vein is sometimes used if the internal jugular vein is stenosed/occluded

b. Fibrous ingrowth around cuff over (~2 weeks) has advantages and disadvantages similar to cuffed PICCs

2. Non-tunnelled

a. May be inserted via the subclavian, internal or external jugular and femoral veins

b. Easily removed at the end of therapy

c. Possible slippage/accidental pull out

d. Ascending infection if patient's dressing not optimally maintained

3. Dialysis versus non-pheresible

a. Dialysable catheters are of larger calibre to ensure adequate flow for dialysis, harvesting of stem cells

iii. Implanted vascular access port system (Port-a-cath)

1. Single or dual port reservoirs

- a. Different sizes and profiles available
- b. Insertion is similar to tunnelled central venous catheters, with additional step of creating a subcutaneous pocket for the port reservoir

2. Different materials
   - a. Silastic/plastic variants with radio-opaque marker base
   - b. Metallic — titanium
3. Surgical incision to create and remove port
   - a. Larger scar than tunnelled central venous catheter
   - b. Infection control considerations
4. Trained personnel to access and manage
5. Skin puncture for every access

c. Modality
   - i. Ultrasound-guided needle access
   - ii. Fluoroscopy to confirm guidewire location in IVC; measuring Mandrel wire tip location helps determine catheter length required
   - iii. Venogram — useful to delineate venous anatomy especially when unable to advance catheter due to stenosis/spasm

d. Routes
   - i. PICC — usually basilic or brachial vein in the arm. Cephalic vein when medial arm veins exhausted;

seldom placed in forearm. Very rarely in the lower limbs veins (great saphenous)

ii. Central venous catheters and ports — internal jugular vein, subclavian vein

e. Preparation

i. Prior discussion of case with Interventional Radiologist

ii. Clearly filled procedure forms with relevant history and details

iii. Informed consent

iv. Fasting — 4 hours (in consideration of potential for contrast reaction and possible need for sedation)

v. Haematology — FBC, PT/PTT (for central venous catheters and ports; not necessary for PICCs)

vi. EMLA (LA) cream applied to skin puncture site 20–30 min before procedure

f. Specific risks

i. Collateral injury to adjacent artery resulting in thromboembolism, pseudoaneurysm, arteriovenous shunt

ii. Pneumothorax

iii. Thrombophlebitis/phlebitis

iv. Haematoma

v. Fibrin sheath formation

vi. Thrombus formation within catheter or in vein around catheter

vii. Catheter slippage/pull out

g. Post-procedure care

i. Weekly change of dressing, or earlier whenever soiled, including Statlock device

ii. Sterile technique when accessing vascular access device

iii. Flush with normal saline before heparinisation/taurolock to clear residual drug from catheter

iv. Urokinase/recombinent tissue plasminogen activator (rTPA) to dissolve fibrin sheath

4. Prophylactic Placement of Bilateral Internal Iliac Artery Balloons

a. Indication

i. Placenta accreta/increta/percreta

ii. Placenta praevia

iii. Any other obstetric or gynaecological condition with potential for severe blood loss

b. Preparation

i. Prior consultation at IR clinic (for thorough explanation of procedure and to obtain informed consent)/Prior discussion of case with Interventional Radiologist

ii. Clearly filled procedure forms with relevant history and details

iii. Blood tests

1. Haemoglobin
2. Platelet count

3. PT/PTT
4. Group and cross match

iv. Cessation of antiplatelet and anticoagulation therapy to reduce risk of prolonged/profuse bleeding
v. Fasting for 6 hours (anaesthesia, contrast reaction)
vi. Shaving (optional in emergent situations)
vii. Bladder catheter (decompress bladder, monitor intake and output)

c. Modalities
   i. Ultrasound-guided access into bilateral common femoral arteries
   ii. Fluoroscopy
      a. low dose, minimal exposure
      b. confirm location of balloon catheter and volume needed to occlude internal iliac arteries
      c. ensure balloons deflated and in good position

d. Outcome
   i. Vascular sheaths and balloon catheter secured to skin
   ii. Patient transferred to operating room for caesarean delivery
   iii. Bilateral occlusion balloons inflated as soon as umbilical cord is ligated
   iv. Balloons deflated after haemostasis is secured to inspect for any residual ooze/bleed
   v. Balloon catheters are then deflated and removed

vi. Left groin sheath is removed, leaving the right groin sheath to maintain access overnight, with a view for emergent angioembolisation should there be unexpected copious bleeding PV/from surgical drain or sudden precipitous/unexplained drop in Hb level

vii. Proceed for angioembolisation if placenta remains *in situ*

viii. Removal of left groin sheath if placenta delivered or subtotal hysterectomy performed. Monitor 24 hours at intensive care unit

ix. IV pump infusion of normal saline at 10 mL/hr to *in situ* right common femoral artery sheath to prevent thromboembolism

x. Monitor dorsalis pedis and posterior tibial pulses

e. Risks

i. Groin haematoma

ii. Infection

iii. Arterial dissection

iv. Contrast allergy/reaction

v. Vascular dissection/rupture

5. Angioembolisation

a. Indication

i. Placenta accreta/increta/percreta with placenta left *in situ* after delivery

ii. Uterine fibroids (as a standalone procedure)
iii. Bleeding tumour (either standalone for palliation or part of staged procedure for large tumour before surgical resection).

b. Preparation
   i. Consultation at IR clinic (for thorough explanation of procedure, counsel on risks and provide alternative treatments before obtaining informed consent)
   ii. Baseline US/MRI scan to document
      1. Size, numbers and viability of fibroids
      2. Confirm placenta accreta/percreta/increta
   iii. Consultation with Women's Pain Anaesthesia team (counselling on pain management after embolisation)
   iv. Fasting for 6 hours (anaesthesia, contrast reaction)
   v. Shaving (optional in emergent situations)
   vi. Bladder catheter (decompress bladder, monitor urine output)

c. Modalities
   i. Ultrasound-guided common femoral artery access
   ii. Fluoroscopy
      a. Angiogram to detail vascular anatomy
      b. Angiogram and fluoroscopy to confirm catheter tip placement in appropriate artery

c. Continuous fluoroscopy during injection of embolic agent to avoid reflux into non-target vessel

d. Embolic agents
   i. Gelfoam slurry
      1. Used in emergency haemorrhage
      2. Temporary, dissolve in days to weeks
      3. Inexpensive
      4. Low risk of non-target collateral embolisation
   ii. Permanent particulate agents
      1. Polyvinyl alcohol (PVA)
         a. Variable size range
         b. Least expensive permanent embolic agent
         c. Some reports of long-term recanalisation of vessel
      2. Embospheres
         a. Uniform size and shape
         b. ? better/closer packing
         c. Costlier than PVA
      3. Drug eluting beads
         a. May be coated with chemotherapeutic agent for slow release into target organ
         b. Currently used for hepatic tumours
   iii. Metallic Coils
      1. Stainless steel coils

2. Nitinol coils — MRI compatible
3. Fibre-lined coils — better thrombogenesis
4. Controlled release coils — able to remove if noted to be unsuitable after initial deployment
5. Amplatzer plugs
   a. Variety of shapes and sizes for different applications
   b. Controlled release — final deployment only when certain
   c. Rapid action
   d. Relative cost may be "cheaper" if multiple coils are required

iv. Glue
1. Liquid agent, radiolucent
2. Mixed with lipiodol or tantalum that affect setting time and provide radio-opacity
3. Sets when in contact with ionic substances
4. Rapid action
5. Ideal for arteriovenous malformations where small vascular feeders are difficult to reach but need to be closed off
6. Leaves a solid cast

v. Onyx
1. Gel-to-paste like agent
2. Sets to become a solid cast

3. Grey colouration — may be useful for tracing vessels during subsequent surgical resection for complex tumours

e. Outcome
   i. Post-embolisation syndrome
      1. First 72 hours
      2. Pain — need for opiate patient controlled analgesia (PCA) pump
      3. Nausea and vomiting
      4. Fever
      5. Per vaginal discharge
   ii. Infection — due to ischaemia and necrosis especially if tissue retained (large polypoidal fibroid)
   iii. Premature menopause — collateral reflux embolisation of ovarian artery
   iv. Bleeding related to tumour necrosis
   v. 6–18 months for fibroid/placenta to resorb

f. Risks
   i. Groin haematoma
   ii. Infection
   iii. Arterial dissection
   iv. Contrast allergy/reaction
   v. Vascular dissection/rupture

6. Percutaneous Nephrostomy (PCN)

a. Indication
   i. Urinary outflow tract obstruction with moderate-to-severe hydronephrosis causing renal impairment
   ii. Pyonephrosis
   iii. Stone removal
b. Preparation
   i. Consultation at IR clinic (for thorough explanation of procedure and to obtain informed consent)
   ii. Fasting for 4 hours (potential contrast reaction)
   iii. Appropriate IV antibiotic prophylaxis
c. Modalities
   i. Ultrasound-guided percutaneous access
   ii. Fluoroscopy
      a. Antegrade nephrostogram to determine level of obstruction
      b. Confirm catheter loop position
d. Risks
   i. Acute sepsis
   ii. Haemorrhage
   iii. Perforation/rupture of renal pelvis/ureter
   iv. Contrast reaction
   v. Urine leakage (catheter drainage holes obstructed)

vi. Urosepsis (if not draining well)

e. Follow-up

i. regular 3–6 monthly change

ii. proceed to antegrade ureteric stenting in 3–7 days when urine clears of blood and no bacterial growth

7. Antegrade Ureteric Stenting

a. Indication

i. Obstruction to ureteric outflow tract (tumour, stones)

ii. Aid surgical resection (palpable and marks ureter position)

iii. Provides patients with "normality" compared to PCN

b. Preparation

i. Fasting for 6 hours (IV sedation, potential contrast reaction)

ii. Appropriate IV antibiotic prophylaxis (same as for PCN)

iii. Urine culture from PCN is negative, no further features of urosepsis

c. Technique

i. Antegrade nephrostogram to determine level of obstruction

ii. Tight stenosis may need balloon plasty

iii. Soft versus stiff (tumour) stent

d. Risks
   i. Pain and discomfort
   ii. Perforation/rupture of renal pelvis/ureter
   iii. Contrast reaction
   iv. Tight tumoural stenosis may result in persistent hydronephrosis, renal impairment and recurrent urosepsis
   v. Obstruction of draining sideholes from crystalline encrustation

e. Follow-up
   i. US kidneys and review in IR clinic at one month
   ii. 3–6 monthly change of ureteric stent

8. Varicose Vein Ablation

a. Indication
   i. Symptomatic varicose veins (see CEAP classification below)
   ii. Cosmesis

b. Classifications
   i. Clinical (C)

C0: no visible or palpable signs of venous disease

C1: telangiectasies or reticular veins

C2: varicose veins

C3: oedema

C4a: pigmentation or eczema

C4b: lipodermatosclerosis or atrophie blanche

C5: healed venous ulcer

C6: active venous ulcer

ii. Aetiologic (E)

Ec: congenital

Ep: primary

Es: secondary (post-thrombotic)

En: no venous cause identified

iii. Anatomic (A)

As: superficial veins

Ap: perforator veins

Ad: deep veins

An: no venous location identified

iv. Pathophysiologic (P)

Pr: reflux

Po: obstruction

Pr,o: reflux and obstruction

Pn: no venous pathophysiology identifiable

c. Preparation

i. Fasting for 6 hours (IV sedation, potential contrast reaction)

d. Modalities
   i. Chemical sclerosant (sodium tetradecyl sulphate)
   ii. Endovascular ablation (laser, radiofrequency)
e. Technique
   i. Ultrasound-guided access into great saphenous vein
   ii. Local and tumescent anaesthetic
   iii. ± IV sedation
f. Outcomes
   i. Bruising
   ii. Skin discolouration
   iii. Pressure bandage or compression stocking to be worn for 7–10 days
g. Risks
   i. Pulmonary embolism
   ii. Phlebitis
h. Follow-up
   i. At 3–7 postoperative day with ultrasound Doppler to exclude deep venous thrombosis and confirm closure of treated vein
   ii. At 6 weeks to confirm closure of treated vein. For sclerotherapy if still patent.

REFERENCES

1. 63810- Guide- 00 15. List of Drugs to Avoid in G6PD Deficiency. Pharmacy Department, KK Women's and Children's Hospital, 2012.
2. 63810-Guide-0042. Women Inpatient Dispensing Guide. Pharmacy Department, KK Women's and Children's Hospital, 2012.
3. Abbassi-Ghanavati M, Greer LG, Cunningham FG. Pregnancy and laboratory studies: a reference table for clinicians. *Obstet Gynecol* 2009; **114**(6):1326–31.
4. Adewuya AO, Ola BA, Dada AO, Fasoto OO. Validation of the Edinburgh Postnatal Depression Scale as a screening tool for depression in late pregnancy among Nigerian women. *J Psychosom Obstet Gynecol* 2006; **27**(4):267–72.
5. Adoni A, Ben Chetrit A. The management of intrauterine devices following uterine perforation. *Contraception* 1991; **43**:77.
6. Arroll B, Khin N, Kerse N. Screening for depression in primary care with two verbally asked questions: cross sectional study. *BMJ* 2003; **327**(7424):1144–6.

7. Azziz R. Epidemiology and pathogenesis of the polycystic ovary syndrome in adults [Internet]. UpToDate. 2012. Available from: http://www.uptodate.com/contents/epidemiology-and-pathogenesis-of-the-polycystic-ovary-syndrome-in-adults
8. Barbieri R, Ehrmann D. Clinical manifestations of polycystic ovary syndrome in adults [Internet]. UpToDate. 2012. Available from: http://www.uptodate.com/contents/clinical-manifestations-of-polycystic-ovary-syndrome-in-adults
9. Barbieri R, Ehrmann D. Diagnosis of polycystic ovary syndrome in adults [Internet]. UpToDate. 2012. Available from: http://www.uptodate.com/contents/diagnosis-of-polycystic-ovary-syndrome-in-adults
10. Barbieri R, Ehrmann D. Treatment of polycystic ovary syndrome in adults [Internet]. UpToDate. 2012. Available from: http://www.uptodate.com/contents/treatment-of-polycystic-ovary-syndrome-in-adults
11. Belgi RH. Epidemiology, clinical manifestations, and diagnosis of tuboovarian abscess [Internet]. UpToDate. 2012. Available from: http://www.uptodate.com/contents/epidemiology-clinical-manifestations-and-diagnosis-of-tuboovarian-abscess
12. Belgi RH. Management and complications of tuboovarian abscess [Internet]. UpToDate. 2012. Available from: http://www.uptodate.com/contents/management-and-complications-of-tuboovarian-abscess
13. Bell KJ., Hayen A, Macaskill P, *et al.* Value of routine monitoring of bone mineral density after starting bisphosphonate treatment: secondary analysis of trial data. *BMJ* [Internet]. 2009 [cited 2012 Dec 13];338. Available from: http://www.ncbi.nlm.nih.gov/pmc/articles/PMC3272655/

14. Benedet J, Pecorelli S, (eds). Staging Classifications and Clinical Practice Guidelines of Gynecologic Cancers. Amsterdam: Elsevier, 2000.
15. Berghella V, Figueroa D, Szychowski JM, *et al.* 17-alpha-hydroxyprogesterone caproate for the prevention of preterm birth in women with prior preterm birth and a short cervical length. *Am J Obstet Gynecol.* 2010 **202**(4):351.e1–351.e6.
16. Bernhard L, Klebba P, Gray D, Mutch D. Predictors of persistence of adnexal masses in pregnancy. *Obstet Gynecol* 1999; **93**(4):585–9.
17. Blechman AN, Mann WJ. Evaluation and management of ruptured ovarian cyst [Internet]. UpToDate. 2011. Available from: http://www.uptodate.com/contents/evaluation-and-management-of-ruptured-ovarian-cyst
18. Briggs GG, Freeman RK, Yaffe SF. *Drugs in Pregnancy and Lactation, 8th ed.* Philadelphia: Lippincott Williams & Wilkins, 2011.
19. Brown J, Josse R. 2002 clinical practice guidelines for the diagnosis and management of osteoporosis in Canada. *CMAJ* 2002; **167**: S1–34.
20. Byrne BMP, Crowley PA, Carrington D. Green-top Guideline No. 13 Chicken Pox in Pregnancy [Internet]. Royal College of Obstetricians and Gynaecologists, 2007. Available from: http://www.rcog.org.uk/files/rcog-corp/uploaded-files/GT13 ChickenpoxinPregnancy2007.pdf
21. Carroll SGM. Green-top Guideline No. 44 Preterm Prelabour Rupture of Membranes [Internet]. Royal College of Obstetricians and Gynaecologists; 2010. Available from: http://www.rcog.org.uk/files/rcog-corp/GTG44PPROM28022011.pdf

22. Casper R, Yonkers K. Treatment of premenstrual syndrome and premenstrual dysphoric disorder [Internet]. UpToDate. 2009. Availablefrom:http://www.uptodate.com/contents/treatment-of-premenstrual-syndrome-and-premenstrual-dysphoric-disorder?source=see_link
23. CDC. General Recommendations on Immunization: recommendations of the Advisory Committee on Immunization Practices (ACIP). *MMWR* 2011; **60**(2):26.
24. CDC. Guiding principles for development of ACIP recommendations for vaccination during pregnancy and breastfeeding. *MMWR* 2008; **57**(21):580.
25. Centers for Disease Control and Prevention, Workowski KA, Berman SM. Sexually transmitted diseases treatment guidelines 2006. *MMWR Recomm Rep* 2006; **55**:1.
26. Centers for Disease Control and Prevention. Morbidity and Mortality Weekly Report -Sexually Transmitted Diseases Treatment Guidelines, 2010. *MMWR* 2010; **59**:1–110.
27. Chee C, Lee D, Chong Y, Tan L, Ng T, Fones C. Confinement and other psychosocial factors in perinatal depression: A transcultural study in Singapore. *J Affect Disord.* 2005; **89**:157–66.
28. Chen C, Hsu T, Wang W. Ileal penetration by a Multiload-Cu 375 intrauterine contraceptive device. A case report with review of the literature. *Contraception* 1998; **58**:295.
29. Cohen K, Rathod M, Ferriman E. Twin pregnancy. *Obstet, Gynaecol Reproduct Medi* 2010; **20**(9):259–64.
30. Cohen LS, Altshuler LL, Harlow BL, *et al.* Relapse of major depression during pregnancy in women who maintain or discontinue antidepressant treatment. *JAMA* 2006; **295**(5):499–507.
31. Cox JL, Holden JM, Sagovsky R. Detection of postnatal depression. Development of the 10-item Edinburgh Postnatal Depression Scale. *Br J Psychiatry* 1987; **150**(6):782–6.

32. Daroszewska A. Prevention and treatment of osteoporosis in women: an update. *Obstet Gynaecol Reproduct Med* 2012; **22**(6):162–9.
33. Delmas PD. Treatment of postmenopausal osteoporosis. *Lancet* 2002; **359**(9322):2018–26.
34. Devaseelan P, Ong S. Twin pregnancy: controversies in management. *Obstet Gynaecol* 2010; **12**(3):179–85.
35. Exacoustòs C, Rosati P. Ultrasound diagnosis of uterine myomas and complications in pregnancy. *Obstet Gynecol.* 1993; **82**(1):97–101.
36. Fine P, Mathé H, Ginde S, *et al.* Ulipristal acetate taken 48–120 hours after intercourse for emergency contraception. *Obstet Gynecol* 2010; **115**(2, Part 1):257.
37. Fonseca EB, Celik E, Parra M, *et al.* Progesterone and the Risk of Preterm Birth among Women with a Short Cervix. *N Engl J Med* 2007; **357**(5):462–9.
38. Fraser IS, Parke S, Mellinger U, *et al.* Effective treatment of heavy and/or prolonged menstrual bleeding without organic cause: pooled analysis of two multinational, randomised, double-blind, placebo-controlled trials of oestradiol valerate and dienogest. *Eur J Contracep Reproduct Health Care* 2011; **16**(4):258–69.
39. Fraser IS, Romer T, Parke S, *et al.* Effective treatment of heavy and/or prolonged menstrual bleeding with an oral contraceptive containing estradiol valerate and dienogest: a randomized, double-blind Phase III trial. *Hum Reprod* 2011; **26**(10):2698–708.
40. Friedman AJ, Barbieri RL, Doubilet PM, *et al.* A randomized, double-blind trial of a gonadotropin releasing-hormone agonist (leuprolide) with or without medroxyprogesterone acetate in the treatment of leiomyomata uteri. *Fertil Steril* 1988; **49**(3):404.

41. Glasier AF, Cameron ST, Fine PM, *et al.* Ulipristal acetate versus levonorgestrel for emergency contraception: a randomised non-inferiority trial and meta-analysis. *Lancet* 2010; **375**(9714):555–62.
42. Gotlib IH, Whiffen VE, Mount JH, *et al.* Prevalence rates and demographic characteristics associated with depression in pregnancy and the postpartum. *J Consult Clin psychol.* 1989; **57**(2):269.
43. Gourlay M, Fine J, Preisser J, *et al.* Bone-density testing interval and transition to osteoporosis in older women. *N Engl J Med* 2012; **366**:225–33.
44. Grimes DA. Intrauterine device and upper-genital-tract infection. *Lancet* 2000; **356**:1013.
45. Growdon WB, Laufer MR. Ovarian and fallopian tube torsion [Internet]. UpToDate. 2011. Available from: http://www.uptodate.com/contents/ovarian-and-fallopian-tube-torsion
46. Hall V, Talbot PR, Stubbs SL, Duerden BI. Identification of Clinical Isolates of Actinomyces Species by Amplified 16S Ribosomal DNA Restriction Analysis. *J Clin Microbiol.* 2001; **39**(10):3555–62.
47. Harden CL, J. Hopp, Ting TY, *et al.* Practice parameter update: management issues for women with epilepsy--Focus on pregnancy (an evidence-based review): Obstetrical complications and change in seizure frequency: Report of the Quality Standards Subcommittee and Therapeutics and Technology Assessment Subcommittee of the American Academy of Neurology and American Epilepsy Society. *Neurology* 2009; **73**(2):126–32.
48. Hay D, Kieran E. Non-HIV sexually transmitted infections. *Obstet, Gynaecol Reproduct Med* 2009; **19**(8):210–4.

49. Hinshaw K, Fayyad A, Munjuluri P. Green-top Guideline No. 26 The Management of Early Pregnancy Loss [Internet]. Royal College of Obstetricians and Gynaecologists; 2006. Available from: http://www.rcog.org.uk/files/rcog-corp/uploaded-files/GT25ManagementofEarlyPregnancyLoss2006.pdf
50. Hoffman M, Sayer R. Adnexal masses in pregnancy. *OBG Management* **19**:27.
51. Hoffman M. Primary ovarian carcinoma during pregnancy. *Clin Consul Obstet Gynecol* 1995; **7**:237.
52. Holmes K, Sparling F, Mardh P, *et al. Sexually Transmitted Disease, 3rd ed.* McGrawHill, 1999.
53. Joint Formulary Committee. *British National Formulary, 62nd ed.* London: BMJ Group and Pharmaceutical Press, 2011.
54. Joint Formulary Committee. Immunological products and vaccines. *British National Formulary, 62nd ed.* London: BMJ Group and Pharmaceutical Press, 2011.
55. Jones D. Triplet pregnancy: Early pregnancy management [Internet]. UpToDate. 2012. Available from: http://www.uptodate.com/contents/triplet-pregnancy-early-pregnancy-management?source=see_link
56. Jones D. Triplet pregnancy: Mid and late pregnancy complications and management [Internet]. UpToDate. 2012. Available from:http://www.uptodate.com/contents/triplet-pregnancy-early-pregnancy-management?source=see_link
57. Kelly AJ, Sowter MC, Trinder J. Green-top Guideline No. 21 The Management of Tubal Pregnancy [Internet]. Royal College of Obstetricians and Gynaecologists; 2004. Available from: http://www.rcog.org.uk/files/rcog-corp/GTG21_230611.pdf
58. Kilpatrick CC, Orejuela FJ. Approach to abdominal pain and the acute abdomen in pregnant and postpartum women

[Internet]. UpToDate. 2011. Available from: http://www.uptodate.com/contents/approach-to-abdominal-pain-and-the-acute-abdomen-in-pregnant-and-postpartum-women

59. KK Department of Gynaecological Oncology. *Treatment Guidelines for Gynaecological Cancers, 2nd ed.* KK Department of Gynaecological Oncology, 2010.
60. Klingensmith ME, Chen LE, Glasgow SC, *et al. The Washington Manual of Surgery, 5th ed.* Saint Louis: Washington University, 2008.
61. Lacey C, Woodhall S. IUSTI: 2010 European Guideline for the Management of Anogenital Warts in Adults [Internet]. IUSTI — International Union Against Sexually Transmitted Infections. 2010. Available from: http://www.iusti.org/regions/europe/Draft_Eurguideline_HPV_2010.pdf
62. Larsson A, Palm M, Hansson L-O, Axelsson O. Reference values for clinical chemistry tests during normal pregnancy. *BJOG* 2008; **115**(7):874–81.
63. Lee H, Chew L, Chow K, *et al.* Singapore Cancer Registry Interim Annual Registry Report Trends in Cancer Incidence in Singapore 2006–2010. Singapore: National Registry of Diseases Office (NRDO).
64. Lee KH, (ed). *Survival Guide to Acute Medicine, 2nd ed.* Singapore: Ridge Books, 2007.
65. Lee NC, Rubin GL, Borucki R. The intrauterine device and pelvic inflammatory disease revisited: new results from the Women's Health Study. *Obstet Gynecol* 1988; **72**(1):1–6.
66. Lee Y-C, Min D, Holcomb K, *et al.* Computed tomography guided core needle biopsy diagnosis of pelvic actinomycosis. *Gynecol Oncol* 2000; **79**(2):318–23.

67. Leiserowitz GS, Xing G, Cress R, *et al.* Adnexal masses in pregnancy: how often are they malignant? *Gynecol Oncol* 2006; **101**(2):315–21.
68. Leone P. Epidemiology, pathogenesis, and clinical manifestations of Neisseria gonorrhoeae infection [Internet]. UpToDate. 2012. Available from: http://www.uptodate.com/contents/epidemiology-pathogenesis-and-clinical-manifestations-of-neisseria-gonorrhoeae-infection
69. Lewis G, Drife J. Why Mothers Die 1997–1999: *The Confidential Enquiries into Maternal Deaths in the United Kingdom*. London: RCOG Press, 2001.
70. Lim BH, Mahmood TA. Pandemic H1N1 2009 (swine flu) and pregnancy. *Obstet, Gynaecol Reproduct Med* 2010; **20**(4):101–6.
71. Lim K, Butt K, Crane JM. SOGC Clinical Practice Guideline. Ultrasonographic cervical length assessment in predicting preterm birth in singleton pregnancies. *J Obstet Gynaecol Can* 2011; **33**(5):486–99.
72. Lippes J. Pelvic actinomycosis: a review and preliminary look at prevalence. *Am J Obstet Gynecol* 1999; **180**(2):265–9.
73. Livengood C, Chacko. Clinical features and diagnosis of pelvic inflammatory disease [Internet]. UpToDate. 2012. Available from: http://www.uptodate.com/contents/clinical-features-and-diagnosis-of-pelvic-inflammatory-disease?source=see_link
74. Livengood C. Pathogenesis of and risk factors for pelvic inflammatory disease [Internet]. UpToDate. 2012. Available from: http://www.uptodate.com/contents/pathogenesis-of-and-risk-factors-for-pelvic-inflammatory-disease?source=see_link

75. Longmore M, Wilkinson IB, Rajagopalan S. *Oxford Handbook of Clinical Medicine, 6th ed*. Oxford: Oxford University Press, 2004.
76. Low-Beer N, Kinghorn G. Green-top Guideline No. 30 Management of Genital Herpes in Pregnancy [Internet]. Royal College of Obstetricians and Gynaecologists; 2007. Availablefrom: http://www.rcog.org.uk/files/rcog-corp/uploaded-files/GT30GenitalHerpes2007.pdf
77. Low-Beer NM, Penn ZJ. Green-top Guideline No. 39 Management of HIV in Pregnancy [Internet]. Royal College of Obstetricians and Gynaecologists; 2010. Available from: http://www.rcog.org.uk/files/rcog-corp/uploaded-files/GtG_no_39_HIV_in_pregnancy_June_2010_v2011.pdf
78. Luesley DM, Baker PN, (eds). *Obstetrics and Gynaecology: An evidence-based text for MRCOG, 2nd ed*. London: Hodder Arnold, 2010.
79. Mahendru A, Gajjar K, Eddy J. Diagnosis and management of tuberculosis in pregnancy. *Obstet Gynaecol* 2010; **12**(3):163–71.
80. Markovitch O, Klein Z, Gidoni Y, *et al*. Extrauterine mislocated IUD: is surgical removal mandatory? *Contraception* 2002; **66**(2):105–8.
81. Martin K, Barbieri R. Treatment of menopausal symptoms with hormone therapy [Internet]. UpToDate. 2012. Available from: http://www.uptodate.com/contents/treatment-of-menopausal-symptoms-with-hormone-therapy
82. McCarthy FP, Jones C, Rowlands S, Giles M. Primary and secondary cytomegalovirus in pregnancy. Obstet Gynaecol 2009; **11**(2):96–100.

83. McGready R, Ashley EA, Nosten F, *et al.* Green-top Guideline No. 54B The Diagnosis and Treatment of Malaria in Pregnancy [Internet]. Royal College of Obstetricians and Gynaecologists; 2010. Available from: http://www.rcog.org.uk/files/rcog-corp/GTG54bDiagnosisTreatmentMalariaPregnancy0810.pdf
84. McGready R, Ashley EA, Nosten F, Rijken M. Green-top Guideline No. 54A The Prevention of Malaria in Pregnancy [Internet]. Royal College of Obstetricians and Gynaecologists; 2010. Available from: http://www.rcog.org.uk/files/rcog-corp/GTG54aPreventionMalariaPregnancy0410.pdf
85. McLearn KT, Minkovitz CS, Strobino DM, *et al.* Maternal depressive symptoms at 2 to 4 months post partum and early parenting practices. *Arch Ped Adolesc Med* 2006; **160**(3):279.
86. Moore Simas TA, Doyle Curiale DK, Hardy J, *et al.* Efforts needed to provide institute of medicine-recommended guidelines for gestational weight gain. *Obstet Gynecol* 2010; **115**(4):777–83.
87. Murray D, Cox J. Screening for depression during pregnancy with the edinburgh depression scale (EDDS). *J Reprod Infant Psychol* 1990; **8**(2):99–107.
88. National Collaborating Centre for Mental Health. *Antenatal and Postnatal Mental Health - The NICE Guideline on Clinical Management and Service Guidance.* Leicester: The British Psychological Society, 2007.
89. National Collaborating Centre for Women's and Children's Health. NICE Clinical Guideline 129 Multiple Pregnancy [Internet]. National Institute for Health and Clinical Excellence (NICE); 2011. Available from: http://www.nice.org.uk/nicemedia/live/13571/56422/56422.pdf

90. National Collaborating Centre for Women's and Children's Health. Hypertension in pregnancy: the management of hypertensive disorders during pregnancy — NICE Clinical Guideline [Internet]. Royal College of Obstetricians and Gynaecologists; 2010. Available from: http://www.nice.org.uk/nicemedia/live/13098/50475/50475.pdf
91. National Institute for Health and Clinical Excellence. Clinical Guideline 44; Heavy menstrual bleeding [Internet]. Royal College of Obstetricians and Gynaecologists; 2007 [cited 2011 May 19]. Available from: http://www.nice.org.uk/nicemedia/pdf/CG44FullGuideline.pdf
92. Neilson J, Kilby M. Green-top Guideline No. 51 Management of Monochorionic Twin Pregnancy [Internet]. Royal College of Obstetricians and Gynaecologists; 2011. Available from: http://www.rcog.org.uk/files/rcog-corp/uploaded-files/T51ManagementMonochorionicTwinPregnancy2008a.pdf
93. Nelson-Piercy C. *Handbook of Obstetric Medicine, 4th ed.* London: Informa Healthcare, 2010.
94. Nonacs R, Cohen L. Depression during pregnancy: diagnosis and treatment options. *J Clin Psychiatry* 2002; **63**(Suppl 7):24–30.
95. O'Hara M, Swain A. Rates and risk of postpartum depression — a meta-analysis. *Int Rev Psychiatry* 1996; **8**(1):37–54.
96. O'Hara M. Social support, life events and depression during pregnancy and the puerperium. *Arch Gen Psychiatry* 1986; **43**:569–73.
97. O'Neill S, Eden J. The pathophysiology of menopausal symptoms. *Obstet, Gynaecol Reproduct Med* 2012; 22(3):63–9.
98. Ong A, Goh K. *A Guide on Infectious Diseases of Public Health Importance in Singapore, 7th ed.* 2011.

99. Oteng-Ntim E, Howard J. Green-top Guideline No. 61 Management of Sickle Cell Disease in Pregnancy [Internet]. Royal College of Obstetricians and Gynaecologists; 2011. Available from: http://www.rcog.org.uk/files/rcog-corp/GTG61_26082011.pdf

100. Owen J, Hankins G, Iams JD, *et al.* Multicenter randomized trial of cerclage for preterm birth prevention in high-risk women with shortened midtrimester cervical length. *Am J Obstet Gynecol* 2009; **201**(4):375.e1–375.e8.

101. Panay N. Management of premenstrual syndrome: Evidence-based guidelines. *Obstet, Gynaecol Reproduct Med.* 2011; **21**(8):221–8.

102. Parker WH, Fu YS, Berek JS. Uterine sarcoma in patients operated on for presumed leiomyoma and rapidly growing leiomyoma. *Obstet Gynecol* 1994; **83**(3):414–8.

103. Pavord S, Myers B, Robinson S, *et al.* UK guidelines on the management of iron deficiency in pregnancy. *Br J Haematol* 2012; **156**(5):588–600.

104. Peipert J, Madden T. Long-term complications of pelvic inflammatory disease [Internet]. UpToDate. 2012. Available from: http://www.uptodate.com/contents/long-term-complications-of-pelvic-inflammatory-disease

105. Pritts EA, Parker WH, Olive DL. Fibroids and infertility: an updated systematic review of the evidence. *Fertil* Sterility. 2009; **91**(4):1215–23.

106. Queenan J, Hobbins J, Spong C. *Protocols for High-Risk Pregnancies, 5th ed.* Chichester: Wiley-Blackwell, 2010.

107. Ross DS. Hyperthyroidism during pregnancy: Treatment [Internet]. UpToDate. 2012 [cited 2012 Aug 18]. Available from: http://www.uptodate.com/contents/hyperthyroidism-during-pregnancy-treatment?source=see_link

108. Ross DS. Hypothyroidism during pregnancy: Clinical manifestations, diagnosis, and treatment [Internet]. UpToDate. 2012 [cited 2012 Aug 18]. Available from: http://www.uptodate.com/contents/hypothyroidism-during-pregnancy-clinical-manifestations-diagnosis-and-treatment?source=see_link
109. Ross J, Stewart P. Green-top Guideline No. 32 Management of Acute Pelvic Inflammatory Disease [Internet]. Royal College of Obstetricians and Gynaecologists; 2008. Available from: http://www.rcog.org.uk/files/rcog-corp/uploaded-files/T32PelvicInflamatoryDisease2008MinorRevision.pdf
110. Schachter SC. Management of epilepsy and pregnancy [Internet]. UpToDate. 2012 [cited 2012 Aug 19]. Available from: http://www.uptodate.com/contents/management-of-epilepsy-and-pregnancy
111. Singapore Ministry of Health. Management of Genital Ulcers and Discharges: Clinical Practice Guidelines Volumes 1–2009 of MOH clinical practice guidelines. Singapore: Ministry of Health, 2009.
112. Sizzi O, Rossetti A, Malzoni M, *et al*. Italian multicenter study on complications of laparoscopic myomectomy. *J Minim Invasive Gynecol* 2007; **14**(4):453–62.
113. Spencer CP, Robarts PJ. Management of adnexal masses in pregnancy. *Obstet Gynaecol* 2006; **8**(1):14–9.
114. Spitzer M, Kaushal N, Benjamin F. Maternal CA-125 levels in pregnancy and the puerperium. *J Reprod Med* 1998; **43**:387.
115. Stagnaro-Green A, Abalovich M, Alexander E, *et al*. Guidelines of the American Thyroid Association for the Diagnosis and Management of Thyroid Disease During Pregnancy and Postpartum. *Thyroid* 2011; **21**(10):1081–125.

116. Strowitzki T, Marr J, Gerlinger C, *et al.* Dienogest is as effective as leuprolide acetate in treating the painful symptoms of endometriosis: a 24-week, randomized, multicentre, open-label trial. *Hum Reprod* 2010; **25**(3):633–41.
117. Taylor D, Paton C, Kapur S. Use of pyschotropic drugs in special patient groups. *The Maudsley Prescribing Guidelines in Psychiatry 11th ed.* Chichester: Wiley-Blackwell, 2012. p. 419–586.
118. Thomson AJ, Ramsay JE. Green-top Guideline No. 63 Antepartum Haemorrhage [Internet]. Royal College of Obstetricians and Gynaecologists; 2011. Available from: http://www.rcog.org.uk/files/rcog-corp/GTG63_05122011APH.pdf
119. To M, Kidd M, Maxwell D. Prenatal diagnosis and management of fetal infections. *Obstet Gynaecol.* 2009; **11**(2):108–16.
120. Van Gelder MMHJ, van Rooij IALM, Miller RK, *et al.* Teratogenic mechanisms of medical drugs. *Hum Reprod Update* 2010; **16**(4):378–94.
121. Vasquez P, Schreiber CA. The missing IUD. *Contraception* 2010; **82**:126–8.
122. Whitecar P, Turner S, Higby K. Adnexal masses in pregnancy: a review of 130 cases undergoing surgical management. *Am J obstet Gynecol* 1999; **181**(1):19–24.
123. WHO Fracture Risk Assessment Tool [Internet]. FRAX. 2011. Available from: http://www.shef.ac.uk/FRAX/
124. WHO Study Group on assessment of fracture risk and its application to screening for postmenopausal osteoporosis. WHO Technical Report Series 843: Assessment of fracture risk and its application to screening for postmenopausal osteoporosis: Report of a WHO Study Group. Geneva: World Health Organisation; 1994.

125. Wiesenfeld H. Treatment of pelvic inflammatory disease [Internet]. UpToDate. 2012. Available from: http://www.uptodate.com/contents/treatment-of-pelvic-inflammatory-disease
126. Woolcock JG, Critchley HOD, Munro MG, Broder MS, Fraser IS. Review of the confusion in current and historical terminology and definitions for disturbances of menstrual bleeding. *Fert Steril* 2008; **90**(6):2269–80.
127. Working Party for Guidelines for the Management of Heavy Menstrual Bleeding. An evidence-based guideline for the management of heavy menstrual bleeding. *N Z Med J* 1999; **112**(1088):174–7.
128. Yao M, Tulandi T. Current status of surgical and nonsurgical management of ectopic pregnancy. *Fertil Steril* 1997, **67**(3):421–33.
129. Yonkers K, Casper R. Clinical manifestations and diagnosis of premenstrual syndrome and premenstrual dysphoric disorder [Internet]. UpToDate. 2012. Available from: http://www.uptodate.com/contents/clinical-manifestations-and-diagnosis-of-premenstrual-syndrome-and-premenstrual-dysphoric-disorder
130. Zakin D, Stern WZ, Rosenblatt R. Complete and partial uterine perforation and embedding following insertion of intrauterine devices. II. Diagnostic methods, prevention, and management. *Obstet Gynecol Surv* 1981; 36:401.
131. Zanetta G, Mariani E, Lissoni A, *et al.* A prospective study of the role of ultrasound in the management of adnexal masses in pregnancy. *BJOG*: 2003; **110**(6):578–83.
132. Zenilman J. Genital Chlamydia trachomatis infections in women [Internet]. UpToDate. 2012. Available from: http://www.uptodate.com/contents/genital-chlamydia-trachomatis-infections-in-women

INDEX